FIRE SUPPORT:
A Veteran's Guide to Health, Healing, and Life Beyond Service

Navigating Physical and Mental Wellness, Overcoming
PTSD, and Thriving in Civilian Life

ERIK LAWRENCE

FIRE SUPPORT: A Veteran's Guide to Health, Healing, and Life Beyond Service

Navigating Physical and Mental Wellness, Overcoming PTSD, and Thriving in Civilian Life

By Erik Lawrence

Copyright ©2025 Erik Lawrence – All Rights Reserved

Published in the United States of America by Erik Lawrence

First printing 2025

ISBN: 978-1-961989-20-7

eBook ISBN: 978-1-961989-21-4

Printed and bound in the United States of America

ATTENTION US MILITARY UNITS, US GOVERNMENT AGENCIES, AND PROFESSIONAL ORGANIZATIONS:

Quantity discounts are available on bulk purchases of this book. For information, please contact:

Erik Lawrence support@vig-sec.com

DISCLAIMER

The information contained in this book is intended for general informational purposes only and is not a substitute for professional medical advice, diagnosis or treatment. The author of this book and the publisher do not assume any liability or responsibility for any errors or omissions in the content.

Please consult with a physician or other healthcare professional before starting any new exercise or nutrition program or if you have any specific concerns about your health. The information in this book is not intended to diagnose, treat, cure or prevent any disease.

The author and publisher of this book make no representations or warranties, express or implied, with respect to the accuracy, completeness or usefulness of the information contained in this book. The author and publisher specifically disclaim any liability, loss or risk, personal or otherwise, that is incurred as a consequence, directly or indirectly, of the use and application of any of the contents of this book.

It is important to note that the information in this book is not intended as a one-size-fits-all approach to health and fitness. Everyone's body is different and it is crucial to consult with a healthcare professional to determine what is best for you. The author and publisher do not recommend any specific tests, products, procedures, opinions or other information that may be mentioned in this book.

Please be aware that the results from following the information in this book may vary from person to person. The author and publisher do not guarantee any specific results or health benefits from following the information in this book.

The author and publisher have attempted to provide accurate information in this book, but the information is subject to change without notice. The author and publisher do not assume any responsibility for errors or omissions or for damages resulting from the use of the information contained in this book.

Before beginning any exercise program, it is important to consult with a physician. This is especially important for individuals over the age of 40 or individuals with pre-existing medical conditions. The exercises outlined in this book may be too strenuous for some people and the reader should use caution and consult with a physician before participating in any of them.

This book is for informational purposes only and is not intended as a substitute for professional medical advice, diagnosis or treatment. If you have any concerns or questions about your health, you should always consult with a physician or other healthcare professional.

By purchasing and using this book, you acknowledge that the author and publisher are not responsible for any injury or harm you may sustain as a result of using the information contained in this book. You assume all risk for any injury or harm that may result from using the information contained in this book.

The author and publisher make no representations or warranties, express or implied, with respect to the information contained in this book and specifically disclaim any liability, loss or risk, personal or otherwise, that is incurred as a consequence, directly or indirectly, of the use and application of any of the contents of this book.

Please be advised that the information in this book is not intended for use as a sole source of information. It should be used in conjunction with other sources and with professional medical advice.

This disclaimer is subject to change without notice.

FOR ORGANIZATIONS OR INDIVIDUALS
PROVIDING CARE FOR VETERANS

To Whom It May Concern,

When it comes to caring for veterans who are suffering, we often see well-meaning efforts that focus on immediate relief—symptom management, emotional support, or temporary aid. While these are vital, they can sometimes act like Band-Aids, addressing the surface without tackling the root causes. To truly serve our veterans and give them a shot at lasting recovery, we need to start with a holistic approach, and that begins with comprehensive diagnostic testing.

Imagine a veteran struggling with chronic fatigue, brain fog, or unexplained pain—issues that could stem from a range of sources. Without knowing what's really going on, we're just guessing at solutions. That's why I urge you to prioritize a full diagnostic workup for every veteran in your care. This should include initial testing for baselines:

- Neurological Testing: From nerve damage to cognitive impairments, thorough neurological assessments can pinpoint issues like neuropathy, seizures, or subtle brain dysfunction that might be mis-attributed to stress or aging.

- Lyme Test: Lyme disease, often contracted from tick bites during service, can mimic other conditions and go undiagnosed for years, causing debilitating symptoms like joint pain and neurological issues.

- Mold Test: Exposure to toxic mold—in barracks, deployment zones, or even post-service housing—can lead to respiratory problems, cognitive decline, and immune system damage.

- TBI Test: Traumatic Brain Injury is a signature wound of modern conflicts, often from blasts or combat trauma, and can underlie mood disorders, headaches, and memory loss if not properly identified.

- Blood Test: A broad panel can reveal deficiencies, inflammation, or infections that might be draining a veteran's health.

- Heavy Metal Test: Exposure to lead, mercury, or other toxins—common in war zones or industrial settings—can accumulate in the body, contributing to everything from fatigue to organ damage.

With these results in hand, you're not just treating symptoms blindly—you're building a roadmap. Say a veteran's primary struggle is PTSD; if a Lyme infection or heavy metal toxicity is also at play, addressing those alongside therapy could amplify the healing process. Or if mold exposure is fueling physical decline, clearing that up might give them the energy to engage in mental health support. It's about working on the whole person, not just one piece at a time.

This isn't a quick fix—it's an investment. Diagnostic testing costs upfront time and money, but it saves resources in the long run by preventing endless trial-and-error treatments. More importantly, it honors our veterans with the dignity of real answers and targeted care. They've given enough; they shouldn't have to settle for patchwork solutions.

I know your resources are stretched thin, but even starting small—partnering with labs, seeking grants, or piloting this with a few veterans—could show the impact. A holistic approach like this doesn't just manage suffering; it aims to end it. Let's give them the full care they deserve, from the ground up.

DEDICATION

To my fellow Veterans

As a Green Beret and Veteran of multiple deployments, I have seen firsthand the toll that military service can take on our physical and mental health. I know how difficult it can be to transition back to civilian life and find a sense of purpose and well-being outside of the military.

That is why I wrote this book on Veterans' health and fitness. I wanted to provide a resource for my fellow Veterans to help them take control of their health and well-being and live their best lives.

In this book, you will find practical strategies for improving your physical health, including nutrition, exercise and sleep. You will also find advice on managing chronic health conditions and addressing mental health issues such as PTSD and anxiety.

I know that it can be overwhelming to make changes to your health and fitness after leaving the military. That is why I have designed this book to be practical and accessible. The strategies and tips in this book are designed to be easily implemented, even with a busy schedule or limited resources.

But this book is about more than just physical health. It is about finding purpose and meaning outside of the military and building a fulfilling life after service. You will find advice on finding community, setting goals and creating a sense of purpose in your post-military life.

I know that it is not easy to ask for help or admit that you are struggling. But I want you to know that you are not alone. There are resources and support available to help you live your best life after military service.

It is my hope that this book will be a valuable resource for my fellow Veterans as we navigate the challenges of post-military life. I am proud to have served with each and every one of you and I am dedicated to supporting your health and well-being in any way that I can.

Sincerely,

ERIK

Erik Lawrence, Green Beret

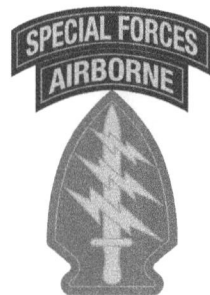

MILITARY OPERATIONS ORDER (OPORD)

Ref: Veteran Health

1. SITUATION:

a. The author recognizes the importance of maintaining physical and mental health for our nation's Veterans. In response, we will be distributing this book specifically tailored to the needs of Veterans.

b. The book will provide valuable information and resources to help Veterans stay active and maintain a healthy lifestyle. It will include information on exercise routines, nutrition and mental health.

2. MISSION:

The mission of this operation is to make this book available to Veterans across the globe and to provide education and support in implementing its content.

3. EXECUTION:

a. <u>Commander's Intent:</u> The commander's intent is to promote healthy lifestyles and wellness among Veterans and to improve their overall quality of life.

b. <u>Concept of Operations:</u>

Phase 1: Preparation and Planning

- Identify local Veterans' organizations and distribution points
- Secure necessary resources (books, promotional materials)

Phase 2: Distribution and Implementation

- Distribute the book to Veterans through local organizations and distribution points.
- Provide education and support to Veterans in implementing the content of the book.

4. SERVICE AND SUPPORT:

a. <u>Logistics:</u> The author will provide the necessary resources for the operation, including copies of this book and promotional materials.

b. <u>Medical:</u> The Veteran will ensure that medical support is available during the implementation phase of the operation.

5. COMMAND AND SIGNAL:

a. <u>Command:</u> The operation will be commanded by the Veteran.

b. <u>Signal:</u> The signal for the start of the operation is having possession of this book.

6. ADMINISTRATION AND LOGISTICS:

a. <u>Personnel:</u> A team of one person will be designated for the operation.

b. <u>Equipment:</u> TBD by Veteran.

7. CONCLUSION:

The author is committed to supporting our nation's Veterans and promoting their health and well-being. By distributing this book and providing education and support, we aim to improve the quality of life for Veterans across the globe.

CONTENTS

V

W

X

Y

Z

ANNEXES

ENDNOTES

ACKNOWLEDGMENTS

This book is dedicated to countless individuals who have selflessly served others, often at great personal cost. Your sacrifices do not go unnoticed, and your experiences are a beacon of light guiding the way toward understanding, healing, and resilience. To those who have suffered consequences from their dedication to service and are now on the path to detoxifying their lives, know that your journey toward wellness is one of courage and inspiration.

I'm sorry to VL and my children for having to learn to live and survive with a father battling PTSD when it really wasn't understood or even thought to be dealt with. You deserved better.

A special thank you to Mrs. C, whose insistence, financial support and guidance were the catalysts for my journey to healing and self-discovery. Your determination to see me thrive led me to take the first, crucial step toward a better life.

To Dr. Sergio Azzolino in San Francisco, I extend my deepest gratitude. Your comprehensive approach, thorough testing, and innovative treatments were instrumental in not only improving my health but also in opening my eyes to the myriads of possibilities for healing. Your work has propelled me to explore further, seeking out doctors and modalities that could extend the same beacon of hope to others that you extended to me.

To JB for her extensive knowledge of exercise physiology, nutrition and self-love giving me the needed start to further discovery and development of much of this book.

To RA for his constant checking up on me and allowing me to vent about the numerous challenges encountered in my life over the years…not bad for a SEAL.

To JK for being a quantumly connected dearest friend for over 30 years. He always shows up when I need to find out I need to live through another life challenge. The best and worst of times.

To JL, the Sapper, for tolerating my rants and insane taskings over decades. Thank you.

To TF and CF for somehow knowing when I needed to speak to, helped and checked up on.

And to all the not mentioned you know who you are and how appreciative I am but cannot express enough.

This journey has been one of transformation, learning, and growth. It has shown me the power of persistence, the value of health, and the importance of seeking and accepting help. To all those who are on similar paths, exploring ways to heal and improve, let this book be a resource, a companion, and a testament to what is possible when we dare to take the first step toward self-improvement. To everyone who has played a part in my journey and to those who are walking their paths of healing and service, thank you. May we all find the strength to continue, the wisdom to seek help when needed, and the courage to embrace the journey ahead.

FOREWORD

There's an old adage, Better to be a Soldier in a garden than a Gardener in a war. Erik Lawrence is the epitome of this saying. Erik, as one might expect from a Green Beret, is always prepared for any eventuality.

He brings a keen insight through experience and preparation to any potential problem. In this case the problem is the health and wellbeing of the United States service member. We've all heard and seen the stats and stories, some of us like Erik firsthand. The current trend for soldiers in transition from duty and service back to civilian life is fraught with pit falls, self-medication, adrenaline seeking and a general feeling of being an outcast with little or no support. It's very apparent that good ole Uncle Sam has his work cut out for him after a long-protracted war on terror and the VA is overwhelmed at best by the number of men and women struggling to successfully navigate that transition.

Where's the help? The guidance? The by the numbers "get this last mission through transition" accomplished successfully? I hope you weren't going to hold your breath while someone answers those questions. The truth of the matter is we are going to have to step up and take care of many of these things ourselves.

Erik has compiled a wealth of knowledge through chasing his own demons and health issues in transition from service and recorded them here in this service manual for any soldier facing the challenge of health and wellness after service to this nation. He has given you and I all the knowledge and access he's acquired from his own journey after service to continue to be all he can be. I can't begin to tell you how much I've learned from Erik in our almost 15 years of friendship. He has helped me with my own transition struggles from professional athletics.

If you are looking for the how-to guide to be happy, healthy and prepared to live a long and prosperous civilian life, then look no more. Erik Lawrence has laid it all out there with Fire Support! I hope you get as much out of it as I did. Soldier on!

Randy Couture

US Army 82-88

Professional fighter 97-2011

INTRODUCTION

I was constantly cranky, easily angered over nothing and obsessing over the most pointless things … I felt like my life was spinning out of control, spiraling down into a no-win situation I couldn't get out of…

I spent over a decade in the United States Army Special Forces and then went on to contract with the US Government in the various conflicts. During my active service, I thought the problems of civilian life were small and insignificant, compared to what I was experiencing during my deployments abroad. What I didn't understand at the time was, that the constant deployments and extreme work load I was going through didn't only affect me right then and there in the moment. They took a toll on my marriage and affected how I was — in civilian life at least as much as in the line of duty.

As a Soldier in the Special Forces, I was trained to survive in combat under the toughest possible circumstances. So, how hard could surviving ordinary civilian life be? I was surprised at how hard the transition from military to civilian really is.

My post-service journey continued the only way I knew how to live. I was always working to be distracted from the demons that came creeping up on me every time I didn't occupy myself with something. I did not pay attention to the physical, mental and emotional health issues that were piling up. The more I tried to "work myself out of my problems," the worse it got.

It got harder and harder to work. I became harder to live with. I didn't see the toll my unresolved issues took on my marriage, my children and my business, before it was too late…

It was only after my youngest daughter was diagnosed with cancer, I was getting divorced, I chose to sell my company to take care of my family situation, and my own physical health was jeopardized by Lyme Disease, I realized how much things had to change. Miraculously, a very wise client of mine saw my deterioration and suggested to me to seek out a particular doctor. That became the beginning of my healing journey and the detox that saved my life.

The doctor's tests was a wakeup call explaining how my lifestyle and the multiple concussions I had suffered, contributed to my destructive behavior. I began a treatment protocol to slowly, but steadily understand what I was dealing with and how make positive changes in my life.

The first step to recovering from delayed-stress syndrome, was admitting to myself that I had a problem and mustering the courage to get help. PTSD is a very real health condition that requires both physical and mental treatment. Without a healthy body, your mind cannot recover and vice versa.

The second step was to create a daily detox schedule to bring my body back to a condition where I had a chance to deal with my mental and physical health problems. Eliminating my Lyme disease was critical, but so was managing my anxiety.

The third step was to rediscover how to find meaning in a civilian world I felt detached from. In the military, everything has a practical purpose; you eat to gain the energy you need, you sleep to be able to stay alert during critical situations... I couldn't find that in civilian life until I realized that I had to control my diet, lifestyle, psyche, here too to be the best version of myself I could possibly be.

 - Erik Lawrence

HOW TO USE THIS BOOK

This book is arranged alphabetically by subject title. Subjects are written as stand-alone entries on a wide variety of topics relating to health in general and items of interest to Veterans in particular. It is not designed to be read cover-to-cover as a narrative, but for use as a reference to the individual topics addressed. Use the book as one would a dictionary or encyclopedia—search through it alphabetically or use the table of contents to locate your subject of interest. You will find references to other authors and books throughout as well as an annex with a list of authors and their works for further reading.

Below is a summary of the included appendices at the back of the guide:

• Annex A

—Daily Activities provides an example of how the author applies the principles of wellness addressed in the guide to his daily schedule.

• Annex B

—Veterans Physical and Mental Health Considerations contains an overview of many topics of specific interest to Veterans and their friends and families without having to navigate thorough many entries.

• Annex C

—Merging Veterans and Players is a detailed account of an organization that assists Veterans and professional athletes through combining their efforts after their respective uniforms come off to support one another in developing and remaining healthy.

• Annex D

—Organizations Supporting Veterans provides a list of organizations—and contact information—that assist Veterans, as well as family members, in a wide variety of health and life situations.

• Annex E

—Alternative Approaches lists entries that are cutting edge or somewhat controversial in the conventional health world. We include them here for the sake of completeness, but the old Roman admonition of, "Caveat Emptor" or "Buyer Beware" applies—do your own due diligence when venturing off the beaten path.

• Annex F

—The First Steps to Healing. Practical advice from a trauma/re-entry counselor on starting your healing journey.

- **Annex G**

  —Further Reading lists other authors and some of their works that provide additional information about selected subjects.

- **Annex H**

  —A list of books that I have personally read on general health and wellness.

- **Annex I**

  —20 Fitness Rules for Men & Women over 40.

As to the structure of the individual entries, there is some repetition in the entries—regarding good practices—which is intentional. The hope is that the reader will gain useful information without having to read many disparate entries to gain common insights that apply to many health subjects. In some cases, the reader will be directed to another entry for more detailed exposition—this has been done to limit the length of individual entries as well as the overall length of the book. The goal is that you find the information you need quickly and that it may be consumed quickly with a minimum of flipping from one place to another.

This book isn't all encompassing in either the breadth of subjects related to health and fitness nor in the depth of knowledge of individual entries—such a tome would run to many volumes and take so long to compile that parts would be obsolete before it could be published. This book is meant as a guide that can provide the first step—or few steps—on a path to wellness. We felt it important to get it out in the world to be used and with the intent to improve it as we go.

Our knowledge of health and fitness is changing and expanding every day. This reference will also change—and likely expand—as new editions are issued. If there are subjects you could not find here that are within the scope of health, and fitness—especially as they pertain to Veterans—please contact the author or publisher with those subjects so we may add them to future editions.

So take a knee, drink water and bon voyage on your path to wellness!

THE ABCs OF GOOD HEALTH FOR VETS

- A -

Acupuncture

An ancient Chinese medicine technique that involves the insertion of thin needles into specific points on the body, acupuncture has been used for thousands of years to treat a range of health conditions, including chronic pain, anxiety and depression. In recent years, acupuncture has gained popularity as a complementary treatment for a range of conditions, including those experienced by Veterans. For Veterans, who may experience physical and mental health concerns related to their service, acupuncture can provide a range of benefits, including:

• *Pain management:* Chronic pain is a common issue for many Veterans, particularly those who have experienced physical injuries or trauma during their service. Acupuncture has been shown to be effective in reducing pain and improving physical function in those with chronic pain conditions, such as back pain, neck pain and joint pain.

• *PTSD symptom reduction:* Post-traumatic stress disorder (PTSD) is a mental health condition that can result from experiencing or witnessing a traumatic event. Acupuncture has been shown to be effective in reducing symptoms of PTSD, including anxiety, depression and hyperarousal.

• *Improved mental health:* In addition to reducing PTSD symptoms, acupuncture has been shown to be effective in improving overall mental health and well-being. It has been shown to reduce symptoms of anxiety and depression and improve overall mood.

• *Reduced medication dependence:* Many Veterans with chronic pain or mental health conditions rely on medication to manage their symptoms. Acupuncture can provide an alternative or complementary treatment that may allow for a reduction in medication use.

• *Improved sleep:* Sleep disturbances are common among Veterans with PTSD and other mental health conditions. Acupuncture has been shown to improve sleep quality and reduce the severity of insomnia.

Acupuncture is generally considered safe when performed by a licensed and trained practitioner. Side effects are typically mild and include soreness or bruising at the needle insertion sites.

To enhance the benefits of acupuncture, Veterans can employ several strategies

• *Seek out a licensed and experienced acupuncturist:* It is important to work with a licensed and experienced acupuncturist who has experience treating Veterans and their unique health concerns.

• *Use acupuncture in combination with other treatments:* Acupuncture is not a standalone treatment for physical or mental health conditions. Veterans should continue to work with their healthcare providers to manage their conditions and may use acupuncture as a complementary treatment.

• *Be open and honest with the acupuncturist:* In order to achieve the best results from acupuncture, Veterans should be open and honest with their acupuncturist about their health concerns, medications and treatment goals.

• *Practice self-care:* Veterans should practice self-care strategies like exercise, healthy eating and stress management to support overall health and well-being in conjunction with acupuncture.

Bottom Line
Acupuncture is a safe and effective complementary treatment option for Veterans who may experience physical and mental health concerns related to their service. By reducing pain, improving mental health and providing an alternative to medication dependence, acupuncture can play.

Addictions

In their various types, addictions pose significant challenges for Veterans' health and well-being. These compulsive behaviors can have debilitating effects, affecting not only the individuals themselves but also their families and communities. In this comprehensive chapter, we will explore different types of addictions that Veterans may face, ranging from substance abuse to behavioral addictions and provide valuable insights into how Veterans can seek help and overcome these issues.

Substance Use Disorders

• *Alcohol:* Alcohol addiction is a prevalent issue among Veterans, often as a way to cope with trauma and stress related to military service. Long-term alcohol abuse can lead to liver disease, heart problems, mental health issues and strained relationships.

- *Treatment and Support:* Veterans can seek help through the VA healthcare system, which offers various treatment options, including detoxification, counseling and support groups. Support from family and friends is crucial and Veterans can also consider rehabilitation programs to address their alcohol addiction.

- *Drugs:* Veterans can become addicted to a range of substances, including opioids, prescription medications and illicit drugs. Drug addiction can lead to financial struggles, legal issues, health problems and strained relationships. Veterans can access treatment through the VA, including detoxification, medication-assisted treatment (MAT) and counseling. Rehabilitation programs, both inpatient and outpatient, offer a structured environment for recovery.

- *Prescription Medications:* Veterans can misuse prescription medications such as opioids, sedatives or stimulants. Signs of prescription medication misuse include increased tolerance, doctor shopping and using medications not as prescribed. Veterans should consult with healthcare professionals to address medication misuse and explore alternative treatments. Mental health support may be essential to manage underlying conditions contributing to misuse.

Behavioral Addictions

- *Gambling:* Gambling addiction can lead to financial ruin, strained relationships and legal troubles. Veterans with gambling addiction may experience severe financial losses and damage to family dynamics. Support groups such as Gamblers Anonymous offer a sense of community and accountability. Cognitive-behavioral therapy (CBT) can help Veterans identify triggers and develop healthier coping strategies.

- *Internet and Gaming:* The allure of online gaming and Internet use can lead to addiction, impacting Veterans' daily lives. Excessive internet and gaming use may exacerbate mental health issues, including depression and anxiety. Veterans can engage in a digital detox, reducing screen time and setting boundaries. CBT techniques help individuals manage excessive internet and gaming use.

- *Food Addiction:* Veterans facing stress might turn to overeating as a coping mechanism. Food addiction can lead to obesity, diabetes and cardiovascular problems. Veterans can seek counseling and support from registered dietitians to address the emotional aspects of food addiction. Developing healthy eating habits and stress management techniques are essential for recovery.

- *Co-occurring Disorders:* Post-Traumatic Stress Disorder (PTSD) and Substance Abuse Veterans with PTSD may turn to substances as a way to self-medicate and alleviate symptoms. Treating both PTSD and substance abuse concurrently, often referred to as integrated treatment, is crucial for recovery. This approach combines therapy, counseling and support.

• **_Depression and Substance Use:_** Comorbidity and Its Impact: Depression and substance use often co-occur, intensifying each other's effects. Comprehensive treatment that addresses both depression and substance use includes medication, therapy and lifestyle changes.

Seeking Help

• **_Recognizing the Problem:_** Veterans and their loved ones should learn to recognize signs of addiction, such as behavioral changes, cravings and social isolation. Acknowledging the problem and being open to seeking help are crucial first steps toward recovery.

• **_Treatment Options:_** Veterans can choose between inpatient programs for intensive support or outpatient programs for more flexibility. Medication-Assisted Treatment (MAT) can help manage withdrawal symptoms and cravings for substances such as opioids. Various therapy approaches, including CBT and motivational interviewing, can be tailored to Veterans' specific needs.

• **_Support:_** Veterans can find solace and understanding in peer support groups where they can share experiences and strategies. The involvement of family and friends in the recovery process can provide essential emotional support. Veterans can access a range of services through the VA, including counseling, healthcare and addiction treatment programs.

• **_Rehabilitation and Recovery:_** Veterans should establish achievable goals for their recovery journey, recognizing that it may involve setbacks. Developing coping skills, identifying triggers and having a relapse prevention plan in place are essential for maintaining sobriety. Building a support network and focusing on a fulfilling, substance-free life are crucial for sustained recovery.

Bottom Line
Addictions, whether related to substances or behaviors, can have a devastating impact on Veterans' lives. However, it's essential to recognize that recovery is possible. By understanding the nature of addictions, recognizing the signs and seeking appropriate help and support, Veterans can embark on a journey towards healthier, addiction-free lives. The road to recovery may be challenging, but with determination and the right resources, Veterans can overcome their addictions and regain control of their well-being.

Amygdalin

Also known as Vitamin B17, Amygdalin is a naturally occurring compound found in various seeds, kernels and fruits, particularly in apricots. Despite controversial claims and limited scientific evidence, some proponents believe amygdalin has potential health benefits and therapeutic uses. It's important to note, however, that the use of amygdalin as a treatment should be approached with caution, as it has risks and potential adverse effects. Let's explore the purported benefits and therapies associated with B17/amygdalin:

• **Cancer Treatment:** One of the primary uses of amygdalin is as an alternative cancer treatment. It is claimed to selectively target and kill cancer cells while leaving healthy cells unharmed. Proponents argue that amygdalin is converted to cyanide in the presence of an enzyme called beta-glucosidase, which is found in higher concentrations in cancer cells. However, scientific evidence supporting these claims is lacking and the use of amygdalin as a standalone cancer treatment is not recommended by medical professionals. It's important to rely on proven and evidence-based cancer treatments, such as chemotherapy, radiation therapy and targeted therapies.

• **Antioxidant Properties:** Amygdalin is believed to have antioxidant properties due to its high content of phenolic compounds. Antioxidants help protect cells from oxidative stress and reduce the risk of chronic diseases. However, the antioxidant potential of amygdalin is not unique to this compound, as many fruits, vegetables and other plant-based foods contain antioxidants. It's crucial to maintain a balanced diet rich in a variety of fruits, vegetables and other whole foods to obtain a wide range of antioxidants.

• **Pain Relief:** Some proponents claim that amygdalin can provide pain relief, particularly in the context of cancer pain. However, scientific evidence supporting this claim is lacking. Pain management for cancer patients should be approached through conventional methods, including medications, palliative care and other evidence-based interventions recommended by healthcare professionals.

• **Blood Pressure Regulation:** Amygdalin has been suggested to have potential blood pressure-regulating effects. However, scientific studies in this area are limited and inconclusive. High blood pressure is a serious medical condition that should be managed under the guidance of a healthcare professional, using evidence-based approaches such as lifestyle modifications and prescribed medications.

• **Immune Support:** Advocates of amygdalin argue that it can boost the immune system and promote overall health. However, scientific evidence supporting these claims is limited. A healthy immune system relies on a balanced diet, regular physical activity, sufficient sleep, stress management and other lifestyle factors. Relying solely on amygdalin for immune support is not recommended.

• **Nutritional Content:** Apricot kernels, which contain amygdalin, also provide certain nutrients, including healthy fats, protein, fiber and vitamins. However, the concentration of amygdalin in these kernels is highly variable and can be potentially toxic in high doses. It's important to note that the nutritional content of apricot kernels does not justify their use as a primary source of nutrition and they should not be considered a substitute for a well-rounded diet.

It's important to highlight that the use of amygdalin carries risks and potential adverse effects, primarily due to its conversion to cyanide. Amygdalin can release cyanide when metabolized, which can be toxic and even fatal in high doses. Symptoms of cyanide toxicity include dizziness, headaches, confusion, shortness of breath and in severe cases, seizures or coma. Ingesting large quantities of apricot kernels or amygdalin supplements can pose significant health risks and their use should be approached with caution.

Furthermore, it's crucial to consult with a qualified healthcare professional before considering amygdalin as a therapeutic intervention. They can provide guidance, assess individual health conditions and needs and offer evidence-based recommendations. They can also provide information on potential interactions with medications and other treatments.

Bottom Line

While some proponents claim potential benefits of B17 amygdalin, such as cancer treatment, antioxidant properties, pain relief, blood pressure regulation, immune support and nutritional content, there is limited scientific evidence to support these claims. The use of amygdalin as a standalone treatment for cancer or other medical conditions is not recommended by medical professionals. It's important to prioritize evidence-based treatments and consult with healthcare professionals for appropriate guidance. The risks associated with amygdalin, including the potential for cyanide toxicity, highlight the importance of caution and informed decision-making.

Anxiety

A normal and often healthy emotion, when anxiety becomes overwhelming and persistent, it can interfere with a person's daily life and well-being. Anxiety disorders are the most common form of mental illness in the United States, affecting over 40-million adults each year.

Anxiety is a feeling of worry, nervousness or unease about something with an uncertain outcome. It is a normal response to stress and it can be beneficial in some situations, such as when it helps a person avoid danger. However, when anxiety becomes excessive, it can interfere with a person's daily activities and relationships, making it difficult to lead a healthy life.

There are several types of anxiety disorders, including generalized anxiety disorder (GAD), panic disorder, social anxiety disorder and specific phobias. A person can also have more than one anxiety disorder at the same time. These disorders can be treated effectively through therapy, medication or a combination of the two. Anxiety can also result from a medical condition or illness like heart disease, diabetes, thyroid problems, irritable bowel syndrome, respiratory illnesses, drug withdrawal (whether via a prescribed medicine or drug abuse) and even rare tumors. In these cases, treatment of the underlying medical issue is important to alleviate the anxiety.

NOTE: Women who have no previous history of anxiety disorders and who abruptly exhibit signs and symptoms of anxiety—especially a 'panic attack'--should immediately seek evaluation in an emergency room or by a cardiologist to rule out a heart attack. Women who are having a heart attack often present with the appearance and signs of a panic attack instead of the traditional signs and symptoms of heart attack associated with males (i.e., tingling or numbness down the left arm and up into the left jaw, chest pain, difficulty breathing—the feeling that "an elephant is sitting on one's chest").

• *Therapy:* Cognitive-behavioral therapy (CBT) is a popular and effective form of therapy for anxiety disorders. CBT helps a person understand and change negative thought patterns and behaviors that contribute to anxiety. The goal of CBT is to help the person develop coping skills that reduce anxiety and prevent future panic attacks.

• *Medication:* Antidepressants and anti-anxiety medications can also be used to treat anxiety disorders. These medications can be helpful in reducing symptoms of anxiety, but they are not a cure. It is important to work with a doctor to determine the best medication and dosage for a specific individual's needs.
In addition to therapy and medication, there are several lifestyle changes that can help reduce symptoms of anxiety and promote overall well-being:

• *Exercise:* Regular physical activity has been shown to reduce symptoms of anxiety and depression. Exercise releases endorphins, which are natural mood-boosters. It also helps reduce stress levels and improve sleep, which can further reduce anxiety.

* *Healthy diet:* Eating a well-balanced diet can help support overall physical and mental health. Reducing caffeine and sugar intake can also be beneficial for individuals with anxiety.

* *Relaxation techniques:* Relaxation techniques, such as deep breathing, meditation and yoga, can help calm the mind and reduce symptoms of anxiety. These techniques can be done anywhere, at any time and can be especially helpful during a panic attack or when feeling overwhelmed.

* *Social support:* Social support is crucial for individuals with anxiety. Connecting with friends and family, joining a support group or seeking counseling can provide a sense of community and reduce feelings of isolation.

* *Limit alcohol and drug use:* Alcohol and drugs may provide temporary relief from anxiety, but they can also make anxiety symptoms worse in the long run. It is important to limit or avoid the use of these substances to promote overall mental health.

* *Get enough sleep:* Getting enough sleep is essential for overall physical and mental health. Lack of sleep can increase anxiety levels, so develop and maintain a healthy sleep routine.

* *Set realistic goals:* Setting realistic goals and expectations for oneself can help reduce feelings of stress and anxiety. Prioritizing tasks and delegating responsibilities can also be helpful in managing stress levels.

Anxiety is a normal emotion that everyone experiences from time to time, but when it becomes persistent and interferes with daily life, it may be time to seek professional help. With proper treatment and lifestyle changes, it is possible to manage anxiety symptoms and lead a healthy, fulfilling life.

Anxiety also is a common mental health issue that can be treated effectively through therapy, medication and lifestyle changes. Some common forms of therapy for anxiety include cognitive-behavioral therapy and exposure therapy, while common medications used to treat anxiety include selective serotonin re-uptake inhibitors (SSRIs) and benzodiazepines.

Lifestyle changes that can help reduce anxiety include:

* Regular exercise
* A healthy diet

- Relaxation techniques
- Social support
- Limiting alcohol and drug use
- Getting enough sleep
- Setting realistic goals

It is important to remember that everyone experiences anxiety differently and what works for one person may not work for another.

Bottom Line

It is important to seek professional help if anxiety is impacting daily life and activities, as left untreated, it can lead to further complications and negatively impact overall well-being. With proper treatment and support, it is possible to manage anxiety and lead a healthy, fulfilling life.

Apple Cider Vinegar (ACV)

Apple Cider Vinegar (ACV) is a fermented liquid made from crushed apples, widely used for its potential health benefits, including digestion support, metabolism regulation, and immune enhancement. Veterans exploring natural wellness solutions may find ACV beneficial for managing weight, blood sugar levels, gut health, and inflammation. Unlike pharmaceutical interventions, ACV provides a holistic approach, though scientific validation varies by claim. This section explores ACV's role, benefits, and practical applications for Veterans.

Understanding Apple Cider Vinegar

ACV is made through a two-step fermentation process, converting apple sugars into acetic acid, the key active compound responsible for its health effects. Raw, unfiltered ACV contains "the mother", a probiotic-rich sediment of enzymes and beneficial bacteria.

Key Components:

- Acetic Acid: Supports metabolism, blood sugar control, and digestion.

- Probiotics & Enzymes: Aid gut health and immune function.

- Polyphenols & Antioxidants: Reduce oxidative stress and inflammation.

The Science Behind ACV's Benefits

Research indicates ACV may improve metabolic and digestive health. A 2018 study in the Journal of Functional Foods found daily ACV consumption reduced blood sugar spikes after meals. A 2019 review in Nutrition Re-views suggested acetic acid enhances fat metabolism and appetite control. While promising, ACV should complement—not replace—medical treatments.

Why Apple Cider Vinegar Matters for Veterans
- Digestive Health: ACV supports gut bacteria balance, easing bloating and acid reflux.

- Metabolic Function: Helps regulate blood sugar and insulin sensitivity, crucial for Veterans managing weight and energy levels.

- Inflammation & Immunity: Polyphenols and acetic acid may reduce inflammation, aiding recovery from service-related wear.

- Cardiovascular Health: Studies suggest ACV may contribute to lower cholesterol and blood pressure.

- Detox & Alkaline Balance: Though the body naturally detoxifies, ACV may support liver function and internal balance.

How to Incorporate ACV into Wellness Practices

1. Digestive Aid (Gut Health, Acid Reflux)

- What: Mix 1 tbsp ACV with warm water before meals.

- Why: Promotes healthy stomach acid levels and digestion.

- How: Drink 5–10 minutes before eating, adjusting dosage if needed.

- Supplies: Organic, raw ACV, filtered water.

2. Metabolism & Weight Management

- What: 1–2 tbsp ACV in water before meals.

- Why: Enhances satiety and fat metabolism.

- How: Dilute with 8 oz water and consume 1–2 times daily.

- Supplies: ACV, measuring spoon, water bottle.

3. Blood Sugar Control

- What: ACV (1 tbsp) with meals high in carbohydrates.

- Why: Slows digestion of sugars, stabilizing glucose levels.

- How: Add to salad dressings, soups, or dilute in water before meals.

- Supplies: ACV, healthy meal plan, glucose monitor (if needed).

4. Anti-Inflammatory Support

- What: ACV mixed with herbal teas (turmeric, ginger).

- Why: Combines anti-inflammatory properties for joint and muscle health.

- How: Stir 1 tbsp ACV into warm tea, drink daily.

- Supplies: ACV, herbal tea, honey (optional).

Precautions & Best Practices

- Dilution is Key: ACV's acidity can erode tooth enamel and irritate the stomach—always mix with water.

- Gradual Introduction: Start with 1 tsp per day and increase gradually.

- Consult a Provider: Veterans with digestive disorders or medications should check with a healthcare professional.

- Use Organic, Unfiltered ACV: Ensures maximum benefits from "the mother" and nutrients.

Veteran-Specific Wellness Integration

- Budget-Friendly Addition: ACV is an affordable wellness tool ($5–$15 per bottle) with long shelf life.

- Easy Travel Solution: Portable and simple to incorporate into daily routines.

- Pair with Other Holistic Approaches: ACV complements balanced nutrition, hydration, and exercise.

- VA-Accessible Support: Discuss potential benefits with VA nutritionists or health coaches.

Bottom Line
Apple Cider Vinegar offers potential wellness benefits for digestion, metabolism, inflammation, and blood sugar control. Veterans can integrate ACV into their routines through simple daily habits, but proper use and dilution are crucial. While research supports some claims, ACV should be part of a broader health strategy, not a sole solution. Starting with small, mindful additions can enhance overall wellness and vitality.

Aromatherapy

A holistic therapy that uses essential oils derived from plants for therapeutic purposes, clinical aromatherapy involves the use of essential oils in a clinical setting to promote healing and well-being. The use of clinical aromatherapy has gained popularity in recent years, especially in the treatment of mental health disorders such as anxiety, depression and post-traumatic stress disorder (PTSD).

Veterans and Mental Health

Veterans are a vulnerable population when it comes to mental health. According to the Department of Veterans Affairs (VA), around 20 percent of Veterans who served in Iraq or Afghanistan have PTSD in a given year. Additionally, Veterans are at a higher risk of depression, anxiety and substance abuse compared to the general population. The VA provides various mental health services to Veterans, including psychotherapy, medication and alternative therapies such as yoga, acupuncture and mindfulness.

Aromatherapy for Veterans

Aromatherapy is a safe and effective complementary therapy that can be used to support Veterans' mental health. Essential oils have been used for centuries for their therapeutic properties, including calming, uplifting and balancing effects on the body and mind. Essential oils can be applied topically, inhaled or ingested (in some cases). The most common method of using essential oils is through inhalation, either by diffusing them in a room or using them in a personal inhaler. The scent of essential oils stimulates the olfactory system, which is linked to the limbic system, the part of the brain responsible for emotions and memories.

Research

Several studies have been conducted on the use of aromatherapy for Veterans with mental health disorders. The following are some of the key findings:

• *Aromatherapy for PTSD:* A study published in the _Journal of Alternative and Complementary Medicine_ in 2012 found that aromatherapy massage using a blend of essential oils (lavender, bergamot and frankincense) significantly reduced symptoms of PTSD in Veterans. The study also found that the aromatherapy massage improved sleep quality and reduced anxiety and depression.

• *Aromatherapy for anxiety and depression:* A randomized controlled trial published in the _Journal of Clinical Nursing_ in 2017 found that inhalation of a blend of essential oils (lavender, bergamot and ylang-ylang) significantly reduced anxiety and depression in Veterans with mild-to-moderate mental health disorders.

• ***Aromatherapy for sleep:*** A study published in the *Journal of Alternative and Complementary Medicine* in 2015 found that inhalation of lavender essential oil improved sleep quality in Veterans with PTSD.

• ***Aromatherapy for pain:*** A study published in the *Journal of Perianesthesia Nursing* in 2016 found that inhalation of a blend of essential oils (lavender, peppermint and helichrysum) reduced pain and anxiety in Veterans undergoing spinal surgery.

NIH Data

The NIH is a federal agency that conducts and supports medical research to improve human health. The NIH has funded several studies on the use of aromatherapy for Veterans. The following are some of the key findings:

• ***Aromatherapy for PTSD:*** A study funded by the NIH and published in the *Journal of Clinical Psychology* in 2016 found that a blend of essential oils (bergamot, frankincense, lavender and vetiver) significantly reduced symptoms of PTSD in Veterans. The study also found that the essential oil blend improved quality of life and reduced depression and anxiety.

• ***Aromatherapy for pain and anxiety:*** A study funded by the NIH and published in the *Journal of Pain and Symptom Management* in 2018 found that aromatherapy with essential oils (lavender, bergamot and frankincense) reduced pain and anxiety in Veterans with chronic pain. The study also found that the aromatherapy improved sleep quality and reduced the need for pain medication.

• ***Aromatherapy for sleep:*** A study funded by the NIH and published in the *Journal of Clinical Sleep Medicine* in 2018 found that inhalation of lavender essential oil improved sleep quality in Veterans with sleep disturbances.

• ***Aromatherapy for cognitive impairment:*** A study funded by the NIH and published in the *Journal of Alzheimer's Disease* in 2016 found that inhalation of rosemary essential oil improved cognitive performance in Veterans with mild cognitive impairment.

Research Limitations

While the research on aromatherapy for Veterans is promising, there are some limitations to consider. First, many of the studies have small sample sizes, which limits the generalizability of the results. Second, some of the studies use different blends of essential oils or different methods of administration, making it difficult to compare results across studies. Third, some of the studies do not have a control group, making it difficult to determine if the effects are due to the essential oils or other factors.

Bottom Line

Clinical aromatherapy is a safe and effective complementary therapy that can be used to support Veterans' mental health. Essential oils have been found to reduce symptoms of PTSD, anxiety, depression, pain and sleep disturbances in Veterans. The NIH has funded several studies on the use of aromatherapy for Veterans, which have provided promising results. While more research is needed to determine the optimal blends and methods of administration, aromatherapy is a valuable tool for healthcare providers to use in conjunction with other treatments for Veterans' mental health disorders.

Arthritis

Arthritis is a common condition that causes inflammation and pain in the joints. Regular exercise can help to improve joint mobility, reduce pain and stiffness. There are multiple types of arthritis with different causes. Some require systemic medications for effective treatment, while others can be managed simply through dietary changes and exercise. Consult with your health care provider to determine if you are suffering from arthritis and what is the best treatment.

For individuals with arthritis, it is important to focus on low-impact exercises, such as swimming, cycling and water aerobics, to reduce the stress on the joints. It is also important to consult with a healthcare professional before starting any new exercise program, as certain medical conditions or medications may affect the types of exercise that are safe and appropriate.

Nutrition is also an important consideration for individuals with arthritis. Diet can affect inflammation in surprising ways. It is best to consult with a nutritionist to systematically identify and eliminate foods that may be the cause of the underlying inflammation.

Asking for Help, Support or Guidance

For Veterans, asking for help isn't just a casual act—it's a deliberate choice to tap into resources, lean on others, and navigate the rough patches of post-service life. Whether it's emotional support, practical assistance, or a bit of direction, reaching out can be a game-changer for wellness and health. This isn't about weakness or passive dependence; it's an active step that takes guts, trust, and a willingness to let others have your six. Veterans face unique challenges—PTSD, isolation, physical wear-and-tear—that make this practice essential for healing and thriving in civilian life. Military culture often drills in self-reliance, but flipping that script can unlock stress relief, resilience, and better days ahead. This section breaks down why it matters, what you gain, and how to make it work, all with a Veteran's lens.

Understanding the Act of Asking

Asking for help means seeking out assistance—be it a listening ear, a hand with bills, or advice on next steps—from people or places you trust. It could be a quick call to a buddy or months of counseling. It's not sitting back and waiting; it's stepping up to say, "I need backup." For Veterans, this might mean countering years of "handle it yourself" training with a new mission: build a team for your well-being.

The Psychology Behind It

Your brain's wired for connection—seeking support taps into that. When stress or trauma hits, like it does for many post-service, your mind craves relief. Asking triggers a release of tension, leaning on social bonds humans have used since tribal days. For Veterans, it's like calling in reinforcements: the load lightens, and your headspace clears. The science says it works—sharing burdens rewires stress responses, making you tougher over time.

The Impact of Asking on Veterans' Health

- Wellness Benefits: Reaching out cuts stress, boosts coping, and opens doors to resources like VA benefits or a vet group's wisdom. It's a lifeline for mental clarity and physical recovery.

- Consequences of Silence: Bottling it up amps anxiety, deepens isolation, and delays healing. Unmet needs—like chronic pain or job struggles—fester without support.

Identifying and Analyzing Your Needs

- Self-Assessment: Take stock—journal how you're feeling, physically or mentally. Spot patterns: sleepless nights, aching joints, or that gnawing loneliness. What's dragging you down most?

- Setting Priorities: Pinpoint what needs help first. Is it PTSD fog, a bad knee, or figuring out civilian life? Rank them—tackle the heavy hitters to get momentum.

Fostering the Habit of Asking

- Set Goals: Make it concrete—SMART style. "Call the VA hotline this week for benefits help" or "Ask my squad mate to check in monthly." Small, clear targets build the habit.

- Building a Support System: Rally your crew—family, fellow vets, or a counselor. Accountability matters; it's like having a spotter in the gym. They keep you honest and moving forward.

Implementation Strategies
- Daily Integration: Weave asking into your routine. A quick text to a friend or a VA call after coffee—make it as regular as PT. Start small—gradual beats overwhelming.

- Habit Stacking: Pair it with what you already do. Call the Veterans Crisis Line while brewing your morning joe or chat with a buddy during your evening wind-down.

Targeted Methods for Veterans' Support
Here's how to ask, who to ask, and what you'll need—tailored to Veterans' real-world needs:

1. Peer-to-Peer Support
- What: Reach out to a fellow vet—squad mate, old CO, or a guy from the VFW—for a call or meetup, 15–60 minutes weekly.

- Why: They get it—no one understands the grind like another vet. It's informal, low-pressure, and builds trust fast.

- How: Text or call: "Hey, can we talk about transitioning?" Meet for coffee or a walk—keep it casual. Weekly check-ins cut isolation and spark ideas. If they're busy, don't sweat it—try another vet.

- Supplies Needed: Phone, maybe a notepad for jotting thoughts, a spot to meet (coffee shop, park).

2. Professional Support
- What: Contact a VA counselor or therapist via Vet Centers (free) for 1–2 hour sessions, weekly or monthly.

- Why: Pros dig into PTSD, pain, or depression with tools vets might not have solo—think therapy or med tweaks.

- How: Call your local Vet Center or 1-877-927-8387, book a slot, show up (in-person or virtual). Ask specific: "I need help with sleep." Stick with it—eight weeks can shift the tide. If it's slow, switch counselors.

- Supplies Needed: Phone or computer, VA contact list (online or pamphlet), quiet space for sessions.

3. Family and Friends

- What: Ask for emotional or practical help—like a listening ear or a ride to the doc—5–30 minutes, one-time or ongoing.

- Why: Your inner circle's a ready resource—less formal, more personal. It eases burdens like juggling family and flashbacks.

- How: Be direct: "Can you listen for a bit?" or "Can you grab my meds?" Keep it short or regular, whatever fits. If they're clueless about vet life, guide them—patience pays.

- Supplies Needed: Phone or face-to-face time, maybe a list of what you need (emotional vent, errand help).

4. VA Resources

- What: Hit up 1-800-827-1000 or VA.gov for benefits, crisis support (Veterans Crisis Line), instant to monthly follow-ups.

- Why: It's your earned backup—cash, health care, or a voice when you're spiraling. Fast access beats waiting.

- How: Dial or click, say, "I need disability help" or "I'm crashing—talk me down." Follow through on forms or callbacks—takes minutes to start, months to max out aid.

- Supplies Needed: Phone or internet, VA ID number (if handy), pen and paper for notes.

5. Community Organizations

- What: Engage VSOs (e.g., American Legion) or nonprofits (e.g., Wounded Warrior Project) for guidance, 1–5 hour sessions or events.

- Why: These groups live for vets—offering mentorship, job leads, or just a crowd that gets you.

- How: Find a local chapter online, attend a meeting, ask: "What's out there for me?" Join events or workshops—three months can net real gains. If one flops, try another.

- Supplies Needed: Internet or phone, transport to events, maybe a notebook for contacts.

Eliminating Barriers to Asking

- Identify Triggers: Spot what stops you—stigma ("Real vets don't ask"), fear of rejection, or "I'll figure it out" pride. Name it, then challenge it.

- Replace Hesitation: Swap silence for action. Instead of stewing, call a hotline. Replace "I'm fine" with "I need a hand"—small swaps, big shifts.

- Veteran-Specific Substitutes:

  - Stigma: Trade "tough it out" for a vet peer chat—normalizes it.

  - Isolation: Swap solo nights for a VSO meetup—connection beats the void.

Mindfulness and Self-Regulation
- Techniques: Pause before dismissing help—focus on your breath (5-5-5 method) or how tense you feel. Awareness cuts knee-jerk "no thanks."

- Benefits: It's like a mental sitrep—knowing when to call for support builds control, a vet's strength.

Seeking Professional Help
- When Needed: If stress, pain, or dark thoughts won't budge, pros (VA counselors, docs) bring heavy artillery—don't wait for a crisis.

- Resources: Vet Centers, VA hotlines, or telehealth are free and vet-ready—start there, escalate as needed.

Maintaining and Sustaining the Habit
- Track Progress: Log who you asked, what you got—better sleep, a benefits check, a lighter mood. Celebrate wins: "Talked to my buddy, slept eight hours."

- Overcome Plateaus: Stuck? Switch sources—peer to VA—or ask bigger: "I need more than a chat." Persistence outlasts ruts.

- Build Resilience: Asking rewires you—each reach-out proves you're not alone, forging a tougher, adaptable mindset.

Bottom Line
Asking for help, support, or guidance is a powerful move for Veterans to cut stress, boost resilience, snag resources, heal faster, and reconnect. It's not about leaning back—it's about stepping up with intent, vulnerability in tow. For vets wrestling PTSD, isolation, or unmet needs, it's a lifeline to wellness, flipping military self-reliance into strategic teamwork. The evidence is clear: reaching out works—stress drops, coping grows, aid flows—though stigma or shaky responses can trip you up. Start simple—hit a hotline, grab a vet buddy, tap the VA—and build it into a habit with clear asks and grit. Consult a doc or VA counselor for big stuff, and stick with trusted sources. It's not the whole answer, but it's a damn good start to a healthier, steadier you.

Ayahuasca

Ayahuasca is a powerful hallucinogenic plant medicine that has been used for centuries by indigenous peoples in the Amazon for spiritual and medicinal purposes. In recent years, ayahuasca has gained attention as a potential treatment for individuals struggling with mental health issues, including Veterans. However, the use of ayahuasca for treating Veterans is a highly controversial topic and there is limited scientific evidence to support its efficacy as a treatment.

While some Veterans and mental health advocates argue that ayahuasca can provide significant benefits, including improved symptoms of depression, anxiety and PTSD, others argue that the substance can have serious adverse effects and that its use as a treatment should be approached with caution.

Studies have shown that ayahuasca can lead to significant reductions in PTSD symptoms, such as re-experiencing traumatic events, avoidance behaviors and hypervigilance. The mechanism of action is not well understood, but it is thought that the plant's active ingredients, such as dimethyltryptamine (DMT), may lead to a change in brain chemistry and help individuals process and integrate traumatic experiences.

However, there are significant risks associated with the use of ayahuasca, including the potential for adverse reactions, such as anxiety, depression and psychosis. There have also been reports of long-lasting negative effects, such as flashbacks and increased susceptibility to future trauma. Additionally, the safety and quality of ayahuasca can be variable, as it is often brewed in unregulated and unsupervised settings.

In general, the use of ayahuasca for treating Veterans is not widely accepted or endorsed by the medical community and the substance remains illegal in many countries, including the United States. This can make it difficult for Veterans to access ayahuasca for treatment purposes, even if they are interested in exploring this option.

Given the lack of scientific evidence and the potential risks associated with ayahuasca use, it is important to approach this issue with caution and to consider alternative, evidence-based treatments for Veterans struggling with mental health issues. This may include evidence-based therapies such as cognitive-behavioral therapy, exposure therapy or mindfulness-based stress reduction.

Bottom Line
While ayahuasca has gained increased attention as a potential treatment option

for Veterans, there is limited scientific evidence to support its efficacy as a treatment. Given the potential risks associated with ayahuasca use, it is important to approach this issue with caution and to consider alternative, evidence-based treatments for Veterans struggling with mental health issues.

B1 Thiamine

The B1 vitamin, also known as thiamine, is a water-soluble vitamin that is essential for the proper functioning of the body. It is one of the eight B vitamins and is necessary for the metabolism of carbohydrates, as well as the proper functioning of the nervous system.

Thiamine is found in a variety of foods, including whole grains, nuts, seeds, legumes and meat. However, many people may not consume enough thiamine through their diet, particularly those who consume a lot of processed or refined foods.

Thiamine deficiency can lead to a range of health problems, including neurological symptoms like confusion and memory loss, muscle weakness and cardiovascular problems. Severe thiamine deficiency can also lead to a condition called beriberi, which can have serious health consequences.

In addition to its role in metabolism and the nervous system, thiamine has been studied for its potential benefits in a range of health conditions, including:

• *Memory and cognitive function:* Thiamine has been studied for its potential to improve memory and cognitive function, particularly in older adults. Some studies have found that thiamine supplements can help to improve memory and cognitive function in those with mild cognitive impairment.

• *Heart health:* Thiamine has been studied for its potential to improve heart health. Some studies have found that thiamine supplements can help to improve heart function and reduce the risk of heart failure in those with heart disease.

• *Energy production:* Thiamine is essential for the metabolism of carbohydrates, which are the body's primary source of energy. Consuming adequate amounts of thiamine can help to support energy production and reduce feelings of fatigue and lethargy.

• *Digestive health:* Thiamine has been studied for its potential to improve digestive health. Some studies have found that thiamine supplements can help to reduce the severity of symptoms in those with irritable bowel syndrome (IBS).

To ensure adequate intake of thiamine, it is important to consume a varied diet that includes sources of thiamine like whole grains, nuts, seeds, legumes and meat. For those who may not consume enough thiamine through their diet, thiamine supplements are also available.

It is important to note that thiamine supplements should be used under the guidance of a healthcare provider, particularly if there are underlying health conditions or concerns. In addition, high doses of thiamine supplements can have negative side effects, including gastrointestinal issues and allergic reactions.

Bottom Line
Overall, thiamine is an essential vitamin that is necessary for the proper functioning of the body. Consuming adequate amounts of thiamine through the diet or through supplements can help to support energy production, improve cognitive and heart health and improve digestive health.

Baking Soda

Baking soda (sodium bicarbonate) is a versatile compound with a long history of medicinal and wellness applications. Beyond its common use in cooking, it has been valued for its alkalizing properties, ability to neutralize acid, and role in supporting overall health. For Veterans, baking soda can serve as an accessible and cost-effective tool for digestive relief, detoxification, muscle recovery, and skin health. This section explores the benefits of baking soda, its impact on the body, and practical ways for Veterans to incorporate it into their wellness routines.

Understanding Baking Soda

Baking soda is a natural alkaline substance that reacts with acids to produce carbon dioxide, which makes it useful for digestion, pH balance, and inflammation reduction. Key wellness applications include:

- Acid Neutralization: Helps relieve heartburn and indigestion.

- Detoxification: Assists in balancing pH levels and removing toxins.

- Muscle Recovery: Reduces lactic acid buildup, easing soreness.

- Skin Health: Soothes irritation, insect bites, and minor burns.

- Oral Care: Freshens breath and supports dental hygiene.

The Science of Baking Soda's Effects

Studies in The Journal of Clinical Pharmacy and Therapeutics (2021) suggest that sodium bicarbonate may help buffer acid in the bloodstream, promoting metabolic balance. Research in Sports Medicine (2020) highlights its role in reducing exercise-induced acidosis, aiding endurance and recovery. Though widely used, proper dosing is essential to prevent overuse effects.

Why Baking Soda Benefits Veterans

- Digestive Relief: Alkalizes stomach acid, reducing heartburn and bloating.

- Post-Exercise Recovery: Buffers lactic acid, minimizing soreness.

- Detoxification Support: Enhances kidney function, supporting natural detox.

- Skin & Oral Care: Addresses minor irritations and enhances dental hygiene.

- Affordable & Accessible: A low-cost, widely available wellness aid.

Identifying When to Use Baking Soda

- Common Signs: Acid reflux, muscle fatigue, skin irritation, oral hygiene concerns.

- Veteran-Specific Triggers: Dietary shifts, high physical exertion, stress-induced acid imbalance.

- Assessment Tools: Track digestion, muscle soreness, and skin reactions.

- Medical Considerations: Monitor sodium intake and kidney function before regular use.

Strategies for Incorporating Baking Soda

- Digestive Aid: 1/2 teaspoon in water after meals for acid relief.

- Muscle Recovery: 1 teaspoon in water post-exercise for soreness reduction.

- Detox Support: 1/4 teaspoon daily in water for pH balance (short-term use).

- Skin Treatment: Paste of baking soda and water applied to irritation or bites.

- Oral Care: Mix with water for a natural mouth rinse or use as toothpaste.

Targeted Uses for Veterans

1. Heartburn & Acid Balance

- What: 1/2 teaspoon baking soda + 8 oz water.

- Why: Neutralizes stomach acid, relieving discomfort.

- How: Drink slowly after meals, use sparingly.

- Supplies: Baking soda, filtered water.

2. Muscle Soreness Recovery

- What: 1 teaspoon baking soda in water.

- Why: Buffers lactic acid, easing post-exercise stiffness.

- How: Consume after intense workouts, not exceeding 2 weeks.

- Supplies: Baking soda, shaker bottle.

3. Detox Bath for Skin & Joints

- What: 1/2 cup baking soda in warm bath.

- Why: Soothes skin, supports detox through pores.

- How: Soak for 20 minutes weekly.

- Supplies: Baking soda, bathtub.

4. Oral Health & Fresh Breath

- What: Baking soda + water mouth rinse.

- Why: Reduces acidity, neutralizes bacteria.

- How: Gargle for 30 seconds, spit out.

- Supplies: Small jar of baking soda, water.

Safety & Considerations

- Daily Intake Limits: High doses can lead to imbalances - moderation is key.

- Medical Conditions: Not recommended for individuals with high blood pressure or kidney disease.

- Avoid Overuse: Prolonged use may alter stomach acid levels, impacting digestion.

- Scientific Evidence: Supported for short-term acid relief and muscle recovery, long-term effects require further research.

Integrating Baking Soda into Daily Life

- Set SMART Goals: Example: "Use baking soda mouth rinse 3x per week for fresher breath."

- Routine Integration: Pair with post-workout recovery or bedtime dental care.

- Leverage Veteran Resources: VA health check-ins, fitness tracking apps, hydration plans.

Bottom Line

Baking soda is a cost-effective, natural remedy for digestion, muscle recovery, detox support, and skin health. Veterans may find it beneficial for balancing pH levels, easing acid-related discomfort, and aiding post-exercise recovery. While research supports its short-term benefits, overuse can pose risks. Simple, controlled applications—like a post-meal acid buffer or detox bath—can enhance wellness. Veterans should consult a healthcare provider before frequent use, especially if managing blood pressure or kidney concerns. When used mindfully, baking soda serves as a valuable addition to a holistic health approach.

Bay Leaves

Many people add bay leaves to foods, especially a bowl of rice (Nigerian), red meat and poultry but do you know why bay leaves are added to food?

When asked why, some reply it's to add flavor to the food. Do you know that if you boil some bay leaves in a glass of water and taste it, it will have little to no flavor?

Now why do you put bay leaves in the meat? The addition of bay leaves to meat converts triglycerides to mono-unsaturated fats and for experimentation and confirmation: cut a chicken in half and cook each half in a separate pan. Place on one half a bay leaf, cook the other half without a bay leaf and observe the amount of fat in both pans.

Recent scientific studies have shown that bay leaves have many benefits & help to get rid of many serious health problems and illnesses.

The benefits of cooking with bay leaf are:

- Bay leaf treats digestive disorders and helps eliminate lumps, heartburn, acidity, & constipation.

- It helps regulate bowel movements by drinking hot bay leaf tea.

- It lowers blood sugar and is also an antioxidant

- It allows the body to produce insulin by eating it or drinking bay leaf tea for a month.

- It eliminates bad cholesterol and relieves the body of triglycerides.

- It's very useful in treating colds, flu and severe cough as it is a rich source of vitamin C; you can boil the leaves and inhale the steam to get rid of phlegm and reduce the severity of cough.

- Bay leaf helps to protect the heart from seizures and strokes as it contains cardiovascular protective compounds.

- It's rich in acids such as caffeic acid, quercetin, eigonol and bartolinide; these substances may prevent the formation of cancer cells in the body.

- It eliminates insomnia and anxiety; if taken before bed, it helps you relax and sleep peacefully.

- Drinking a cup of boiled bay leaves twice a day breaks kidney stones and cures infections.

Just like garlic and ginger are a must find amongst my collection of spices, Bay leaves are a must see in my collection of spices too (my little spice secrets to good aroma and flavor)

Beets

A beet is a root vegetable that is not only delicious but also highly nutritious. Beets belong to the same family as chard and spinach and have been enjoyed as a food source for thousands of years. Beets come in a variety of colors, including red, yellow and candy cane (striped) and have a sweet, earthy flavor.

One of the main benefits of beets is their high nutrient content. They are an excellent source of vitamins and minerals, including folate, potassium and vitamin C. Folate is important for cell growth and development and is particularly important for women who are pregnant or planning to become pregnant. Potassium is an electrolyte that helps regulate fluid balance in the body and is important for heart health and maintaining a healthy blood pressure. Vitamin C is an antioxidant that helps boost the immune system and protect against oxidative damage.

In addition to vitamins and minerals, beets are also high in antioxidants, particularly anthocyanins, which give beets their rich, red color. Antioxidants help protect against damage from free radicals, which are unstable molecules that can cause oxidative stress and contribute to the development of chronic diseases like cancer and heart disease.

Another benefit of beets is their high fiber content. Beets are a good source of both soluble and insoluble fiber, which help to promote digestive health and regulate blood sugar levels. Insoluble fiber helps keep the digestive system moving, while soluble fiber helps slow the absorption of sugar into the bloodstream, which helps to prevent spikes in blood sugar levels.

In addition to their high nutrient content, beets also have potential health benefits for specific health conditions. For example, beets have been shown to improve cardiovascular health by increasing nitric oxide levels in the blood. Nitric oxide helps to relax and dilate blood vessels, which improves blood flow and can help lower blood pressure. Beets have also been shown to have anti-inflammatory properties, which may help to reduce the risk of chronic diseases like heart disease and cancer.

Bottom Line
Beets are a delicious and nutritious vegetable that are an excellent source of vitamins, minerals and antioxidants. Whether you enjoy them roasted, grated in a salad, blended into a smoothie or in a soup, beets are a great way to add nutrition and flavor to your diet.

Blood Detoxification

Blood detoxification is the process of removing harmful toxins and substances from the bloodstream. The body's natural detoxification process is primarily carried out by the liver, which filters the blood and removes toxins. However, due to factors such as poor diet, stress and exposure to environmental toxins, the liver can become overwhelmed and in need of support.

There are several ways to support the body's natural blood detoxification process:

- **Diet:** Eating a diet rich in fruits and vegetables, lean protein and healthy fats can help to support the liver in its detoxification process. Avoiding processed foods, sugar, alcohol and caffeine can also help to reduce the load on the liver.

- **Supplements:** Certain supplements, such as Milk Thistle, N-Acetyl Cysteine and Alpha Lipoic Acid, can help to support the liver in its detoxification process. These supplements can help to protect the liver from damage, increase the production of antioxidants and promote the elimination of toxins.

- **Vitamins:** B-complex vitamins—especially B9 and B12—help reduce liver inflammation and supplements may help if dietary sources are insufficient

- **Physical activity:** Regular physical activity can help to improve circulation, which can aid in the removal of toxins from the bloodstream.

- **Hydration:** Drinking plenty of water can help to flush toxins out of the body and support the kidneys in their detoxification process.

- **Sweat:** Sweating is another way the body gets rid of toxins. Sauna, hot yoga and other activities that make you sweat can be beneficial for blood detoxification.

Bottom Line
It's important to remember that the body is constantly detoxifying and the liver is working 24/7 to filter the blood and remove toxins. However, by supporting the body's natural detoxification process, you can help to reduce the load on the liver and improve overall health and well-being. It's also important to seek guidance from a healthcare professional before starting any detox program and to approach it gradually.

BrainTap System

For Veterans, wellness often means finding tools to quiet the noise—mental, physical, or emotional—that lingers after service. The BrainTap system, a brain fitness gadget from BrainTap Technologies, steps into that gap. It's a mobile app packed with guided audio sessions, paired with an optional headset that uses light and sound to nudge your brain into calmer, sharper states. This isn't your standard meditation—it's a tech-driven way to tackle stress, sleep troubles, and foggy focus, all without popping a pill. For Veterans wrestling with the aftermath of deployments or tough transitions, BrainTap offers a hands-on, non-invasive path to re-balance and recharge. This section digs into what it is, why it matters, and how to make it work, all tailored to the Veteran experience.

Understanding the BrainTap System
BrainTap combines a smartphone app with over 2,000 audio tracks—think guided relaxation or focus boosters—with an optional Bluetooth headset that flashes LED lights and pumps sound through earphones. It's built to shift your brainwaves into states like alpha (relaxed alertness) or theta (deep calm) using a mix of tones and pulses. Sessions run 8–42 minutes, making it a quick hit or a deeper dive, depending on your day. For Veterans, it's a portable ally against the chaos of post-service life.

The Science Behind It
Your brain runs on waves—electrical patterns that shift with your mood or focus. Stress keeps you stuck in high-alert beta; sleep loves slow delta. BrainTap uses binaural beats (dual-ear tones), isochronic pulses, and light flickers to guide those waves where you want them. The idea's rooted in biofeedback—training your nervous system to chill out or lock in. For Veterans, it's like recalibrating after years of high-stakes ops: soothing an overactive fight-or-flight response or clearing mental static. The science isn't ironclad yet—user stories outpace big research—but the concept tracks with how sound and light can tweak your headspace.

The Impact of BrainTap on Veterans' Health
- Wellness Benefits: It's a reset button—easing tension, sharpening your edge, and helping you sleep like you mean it. Veterans get a drug-free shot at feeling steadier.
- Consequences of Ignoring It: Skip it, and stress, restless nights, or brain fog can dig in deeper—piling onto service-worn bodies and minds.

Identifying and Analyzing Your Needs
- Self-Assessment: Check in with yourself—journal it or just think it through. Struggling to unwind? Waking up wired? Can't focus on the day's mission? Pinpoint where you're off.
- Setting Priorities: Rank your battles—stress first if you're wound tight, sleep if nights are a fight, focus if civilian tasks blur. Start where it hurts most.

Fostering BrainTap Use
- Set Goals: Keep it SMART—e.g., "Use a 20-minute sleep session every night for two weeks to crash better." Clear targets turn it into a habit, not a chore.
- Building a Support System: Loop in a buddy or family—tell them you're trying

it, let them nudge you to stick with it. Accountability's a vet's old friend.

Implementation Strategies
- Daily Integration: Slot BrainTap into your routine—post-PT, pre-bed, or during a coffee break. Start with one session; ease beats overload.
- Habit Stacking: Pair it with what's already locked in. Run a focus session while stretching or a calm one with your evening wind-down.

Targeted Protocols for Veterans' Wellness
Here's how to use BrainTap for specific needs, with supplies for each:

1. Stress Relief
- What: Run a 20-minute "Stress Less" session from the app, with or without the headset, once daily.

- Why: Long tours or tough transitions keep your stress dial cranked—BrainTap's tones and lights dial it back, soothing that wired feeling.

- How: Sit or lie back, pop on headphones (headset if you've got it), pick "Stress Less" in the app, and let the voice and pulses guide you. Daily—midday works if you're fraying. If lights bug you, skip the visor. Takes a week to feel lighter.

- Supplies Needed: BrainTap app ($9.99/month basic), headphones (any), optional headset ($647), quiet spot.

2. Improved Sleep
- What: Use a 20–30-minute "Deep Sleep" session nightly, headset preferred.

- Why: Restless nights from hypervigilance or pain? This guides your brain into slow waves, cutting the toss-and-turn cycle.

- How: Before bed, dim the room, wear the headset (or earbuds), select "Deep Sleep," and drift off—20 minutes minimum. Stick with it—sleep deepens over days. If you wake mid-night, rerun it.

- Supplies Needed: BrainTap app, headphones or headset, dark room, comfy spot (bed or chair).

3. Enhanced Focus
- What: Hit a 15–20-minute "Performance Boost" session mid-morning, headset optional.

- Why: Foggy focus from TBI or burnout? This perks up alert brainwaves, sharpening you for work or family.

- How: Grab headphones, sit upright, pick "Performance Boost," and follow the cues—20 minutes max. Daily—pair with coffee if you're dragging. If it's too much, cut to 15. Clarity kicks in fast.

- Supplies Needed: BrainTap app, headphones or headset, chair or desk.

4. Emotional Balance
- What: Run a 20–30-minute "Emotional Mastery" session, 2–3 times weekly, headset enhances it.

- Why: Carrying old weight—grief, anger? Guided visuals and sound reframe it, easing the load.

- How: Find a quiet corner, use the headset or earbuds, select "Emotional Mastery," and let it roll—30 minutes if you're raw. Twice weekly minimum; add a third if it's heavy. Takes weeks to shift.

- Supplies Needed: BrainTap app, headphones or headset, private space.

5. Energy Boost
- What: Use a 15–20-minute "Energy Recharge" session post-lunch, headset optional.

- Why: Afternoon slumps hit hard after years of pushing—this lifts the fog, recharges you naturally.

- How: Sit back, plug in headphones, choose "Energy Recharge," and soak it in—20 minutes tops. Daily when you're wiped. If it's too peppy, switch to "Focus." Energy ticks up same-day.

- Supplies Needed: BrainTap app, headphones or headset, comfy seat.

Eliminating Barriers to Use
- Identify Triggers: Spot what stalls you—cost ("$647's steep"), doubt ("Does it work?"), or time ("I'm busy"). Call it out, then counter it.

- Replace Hesitation: Swap "I'll try later" for a 10-minute app test—free trial's there. Trade screen scrolling for a session—same downtime, better payoff.

- Veteran-Specific Substitutes:

  - Skepticism: Swap "It's BS" for a week's trial—judge it yourself, like testing gear.

  - Fatigue: Trade naps for a quick "Energy" hit—less crash, more juice.

Mindfulness and Self-Regulation
- Techniques: Focus on the tones or lights—tune into how your breathing slows. It's a mental anchor, cutting knee-jerk "I don't need this."

- Benefits: Awareness grows—you'll spot when stress or fog creeps in, cueing a session. It's control, vet-style.

Seeking Professional Help
- When Needed: If sleep, stress, or focus won't budge—or if lights trigger headaches—tap a VA doc or therapist. BrainTap's a boost, not a fix.

- Resources: VA clinics, Vet Centers, or telehealth can pair it with therapy or meds—free and vet-ready.

Maintaining and Sustaining Use
- Track Progress: Note shifts—better sleep, less edge, clearer head—in a log or app. Celebrate a solid night or sharp day; it fuels the grind.

- Overcome Plateaus: Flatlining? Swap sessions—stress to sleep—or add a second daily hit. Persistence beats the wall.

- Build Resilience: Each session's a small win—stack them, and you're tougher, steadier, ready for what's next.

Bottom Line
The BrainTap system is a Veteran-friendly shot at cutting stress, sleeping sound, sharpening focus, balancing emotions, and boosting energy. It's an app ($9.99/ month) with guided audio and an optional headset ($647) that uses light and sound to tweak your brainwaves—tech, not magic. For vets battling restless nights, mental haze, or tension, it's a drug-free tool to reset and roll forward. Users swear by the calm and clarity; science hints it's legit—though it's more buzz than proof so far. Risks? Lights might annoy, and the headset's price stings if cash is tight. It's not a lone cure—pros say pair it with real care—so check with a VA doc, start with the app, and weave it into your routine. It's a solid assist for wellness, not a silver bullet, paying off with steady use.

Breathwork

Breathwork therapy is an alternative treatment modality that focuses on breathing techniques to improve physical and mental health. The practice involves controlled breathing exercises that can help regulate the body's physiological response to stress, anxiety and trauma. Breathwork therapy has been increasingly used as a complementary therapy for Veterans to help alleviate symptoms of post-traumatic stress disorder (PTSD) and other mental health conditions.

Why Breathwork
Military service can lead to traumatic experiences that can cause long-lasting physical and mental health problems. Veterans are at a higher risk of developing PTSD, depression, anxiety and substance abuse compared to the general population. Traditional treatments for these conditions include medication, psychother-

apy and other interventions. However, these treatments may not be effective for everyone and many Veterans may experience side effects or feel reluctant to seek care due to stigma or other reasons.

Breathwork therapy offers a non-invasive and natural approach to managing symptoms of PTSD and other mental health conditions. Breathwork can help regulate the body's response to stress and trauma by activating the parasympathetic nervous system, which controls the "rest and digest" response. Breathing exercises can help reduce heart rate, blood pressure and muscle tension, promoting a sense of calm and relaxation. Additionally, breathwork can improve oxygenation and circulation, which can support physical healing and reduce chronic pain.

Benefits of Breathwork

Breathwork therapy can provide a range of benefits for Veterans, including:

- **Reduced symptoms of PTSD:** Studies have shown that breathwork therapy can help reduce symptoms of PTSD in Veterans, including intrusive thoughts, hyperarousal and avoidance. A study published in the _Journal of Traumatic Stress_ in 2017 found that Veterans who participated in a breathwork program had significant improvements in PTSD symptoms, compared to those who received a control intervention.

- **Improved mood and well-being:** Breathwork therapy can help improve mood and overall well-being in Veterans. A study published in the _Journal of Psychiatric Research_ in 2015 found that Veterans who participated in a breathwork program had significant reductions in symptoms of depression and anxiety, as well as improvements in quality of life.

- **Increased resilience:** Breathwork therapy can help improve resilience and coping skills in Veterans, allowing them to better manage stress and trauma. A study published in Military Medicine in 2016 found that Veterans who participated in a breathwork program had significant improvements in perceived stress and resilience, compared to those who received a control intervention.

- **Improved sleep:** Breathwork therapy can help improve sleep quality and reduce sleep disturbances in Veterans. A study published in Military Medicine in 2019 found that Veterans who participated in a breathwork program had significant improvements in sleep quality and reduced symptoms of insomnia, compared to those who received a control intervention.

Types of Breathwork

There are several types of breathwork techniques that can be used for Veterans' therapy, including:

• *Diaphragmatic breathing:* This is a simple technique that involves breathing deeply into the belly, using the diaphragm muscle. This technique can help reduce muscle tension and promote relaxation.

• *Coherent breathing:* This technique involves breathing at a consistent rate, such as inhaling for four seconds and exhaling for four seconds. Coherent breathing can help regulate the body's response to stress and promote a sense of calm.

• *Alternate nostril breathing:* This technique involves breathing in through one nostril and out through the other nostril in a cyclical pattern. Alternate nostril breathing can help balance the body's energy and promote relaxation.

• *Sudarshan Kriya Yoga (SKY):* SKY is a specific type of breathwork that involves a series of rhythmic breathing exercises that are performed in a specific sequence. SKY has been studied extensively for its effects on mental health and has been found to be effective in reducing symptoms of PTSD, depression and anxiety in Veterans. SKY also involves meditation and yoga postures, making it a more comprehensive approach to healing.

• *Wim Hof Method:* This technique involves a combination of deep breathing exercises and exposure to cold temperatures. The Wim Hof Method has gained popularity in recent years for its purported health benefits, including improved immunity and reduced inflammation. While there is limited research on the use of the Wim Hof Method for Veterans' therapy specifically, some Veterans have reported positive results from the practice.

Research

Several studies have investigated the effectiveness of breathwork therapy for Veterans' mental health. The following are some of the key findings:

• *Breathwork for PTSD:* A study published in the _Journal of Traumatic Stress_ in 2017 found that Veterans who participated in a 12-week breathwork program had significant reductions in PTSD symptoms, compared to those who received a control intervention. The study also found that breathwork was associated with improvements in anxiety, depression and overall quality of life.

• *Breathwork for depression and anxiety:* A study published in the _Journal of Psychiatric Research_ in 2015 found that Veterans who participated in a 12-week breathwork program had significant reductions in symptoms of depression and anxiety, compared to those who received a control intervention. The study also found that breathwork was associated with improvements in perceived stress and resilience.

- **Breathwork for sleep:** A study published in Military Medicine in 2019 found that Veterans who participated in a 6-week breathwork program had significant improvements in sleep quality and reduced symptoms of insomnia, compared to those who received a control intervention.

- **Breathwork for chronic pain:** A study published in the _Journal of Alternative and Complementary Medicine_ in 2020 found that Veterans who participated in a 4-week breathwork program had significant reductions in chronic pain, compared to those who received a control intervention. The study also found that breathwork was associated with improvements in sleep quality and quality of life.

Bottom Line
Breathwork therapy is a safe and effective complementary therapy for Veterans' mental health. The practice can help regulate the body's response to stress and trauma, improve mood and well-being and increase resilience and coping skills. There are several types of breathwork techniques that can be used in Veterans' therapy, including diaphragmatic breathing, coherent breathing, alternate nostril breathing, SKY and the Wim Hof Method. While more research is needed to determine the optimal duration and frequency of breathwork interventions, breathwork is a valuable tool for healthcare providers to use in conjunction with other treatments for Veterans' mental health conditions.

Burn Sheet (Emotional Release List)

Veterans carry weight—memories of tough missions, habits born from stress, emotions that stick like burrs. A burn sheet is a way to offload that load: you write down what's dragging you down, then burn it to let it go. It's not just scribbling thoughts—it's a deliberate purge, a ritual to clear out the junk and move forward. For Veterans wrestling with trauma, guilt, or the grind of civilian life, this simple act can cut through the noise and lighten the pack. Rooted in writing therapy and old-school traditions, it's about release, not reflection. This section breaks down what a burn sheet is, why it's worth a shot, and how to do it right, all with a Veteran's edge.

Understanding the Burn Sheet
A burn sheet is a list—handwritten or typed—of the stuff you want out of your head or life: regrets, bad habits, nagging fears. Once it's down, you torch it—literally—watching it turn to ash as a signal you're done with it. Unlike journaling's open-ended ramble, this is a targeted strike: name the enemy, eliminate it. For Veterans, it's a chance to unload service scars or post-service struggles in a way that feels final.

The Psychology Behind It

Your brain holds onto things—good and bad—like a rucksack you can't drop. Writing it out pulls those burdens into the light; burning them sends a message: "I'm cutting you loose." It's a mental reset, tapping into how humans have used rituals for centuries to mark change. For Veterans, it's like debriefing a mission—acknowledge it, then leave it behind. The act doesn't erase the past, but it can shift how it sits with you, easing the grip of old ghosts.

The Impact of Burn Sheets on Veterans' Health

- Wellness Benefits: It clears mental clutter, soothes raw emotions, and sparks a sense of control—key for vets rebuilding after service. It's a DIY tool for calm and clarity.
- Consequences of Holding On: Skip it, and that weight festers—stress builds, habits stick, and the past keeps calling shots. Silence can turn a burden into a barricade.

Identifying and Analyzing Your Burdens

- Self-Assessment: Take inventory—what's eating at you? Jot it in a notebook: sleepless nights, a grudge from deployment, that fifth beer every night. Be honest—patterns show what's loudest.
- Setting Priorities: Pick the heavy hitters—trauma keeping you up, guilt over a call you made, or a habit tanking your health. Start with what's blocking your path most.

Fostering the Burn Sheet Habit

- Set Goals: Make it clear—e.g., "Write and burn one sheet this month to ditch deployment regrets." Keep it simple, measurable, like a mission objective.
- Building a Support System: Tell a trusted vet buddy or family member you're doing it—they can check in, keep you on track, like a wingman on patrol.

Implementation Strategies

- Daily Integration: Fit it into your flow—maybe after a rough day or a trigger flares. Start with one sheet; gradual beats overkill, like pacing a long march.
- Habit Stacking: Pair it with routine—write while coffee brews, burn it during your evening sitrep. Ties it to what's already locked in.

Targeted Techniques for Veterans' Release

Here's how to build and burn a sheet, with supplies for each step:

1. Listing the Load

- What: Spend 10–20 minutes writing what you want gone—e.g., "anger at losing my team," "smoking to forget," "fear I'm broken."

- Why: Naming it pulls it out of your head—makes it real, not a shadow. For vets, it's like ID'ing the enemy before engaging.

- How: Grab paper, sit somewhere quiet, let it rip—no filter. "Guilt over that last op" or "nights I can't shut off." Specifics hit harder. Don't overthink—just dump it.

- Supplies Needed: Notebook or loose paper, pen, private spot.

2. Reflection Before Release

- What: Sit with your list 5–10 minutes, feeling each item's weight, then decide to let it go.

- Why: Acknowledging it gives it a moment—then you cut ties. It's a vet's nod to the past without living in it.

- How: Read it slow—out loud if you're alone. Feel the sting, then say, "I'm done." No planning, just release. If it's heavy, breathe deep (5-5-5) to steady up.

- Supplies Needed: Your list, quiet space, maybe a timer.

3. Burning the Sheet

- What: Burn the list in a fireproof container—metal bowl, sink—watching it ash out.

- Why: Fire transforms—paper to nothing. For vets, it's a symbolic frag out: blow it up, move on.

- How: Outside or over a sink, light it with a match or lighter—safe spot, no wind. Watch it curl and fade; takes 30 seconds. Douse with water if embers linger. If fire's a no-go, shred it—but burning's the punch.

- Supplies Needed: List, fireproof container (bowl, can), lighter or matches, water cup for safety.

4. Post-Ritual Reset

- What: Take 5–10 minutes quiet—breathe, sit, maybe say, "I'm free."

- Why: Seals the deal—lets your mind settle after the purge. Vets know the calm after action; this is it.

- How: Sit still, focus on your breath (4-7-8 if you're wired), or speak an affirmation—"That's gone." Keep it personal—no log, just closure. If tears hit, let 'em roll.

- Supplies Needed: Comfy spot, maybe a watch for timing.

5. Frequency of Use

- What: Do it monthly or when triggers spike—e.g., after a flashback or bad week.

- Why: Keeps it intentional—not a daily grind, but a tool for big moments. Vets thrive on purpose; this fits.

- How: Mark a day—full moon, end of month—or hit it when you're drowning. One sheet, one burn, then rest. If it's too often, dial back—obsession's a trap.

- Supplies Needed: Same as above, calendar (optional).

Eliminating Barriers to Release
- Identify Triggers: Spot what stops you—"It's dumb," "I'll look weak," or "It won't work." Call it out—then prove it wrong.

- Replace Hesitation: Swap "I'll hold it in" for a quick list—five minutes, done. Trade brooding for burning—action beats stewing.

- Veteran-Specific Substitutes:

  - Guilt: Swap "I deserve this" for "I'll burn it"—write it, torch it, walk away.

  - Numbing: Trade a drink for a sheet—list "booze to sleep," burn it, breathe.

Mindfulness and Self-Regulation
- Techniques: Focus on the pen, the flame—stay present. It's a mental anchor, cutting the spiral of "what ifs." Vets know focus saves; this channels it.

- Benefits: You'll spot when you're sinking—cue the sheet. Awareness builds grit, one burn at a time.

Seeking Professional Help
- When Needed: If trauma or habits (booze, pills) run deep, pair this with a VA shrink—don't solo the big stuff.

- Resources: VA therapy, Vet Centers, or hotlines are free—back up your burn with pros who get vets.

Maintaining and Sustaining the Practice
- Track Progress: Note how you feel post-burn—lighter head, quieter nights? Mark a win: "Burned the guilt, slept solid."

- Overcome Plateaus: Stalled? Add a new item or burn more often—push through like a ruck march plateau.

- Build Resilience: Each sheet's a step—stack 'em, and you're tougher, shedding what doesn't serve you.

Bottom Line

A burn sheet's your chance to list the crap—trauma, habits, fears—and burn it gone, aiming for clearer thoughts, healed wounds, less stress, new patterns, closure, and control. For vets hauling PTSD, guilt, or adjustment baggage, it's a hands-on way to dump the load, rooted in writing and ritual. It's not journaling—it's a purge with fire. Users say it works; science backs the writing part—burning's more gut than proof. Risks? Overdoing it can backfire, especially on heavy stuff—keep it balanced. It's not a fix-all—pros say tie it to real care—so check with a VA doc, use it as a sidekick, and burn safe. Simple, cheap, and vet-ready, it's a release worth trying, one sheet at a time.

Cancer

A disease that affects millions of people worldwide – and Veterans are no exception – Veterans are at increased risk for certain types of cancer, including lung, prostate and colorectal cancer, due to exposure to toxic substances and other environmental factors. Preventing, detecting and treating cancer is crucial for Veterans, as it can help to improve overall health and quality of life.

Here is a guide for Veterans on preventing, detecting and treating cancer:

Prevention

- *Maintain a healthy lifestyle:* Maintaining a healthy lifestyle, including eating a balanced diet, getting regular exercise and avoiding tobacco and excessive alcohol consumption, can help to reduce the risk of cancer.

- *Get vaccinated:* Certain vaccines, such as the HPV vaccine, can help to reduce the risk of certain types of cancer.

- *Get regular check-ups:* Regular check-ups, including screenings for cancer, can help to detect cancer early, when it is most treatable.

Detection

- *Know your family history:* Understanding your family history of cancer can help to determine your risk for certain types of cancer and guide your screening schedule.

- *Get regular screenings:* Regular screenings, such as mammograms, prostate exams and colonoscopies, can help to detect cancer early, when it is most treatable.

- *Pay attention to changes in your body:* Paying attention to changes in your body, such as unusual lumps or changes in bowel habits, can help to detect cancer early.

Treatment

- *Seek medical attention:* If you suspect that you have cancer, it is important to seek medical attention as soon as possible to determine the best course of treatment.

- **Consider all treatment options:** There are a variety of treatment options available for cancer, including surgery, radiation therapy, chemotherapy and immunotherapy. It is important to consider all options and work with your healthcare provider to determine the best course of treatment for you.

- **Manage side effects:** Cancer treatment can cause a range of side effects, including fatigue, pain and nausea. It is important to work with your healthcare provider to manage these side effects and improve overall quality of life.

- **Participate in support groups:** Participating in support groups, such as those offered by cancer organizations, can provide a sense of community and support during treatment.

- **Get enough sleep:** Getting enough sleep is important for managing the side effects of cancer treatment and improving overall health.

- **Exercise regularly:** Regular exercise can help to reduce the side effects of cancer treatment and improve overall health.

- **Eat a balanced diet:** Eating a balanced diet, including foods high in antioxidants, can help to reduce the side effects of cancer treatment and improve overall health.

Cancer is a serious concern for Veterans and it is important to take steps to prevent, detect and treat this disease. By maintaining a healthy lifestyle, getting regular check-ups and screenings and seeking medical attention if you suspect that you have cancer, Veterans can improve their chances of detecting and treating cancer early, when it is most treatable. Additionally, by managing side effects, participating in support groups, getting enough sleep, exercising regularly and eating a balanced diet, Veterans can improve their overall health and quality of life during cancer treatment.

In addition to traditional medical treatments, such as surgery, radiation therapy and chemotherapy, there are several non-traditional methods for treating cancer that some individuals may choose to explore. These methods include holistic medicine and spooky2.

Holistic Medicine

Holistic medicine is a type of alternative medicine that takes a whole-person approach to health and wellness, considering physical, emotional, spiritual and environmental factors. Holistic medicine for cancer treatment may include:

- **Nutrition:** A healthy diet that is rich in vitamins, minerals and antioxidants is important for supporting the body during cancer treatment. Some holistic practitioners may recommend specific diets, such as the alkaline diet, to help reduce the risk of cancer and improve overall health.

• **Supplements:** Certain supplements, such as vitamins and minerals, may be recommended by holistic practitioners to support the body during cancer treatment.

• **Mind-body therapies:** Mind-body therapies, such as meditation, yoga and acupuncture, can help to reduce stress and improve overall health.

• **Herbs and botanicals:** Some holistic practitioners may recommend herbs and botanicals, such as turmeric and green tea, to help reduce the risk of cancer and improve overall health.

It is important to note that while holistic medicine can provide support and relief for some individuals, it should not be used as a substitute for traditional medical treatment for cancer. It is also important to discuss any holistic treatments with your healthcare provider to ensure that they are safe and appropriate for your individual needs.

Spooky2

Spooky2 is a type of alternative therapy that uses electromagnetic frequencies to treat a variety of conditions, including cancer. The therapy involves using a device that generates specific frequencies, which are then applied to the body to help reduce the risk of cancer and improve overall health.

While the use of spooky2 is considered alternative, there is scientific evidence to support its effectiveness for treating cancer. It is important to discuss the use of spooky2 with your healthcare provider to determine if it is safe and appropriate for your individual needs.

Bottom Line
There are several non-traditional methods for treating cancer, including holistic medicine and spooky2. While these methods may provide support and relief for some individuals. It is important to discuss any alternative treatments with your healthcare provider to ensure that they are safe and appropriate for your individual needs.

Cardiovascular Disease

Cardiovascular disease (CVD) is a broad term that includes conditions such as heart disease, stroke and hypertension. Regular exercise can help to improve cardiovascular health by lowering blood pressure, improving cholesterol levels and reducing the risk of heart disease and stroke. *It is critical to consult with a healthcare professional before starting any new exercise program, as certain medical conditions or medications may affect the types of exercise that are safe and appropriate.*

For individuals with CVD, it may be important to focus on aerobic exercises, such as walking, cycling and swimming, as well as resistance training to build muscle mass.

Nutrition is also an important consideration for individuals with CVD. A diet that is high in fruits, vegetables, whole grains, lean proteins and healthy fats can help to lower cholesterol levels and improve overall cardiovascular health. It is also important to limit or avoid foods that are high in saturated and trans fats, as well as added sugars.

Castor Oil

Derived from the seeds of the plant known as *Ricinus communis*, castor oil has been used for centuries as a versatile remedy for various health issues. One of its notable applications is detoxification, aiding the body in eliminating toxins and promoting overall well-being. By understanding the potential advantages and proper use, individuals can harness the power of castor oil to support their health journey.

Benefits of Castor Oil for Detoxification

• *Stimulating the lymphatic system:* Castor oil possesses lymphatic-stimulating properties, facilitating the removal of waste and toxins from the body.

• *Enhancing digestive health:* Castor oil promotes regular bowel movements, helping to alleviate constipation and support a healthy digestive system.

• *Liver detoxification support:* The liver plays a crucial role in detoxification and castor oil can aid in promoting liver health and function.

• *Anti-inflammatory effects:* Castor oil possesses anti-inflammatory properties, which can help reduce inflammation within the body, supporting the detoxification process.

• **Skin health benefits:** Topical application of castor oil can improve skin health by drawing out impurities, reducing inflammation and moisturizing the skin.

Castor Oil for Detoxification

• **Castor oil packs:** Applying a castor oil pack to the abdomen is a popular method for detoxification. The pack helps stimulate circulation, reduce inflammation and support detoxification processes in various organs.

• **Oral consumption:** Consuming small amounts of castor oil orally can promote bowel movements, aiding in detoxification and relieving constipation. It is essential to follow proper dosage guidelines and consult a healthcare professional.

• **Massage and topical application:** Massaging castor oil onto the skin can promote lymphatic drainage and facilitate detoxification. It is commonly used for lymphatic massage and addressing skin conditions such as acne, rashes and inflammation.

• **Oil-pulling:** Swishing a small amount of castor oil in the mouth (oil pulling) can help eliminate toxins, reduce bacteria and improve oral health.

Preparing a Castor Oil pack

• Choose an organic, cold-pressed and hexane-free castor oil to ensure purity and retain its beneficial properties.

• Gather supplies: Castor oil, a soft cloth, plastic wrap and a heating pad.

• Soak the cloth in castor oil and place it on the desired area (usually the abdomen).

• Cover the cloth with plastic wrap and apply the heating pad for 30-60 minutes.

• Cleanse the skin afterward and store the pack in an airtight container for future use.

Oral Consumption Guidelines

- Start with a small dose (1-2 teaspoons) to test tolerance and ensure no adverse reactions.

- Mix the castor oil with a small amount of juice or water to mask its taste.

- Consume the mixture on an empty stomach, preferably in the morning.
- Gradually increase the dosage if needed but do not exceed recommended amounts.

Topical Application and Massage

- Apply castor oil to the desired area and gently massage it into the skin.

- For lymphatic massage, use upward strokes towards the heart to promote lymphatic flow.

- Use circular motions to massage the oil into the skin and facilitate absorption.

Oil-Pulling

- Take a small amount of castor oil and swish it around in the mouth for 10-15 minutes.

- Spit out the oil into a disposable bag or tissue, avoiding the sink to prevent clogging.

- Rinse the mouth thoroughly with water and brush your teeth as usual.

Duration and Frequency

- The frequency and duration of castor oil detoxification methods can vary based on individual needs and tolerance.

- Start with a lower frequency (e.g., once a week) and gradually increase if well-tolerated.

- Listen to your body and adjust the frequency as needed.

Bottom Line
Castor oil offers numerous benefits and versatile applications for detoxification and promoting overall health. Whether through castor oil packs, oral consumption, topical application or oil pulling, individuals can harness the power of this natural

remedy to support their detoxification journey. However, it is crucial to consult a healthcare professional before starting any detoxification regimen, especially if you have pre-existing medical conditions or are on medication. By following proper guidelines and understanding the process, individuals can integrate castor oil into their health routines and experience its potential benefits for detoxification and improved well-being.

Chaga Mushrooms

Chaga mushrooms (*Inonotus obliquus*) are a type of medicinal mushroom that grows primarily on the bark of birch trees in cold climates. They are found in many countries, including Russia, Poland, Sweden, Finland, Canada and the northeastern United States. In Russia and the Baltic States, chaga mushrooms have been traditionally used for medicinal purposes for centuries. It is most commonly found in the northern hemisphere, primarily in the boreal forest regions of North America and Eurasia.

Chaga mushrooms should be harvested from a living and healthy birch tree and should be properly cleaned, dried and prepared before use. Chaga mushrooms should not be consumed in large amounts and should only be used under the guidance of a healthcare professional, especially if you have a medical condition or are taking any medications.

Chaga mushrooms have been used for centuries for their medicinal properties. It's important to note that most of the benefits of chaga mushrooms are not yet fully researched and proven by scientific studies, but traditional use and some preliminary studies suggests potential benefits. Some potential benefits include:

• *Antioxidant properties:* Chaga mushrooms contain high levels of antioxidants, which can help protect cells from damage caused by free radicals.

• *Immune system support:* Chaga mushrooms may help boost the immune system and fight off infections.

• *Anti-inflammatory properties:* Chaga mushrooms may help reduce inflammation in the body, which can help alleviate symptoms of certain conditions such as arthritis.

• *Cancer prevention:* Some studies suggest that chaga mushrooms may have anti-tumor properties and may help prevent the growth of cancer cells.

• *Cardiovascular health:* Chaga mushrooms may help lower cholesterol levels and improve heart health.

Chaga mushrooms can be consumed in a variety of forms. For example:

- **Tea:** One of the most popular ways to consume chaga mushrooms is by brewing them into a tea. To make chaga tea, simply break off a piece of the mushroom, grind it into a powder and steep it in hot water for 10-15 minutes.
- **Tincture:** You can also make a tincture by steeping chaga mushrooms in alcohol for several weeks, then strain the liquid and take it in small doses as a supplement.

- **Powder:** You can also purchase chaga mushroom powder and add it to smoothies, coffee or other drinks.

- **Capsules:** You can also purchase chaga mushroom in capsule form, as a dietary supplement.

- **Extracts:** Chaga mushroom extracts are also available, usually in liquid form and can be added to tea or coffee.

Clean Air

Clean air is essential for human health and well-being. Our bodies rely on oxygen from the air we breathe to fuel our cells and keep us alive. However, air pollution is a growing problem in many parts of the world and it's becoming increasingly clear that exposure to dirty air can have serious health consequences.

Supports Respiratory Health
Breathing clean air is crucial for respiratory health. Exposure to air pollution, especially fine particulate matter, can cause serious health problems such as asthma, bronchitis and even lung cancer. In addition, air pollution can exacerbate existing respiratory conditions such as chronic obstructive pulmonary disease (COPD) and make it harder for people with asthma to breathe.

Protects Cardiovascular Health
Air pollution can also have serious impacts on cardiovascular health. Exposure to fine particulate matter has been linked to an increased risk of heart attacks, stroke and other cardiovascular problems. This is because particulate matter can penetrate deep into the lungs and cause oxidative stress that results in inflammation that can damage blood vessels and increase the risk of heart disease.[12345]

Boosts Immune System Function

Clean air is essential for maintaining a healthy immune system. Exposure to air pollution can weaken the immune system, making it harder for the body to fight off infections and illnesses. In addition, air pollution has been linked to increased levels of inflammation, which can disrupt the normal functioning of the immune system.

Improves Mental Health

Clean air is also important for mental health. Studies have shown that exposure to air pollution can increase the risk of anxiety, depression and other mental health problems. Additionally, air pollution can exacerbate existing mental health conditions, making it harder for people to manage their symptoms.

Promotes Cognitive Function

Air pollution can also have serious impacts on cognitive function, especially in children. Studies have shown that exposure to air pollution during early life can cause long-term changes in the brain that can lead to problems with memory, attention and learning. Additionally, exposure to air pollution has been linked to increased risk of dementia in older adults.

Supports Fertility and Reproductive Health

Air pollution can also have serious impacts on fertility and reproductive health. Exposure to air pollution has been linked to decreased sperm count and motility, making it harder for couples to conceive. Additionally, exposure to air pollution during pregnancy can increase the risk of premature birth, low birth weight and other pregnancy-related complications.

Reduces Risk of Cancer

Exposure to air pollution has also been linked to an increased risk of cancer, especially lung cancer. This is because air pollution can cause oxidative stress and inflammation that can damage DNA and increase the risk of cancer. Additionally, air pollution can cause changes in hormone levels that can disrupt normal cellular function and increase the risk of cancer.

Bottom Line

Clean air is essential for human health and well-being. From supporting respiratory health to promoting cognitive function and reducing the risk of cancer, exposure to clean air is critical for optimal health. However, air pollution is a growing problem in many parts of the world and it's becoming increasingly clear that exposure to dirty air can have serious health consequences. To protect our health and well-being, it's important that we take steps to reduce air pollution and ensure that we have access to clean air. This can include things like reducing emissions of particulate matter from cars and industry. By taking these steps, we can work towards a future where everyone has access to clean air and can enjoy the numerous health benefits that come with it. By investing in clean air, we can create a healthier and more sustainable world for generations to come. Ensure proper ventilation and use air purifiers in homes and workplaces to reduce indoor air pollution. Ozone generators can be used to clean lingering smells and germs but fully ventilate the space after the generator has been used. Get out and enjoy nature when you have access to areas that have clean and pollen-free air!

Coconut Oil

A highly versatile and popular ingredient used for a variety of purposes for thousands of years, coconut oil is extracted from the meat of mature coconuts and is rich in medium-chain fatty acids, which make it unique compared to other types of oils.

Here are some of the most significant health uses and benefits of coconut oil:

• *Heart Health:* Coconut oil is composed mainly of medium-chain triglycerides (MCTs), which have been shown to have a beneficial effect on cholesterol levels. MCTs can raise levels of good cholesterol (HDL) while decreasing levels of bad cholesterol (LDL), potentially reducing the risk of heart disease.

• *Weight Management:* Coconut oil is rich in MCTs, which are metabolized differently than other types of fatty acids. Unlike long-chain fatty acids, MCTs are rapidly metabolized by the liver and can increase energy expenditure, making them a useful tool for weight management.

• *Skin and Hair Care:* Coconut oil is a popular ingredient in many skin and hair care products due to its moisturizing and nourishing properties. When applied topically, it can help to soothe dry skin and hair, reducing itching and flaking.

• *Brain Health:* Coconut oil has been shown to have a positive impact on brain function, particularly in individuals with Alzheimer's disease. It is thought to help the body produce ketones, which can provide energy for the brain and potentially improve cognitive function.

• *Anti-Inflammatory:* Coconut oil has anti-inflammatory properties that make it useful for reducing pain and swelling in the body. It is particularly beneficial for individuals with conditions such as arthritis and osteoporosis.

• *Dental Health:* Coconut oil is commonly used as an ingredient in toothpastes and mouthwashes due to its antibacterial properties. It has been shown to reduce the growth of harmful oral bacteria, potentially reducing the risk of tooth decay and gum disease.

• **Improved Digestion:** Coconut oil has been shown to have a positive impact on digestive health, potentially reducing symptoms of digestive disorders such as Crohn's disease and irritable bowel syndrome.

• **Boosts Immunity:** Coconut oil is rich in lauric acid, which has been shown to have antiviral, antibacterial and antifungal properties. This makes it a useful tool for boosting the immune system and reducing the risk of illness and infection.

It is important to note that not all coconut oil is created equal. It is recommended to choose cold-pressed organic and unrefined coconut oil to maximize its health benefits. Additionally, while coconut oil is generally considered safe for consumption, excessive consumption can lead to weight gain and elevated cholesterol levels. As with any food, moderation is key.

Bottom Line
Coconut oil is a highly versatile and nutrient-dense ingredient that offers numerous health benefits. Its unique composition of medium-chain fatty acids makes it a useful tool for improving heart health, promoting weight management and boosting immunity, among other benefits. When used in moderation and in conjunction with a balanced diet and regular physical activity, coconut oil can be an effective tool for promoting overall health and wellness.

Codependency

A behavioral and emotional condition that can affect individuals in a variety of ways, from personal relationships to work and everyday life, codependency is often characterized by a strong need to please others, a tendency to put the needs of others ahead of one's own needs and a fear of rejection or abandonment.

Melody Beattie, a leading expert on codependency, defines codependency as "a psychological condition or a relationship in which a person is controlled or manipulated by another who is affected with a pathological condition, such as addiction, alcoholism or other behavioral problems."

Chris S Jennings, a therapist specializing in codependency, suggests that codependency can manifest as a "chronic pattern of avoiding or minimizing one's own feelings and needs in order to accommodate or take care of the feelings and needs of others."

There is a variety of methods and approaches to treating codependency, including therapy, self-help and support groups. Here, we will explore some of the most common and effective methods for treating codependency.

Therapy

Therapy is often the first line of treatment for codependency, as it can help individuals gain insight into their patterns of behavior and develop new coping skills. Cognitive-behavioral therapy (CBT) is one approach that has been found to be effective for treating codependency. CBT is a type of therapy that helps individuals identify and change negative thoughts and behaviors.

Another approach is dialectical behavior therapy (DBT), which focuses on teaching individuals skills for managing emotions and improving relationships. DBT incorporates mindfulness practices, which can be helpful for individuals who struggle with codependency.

Other types of therapy that may be effective for treating codependency include psychodynamic therapy, which explores the root causes of codependency and group therapy, which allows individuals to connect with others who are struggling with similar issues.

Self-Help

Self-help techniques can be effective for individuals who are not ready or able to seek therapy. Self-help approaches may include reading books on codependency, practicing mindfulness and meditation and journaling to reflect on thoughts and emotions.

Melody Beattie has written several books on the subject, including Codependent No More and Beyond Codependency. Codependency, by Chris Jennings, is another valuable resource. These books offer practical advice and guidance for individuals who are struggling with codependency.

Support Groups

Support groups can be a valuable resource for individuals who are struggling with codependency. Support groups offer a safe and non-judgmental environment where individuals can connect with others who are struggling with similar issues. Al-Anon, a support group for friends and family members of individuals with alcohol addiction, is one of the most well-known support groups for codependency. Other support groups for codependency include Co-Dependents Anonymous and Adult Children of Alcoholics.

Bottom Line

Codependency is a behavioral and emotional condition that can have a significant impact on an individual's well-being and quality of life. However, there are effective methods for treating codependency, including therapy, self-help and support groups. Therapeutic approaches such as cognitive-behavioral therapy and dialectical behavior therapy can help individuals gain insight into their patterns of behavior and develop new coping skills. Self-help techniques such as reading books on codependency and practicing mindfulness can also be effective. Support groups can offer a safe and non-judgmental environment for individuals to connect with others who are struggling with similar issues. Melody Beattie and Chris S Jennings are leading experts in the field of codependency and their work can be a valuable resource for individuals who are struggling with codependency.

Cold Plunges

The "cold plunge" is a technique made popular by Wim Hof, also known as the "Iceman," who has gained fame for his ability to withstand extreme cold temperatures. The cold plunge involves immersing oneself in cold water, typically for brief periods of time, with the goal of improving physical and mental well-being.

Proponents of the cold plunge technique claim that it can improve circulation, boost the immune system and increase energy levels. Cold water immersion has been shown to cause constriction of blood vessels, which can lead to improved blood flow and oxygenation. This can help to reduce inflammation and improve overall physical performance. Additionally, cold water immersion can also lead to the release of endorphins, which can provide a sense of euphoria and improve mood.

Wim Hof and his followers also claim that cold immersion can have a positive impact on mental health and well-being. Cold water immersion can lead to increased activity in the hippocampus, which is the part of the brain that is associated with learning, memory and emotion regulation. This can lead to improved mood, reduced stress and a greater sense of overall well-being.

It's important to note that while cold water immersion can have some benefits, it's also not suitable for everyone. Individuals with certain medical conditions, such as Raynaud's disease or cold urticaria, should avoid cold immersion. Also, it's important to start with shorter immersion time and gradually increase the duration. People who are not used to cold immersion should start with warm water and gradually decrease the temperature. Consult with a healthcare professional before starting any new exercise or health regimen, including cold immersion.

There are several potential benefits of taking a cold plunge or cold shower, including:

- *Improved circulation:* Cold water can constrict blood vessels, causing blood to circulate more efficiently throughout the body.

- *Increased metabolism:* Cold water can also increase the body's metabolic rate, which can lead to weight loss.

- *Improved mood:* Cold water can trigger the release of endorphins, which can lead to an improved mood and a sense of well-being.

- *Increased immunity:* Cold water can also stimulate the immune system, making it more effective at fighting off illness and disease.
- *Reduced muscle soreness and recovery time:* Cold water can also reduce muscle soreness and recovery time after exercise by decreasing inflammation and swelling.

- *Increased alertness:* Cold water can help you to become more alert and awake, making you more productive during the day.

- *Improved skin and hair:* Cold water can make your skin and hair look healthier by closing the pores and making the cuticles of hair lie flat.

Cold plunging, also known as cold water immersion, is the practice of submerging the body in cold water for a short period of time. Here is a general guide on how to do a cold plunge:

Gradually acclimatize yourself to cold water by starting with lukewarm water and gradually decreasing the temperature over time.

- Fill a tub, pool or lake with cold water. The ideal temperature for a cold plunge is around 50-60°F.

- Before submerging, take a few deep breaths to prepare yourself mentally and physically for the cold.

- Slowly lower yourself into the water, starting with your feet and gradually submerging your entire body.

- Stay in the water for about 30 seconds to a minute, gradually increasing the duration over time.

- Once you're finished, quickly get out of the water and dry off. It's important to not stay in the cold water for too long as it can cause hypothermia.

- Try to take a cold shower after the cold plunge as well, this will help to increase the circulation in the body and will make you feel more refreshed.

Repeat the process every day, increasing the duration of the plunge each time.

It's important to note that you should always be cautious when immersing yourself in cold water and that you should not do this if you have any medical conditions that may be affected by cold water. It's always best to consult with your doctor first.

It's also important to note that cold water immersion is not recommended for everyone, especially those with cardiovascular problems or Raynaud's disease. People with these conditions should consult their doctor before attempting any cold water immersion.

Bottom Line
The cold plunge, popularized by Wim Hof, is a technique of immersing oneself in cold water with the goal of improving physical and mental well-being. While there are some potential benefits, it's important to be cautious and consult with a healthcare professional before trying it out.

Colonic (Colon Hydrotherapy)

Veterans know the body takes a beating—years of MREs, stress that knots your gut, maybe even toxins from burn pits or field ops. Colonics, or colon hydrotherapy, steps up as a way to flush that out: warm water pumped through your large intestine to clear waste, mucus, and whatever else might be hanging around. It's not a barracks rumor—it's a real procedure, done by pros with gear built for the job. For Veterans dealing with digestive gripes or just feeling bogged down, colonics pitch a cleanse that's more than a quick fix. This isn't mainstream medicine—science is skeptical—but some swear it's a reset worth trying. This section lays out what colonics are, why they might click for vets, and how to approach them smart, with your health in the crosshairs.

Understanding Colonics
Colonics mean running filtered, warm water—think 5–15 gallons—through your colon over 30–60 minutes via a small tube in your rectum. A certified hydrotherapist controls the flow, and waste exits through a separate line in a closed system—no mess, no fuss. It's not an enema, which just hits the lower end; this goes deep, softening and flushing what's stuck. Rooted in old-school cleansing ideas, it's now a staple in alternative health circles, promising a gut overhaul for those willing to give it a shot.

The Science Behind It

Your colon's a workhorse—moving waste out through muscle waves called peristalsis. Colonics jump in, flooding it with water to loosen buildup and push it along. The pitch? Clear the pipes, lighten the load on your system. Some say it scrubs out toxins or bacteria; others argue your liver and kidneys already handle that. For Veterans, it's less about lab proof and more about feel—does it leave you steadier? Science leans cautious—your body's built to detox itself—but the hands-on appeal keeps it in play.

The Impact of Colonics on Veterans' Health

- Wellness Benefits: A cleaner gut could ease digestion, boost energy, maybe even cut inflammation—stuff vets need when the body's been through the wringer.

- Consequences of Skipping It: Ignore gut woes, and you're stuck with bloating, fatigue, or that heavy feeling—piling onto service scars.

Identifying and Analyzing Your Gut Needs

- Self-Assessment: Check your sitrep—constipated after years of field chow? Bloated from stress? Tired no matter what? Write it down—spot what's off.

- Setting Priorities: Zero in on the big ones—digestion if you're backed up, energy if you're dragging, detox if burn pit ghosts linger. Hit the loudest first.

Fostering the Colonics Habit

- Set Goals: Keep it tight—e.g., "Try one session this month to shake the sluggishness." Clear, doable, like a recon plan.

- Building a Support System: Tell a battle buddy or your doc you're testing it—they can weigh in, keep you grounded, like a squad watching your flank.

Implementation Strategies

- Occasional Use: Slot it in when you need a reset—monthly or yearly, not daily. Ease in; it's a tool, not a lifestyle.

- Habit Stacking: Pair it with a cleanse day—light eats, extra water, then the session. Ties it to what's already in your kit.

Targeted Protocols for Veterans' Wellness

Here's how to use colonics for specific needs, with supplies for each:

1. Digestive Health

- What: Book a 45-minute session with a hydrotherapist to flush the colon, once as a trial.

- Why: MREs and stress can jam your gut—colonics aim to clear the backlog, easing bloating or irregularity.

- How: Find a pro, lie back, let 5–10 gallons flow through—mild cramps might hit, but they pass. Prep with light food (veggies, broth) the day before, hydrate after. Try it once—see if your gut feels freer in a day or two.

- Supplies Needed: Certified hydrotherapist ($75–$150), water bottle for pre/post, loose clothes.

2. Detoxification

- What: Schedule a 60-minute session with optional herbal infusion, post-exposure or yearly.

- Why: Burn pits, chemicals—vets carry that load. Colonics pitch a flush for what might stick inside, even if your liver's on it.

- How: Ask for herbs (e.g., chamomile) in the water—takes an hour. Fast lightly before, rest after. Once a year or after a trigger—judge by how you feel. If it's too much, skip the add-ins.

- Supplies Needed: Hydrotherapist with herbal options, fasting plan (paper list), comfy spot for recovery.

3. Energy Boost

- What: Hit a 30–45-minute session when fatigue drags, monthly max.

- Why: Feeling heavy from old injuries or mental grind? Flushing waste might lift that fog—placebo or not, vets need the edge.

- How: Book it, hydrate well (32 oz water pre/post), take it easy after—45 minutes tops. Monthly if it works; skip if you're still wiped. Energy might tick up same-day.

- Supplies Needed: Hydrotherapist, water bottle, rest spot (couch, bed).

4. Pain and Inflammation Relief

- What: Try a 45-minute session targeting inflammation, once to test.

- Why: Joints ache from rucks, head pounds from stress—colonics claim to cut that by lightening your system's load.

- How: Go standard—no add-ins—lie still, let it run. Pair with rest and anti-inflammatory eats (fish, greens) after. One shot—check pain levels next day. If it's bunk, stick to PT.

- Supplies Needed: Hydrotherapist, post-session meal plan, quiet space.

5. Immune Support

- What: Use a 60-minute session with probiotics in the water, quarterly or post-illness.

- Why: Gut's your immune hub—colonics with good bacteria might shore it up, handy for vets fighting wear-down.

- How: Request probiotic infusion, take an hour, follow with yogurt or kefir. Quarterly if you're prone to bugs—see if colds drop. Too pricey? Skip the extras.

- Supplies Needed: Hydrotherapist with probiotics, post-session probiotic food, water.

Eliminating Barriers to Use
- Identify Triggers: Spot what holds you back—"Sounds weird," "Too risky," "No time." Name it, then gut-check it.

- Replace Hesitation: Swap "I'll pass" for a single trial—scout it like a new AO. Trade doubt for "What's it do?"—test, assess, decide.

- Veteran-Specific Substitutes:

  - Skepticism: Swap "BS cleanse" for "One and done"—try it, call it.

  - Fatigue: Trade "Too tired" for "Energy shot"—flush it, feel it.

Mindfulness and Self-Regulation
- Techniques: Focus on the water's flow or your breath during—stay in the moment. It's a mental anchor, cutting "this won't work" chatter.

- Benefits: You'll know when your gut's screaming—cue the session. Awareness keeps you in command, vet-style.

Seeking Professional Help
- When Needed: Got IBS, heart issues, or kidney trouble? Hit your VA doc first—colonics aren't for everyone.

- Resources: VA gastro pros, clinics, or telehealth can green-light it—free and vet-savvy.

Maintaining and Sustaining the Practice
- Track Progress: Log how you feel post-flush—less bloat, more pep? Mark a win: "Gut's quiet, energy's up."

- Overcome Plateaus: No change? Tweak timing—monthly to quarterly—or skip if it's flat. Push like a stalled op.

- Build Resilience: Each flush builds grit—shedding what slows you keeps you mission-ready.

Concussions

A concussion is a type of traumatic brain injury (TBI) caused by a blow or jolt to the head. It can also be caused by a hit to the body that causes the head to move rapidly back and forth. Concussions can range in severity, from mild to severe, and can have a variety of symptoms, including headache, confusion, dizziness, nausea and loss of consciousness. The diagnosis and treatment of TBI is an ongoing area of study and innovation. New approaches to treatment and diagnostic modalities are being developed and examined for use from the battlefield to the clinic.

The current state-of-the-art is changing rapidly with trials and studies being conducted by private and public organizations. An example of a partnership in research is the Acute Effects of Neurotrauma Consortium (AENC) which includes Phelps Health, the Leonard Wood Institute, the Missouri University of Science and Technology, University of Missouri and Washington University in St. Louis, Missouri who work together to prevent, detect and treat "acute" (short-term) TBI.[6]

The treatment of concussions typically involves a combination of rest and symptom management. The most important aspect of treatment is allowing the brain time to heal, which means limiting physical and cognitive activities that could exacerbate symptoms. This may include avoiding sports or other physical activities and limiting or avoiding activities that require concentration, such as reading, watching TV or using a computer.

Rest and symptom management are the mainstay of treatment for concussion. However, there are also a number of other interventions that can be used to help manage symptoms and speed up recovery. New approaches using functional magnetic resonance imaging (fMRI) to guide treatments have shown great promise in the treatment of concussions. One organization in the US known for this technique is Cognitive FX in Provo, Utah. The Functional Neurological Center in Minnetonka, Minnesota uses a number of technological assessments to obtain a baseline diagnosis and to monitor improvements during the course of treatment.

For headaches, over-the-counter pain medications such as ibuprofen and acetaminophen can be used. For nausea, anti-nausea medication may be prescribed. For dizziness, vestibular therapy may be recommended. This type of therapy is designed to help retrain the brain to process information from the inner ear, which can help reduce dizziness and balance problems.

Another important aspect of concussion treatment is rehabilitation. Rehabilitation can help individuals regain their cognitive, physical and emotional functioning. It typically includes exercises to improve balance, coordination and strength, as well as cognitive exercises to improve memory, attention and other cognitive skills.

In addition, cognitive-behavioral therapy (CBT) may be recommended to help individuals cope with the emotional and psychological effects of a concussion. This type of therapy can help individuals manage feelings of anxiety, depression and stress and can also help them develop strategies for coping with symptoms and managing their recovery.

In some cases, medications may be prescribed to help manage symptoms. For example, antidepressants may be prescribed to help manage symptoms of depression or anxiety and sleep aids may be prescribed to help individuals who are having difficulty sleeping.

It is also important to follow up with a healthcare provider after a concussion, to monitor symptoms and ensure that the individual is recovering properly. If symptoms persist or worsen, additional tests may be done to rule out any underlying conditions or complications.

In severe cases, a prolonged period of rest and rehabilitation may be required. In some cases, individuals may need to take time off work or school and may require additional support to manage daily activities.

Bottom Line
The treatment of concussions typically involves a combination of rest and symptom management. Medications may be used to help manage symptoms such as headaches and nausea. Rehabilitation can help individuals regain their cognitive, physical and emotional functioning. Cognitive-behavioral therapy (CBT) may be recommended to help individuals cope with the emotional and psychological effects of a concussion. And it is important to follow up with a healthcare provider after a concussion, to monitor symptoms and ensure that the individual is recovering properly.

Techniques to treat concussions

There are a number of techniques that can be used to treat concussions, including:

• *Rest:* The most important aspect of concussion treatment is allowing the brain time to heal. This means limiting physical and cognitive activities that could exacerbate symptoms. It's important to avoid sports or other physical activities and limit or avoid activities that require concentration, such as reading, watching TV or using a computer.

• *Symptom management:* Over-the-counter pain medications such as ibuprofen and acetaminophen can be used to manage headaches, anti-nausea medication may be prescribed for nausea and vestibular therapy may be recommended for dizziness.

• *Rehabilitation:* Rehabilitation can help individuals regain their cognitive, physical and emotional functioning. It typically includes exercises to improve balance, coordination and strength, as well as cognitive exercises to improve memory, attention and other cognitive skills.

• *Medications:* In some cases, medications may be prescribed to help manage symptoms. For example, antidepressants may be prescribed to help manage symptoms of depression or anxiety and sleep aids may be prescribed to help individuals who are having difficulty sleeping.

• *Cognitive-behavioral therapy (CBT):* CBT may be recommended to help individuals cope with the emotional and psychological effects of a concussion. This type of therapy can help individuals manage feelings of anxiety, depression and stress and can also help them develop strategies for coping with symptoms and managing their recovery.

• *Hyperbaric Oxygen Therapy (HBOT):* Hyperbaric Oxygen Therapy is a medical treatment that provides the patient with 100% pure oxygen in a pressurized chamber. This treatment increases the oxygen level in the body, which can help to reduce inflammation and promote healing.

• *Chiropractic care:* Chiropractic care is the treatment of the neuromuscular system through the use of manual techniques. Chiropractic adjustments can improve the function of the spine, which in turn can improve the function of the nervous system.

• *Nutrition and supplements:* Certain vitamins and minerals may be recommended to help with the healing process. Vitamins such as Vitamin D, Vitamin B12 and Vitamin C have been shown to have a positive effect on the brain. Omega-3 fatty acids and antioxidants may also be recommended to reduce inflammation and promote brain function.

It's important to note that not all treatments may be suitable for everyone and that the best course of treatment will vary depending on the individual's symptoms and needs. It's always best to consult with a healthcare professional to determine the best course of treatment for a concussion.

Support organizations for concussions

There are a number of organizations that provide support and resources for individuals who have experienced a concussion, as well as for their families and caregivers. Some of the most notable organizations include:

• *The Brain Injury Association of America (BIAA):* The BIAA (https://www.biausa.org/) is a national organization that provides support and resources for individuals with brain injuries and their families. They offer information and resources on the prevention, recognition and management of concussions, as well as support groups and advocacy services.

• *The American Academy of Neurology (AAN):* The AAN (https://www.aan.com/) is a professional organization of neurologists and other healthcare professionals that provides information and resources on the recognition and management of concussions. They also provide guidelines on when it is safe for an individual to return to physical activities following a concussion.

• *The Concussion Legacy Foundation (CLF):* The CLF (https://concussionfoundation.org/) is a nonprofit organization that focuses on the study and prevention of brain injuries, including concussions. They provide information and resources on the prevention, recognition and management of concussions, as well as support groups and educational programs.

• *The Center for Postconcussion Syndrome (PCS) & Post Traumatic Stress Disorder (PTSD) Treatment:* The Center for PCS and PTSD Treatment (formerly Sports Concussion Institute) (https://concussiontreatment.com/) is a leading organization in the field of sports-related concussions, providing education and resources to athletes, coaches and healthcare professionals. They also conduct research on the causes and effects of sports-related concussions and provide guidelines on when it is safe for an athlete to return to physical activities following a concussion.

• *The National Institute of Neurological Disorders and Stroke (NINDS):* The NINDS (https://www.ninds.nih.gov/) is a division of the National Institutes of Health that conducts research on the causes, prevention and treatment of neurological disorders, including concussions. They provide information and resources on the latest research on concussions and brain injuries, as well as clinical trials on the treatment of concussions.

• **Concussion Alliance:** Concussion Alliance (https://www.concussionalliance.org/) is a 501(c)(3) non-profit science-based patient advocacy organization founded in 2018.Their mission is to support concussion patients in their recovery with educational resources, keep providers up-to-date on new research, educate the next generation of healthcare professionals and change the public perception of concussions to reflect the seriousness of the injury. They also have a page dedicated to Service Members and Veterans at https://www.concussionalliance.org/Veterans.

These organizations can be a valuable resource for individuals who have experienced a concussion, as they provide information and resources on the latest research, as well as support and guidance on how to manage symptoms and recover from a concussion.

Connecting Consciousness, Mind, and Body for Healing and Growth with Plants

The integration of consciousness, mind, and body offers a holistic framework for healing trauma and fostering personal growth, uniting awareness, thoughts, and physicality into a cohesive system. Consciousness is our state of presence and perception, the mind encompasses thoughts and emotions, and the body serves as the physical foundation—each interacting dynamically. Trauma—whether from physical injury, emotional loss, or psychological stress—can fracture this unity, leading to disconnection, anxiety, or chronic ailments. Traditional practices like meditation, therapy, and exercise align these domains, but plant medicines and DMT-like substances introduce a potent, experiential dimension, used historically and increasingly today to purge suppressed burdens, deepen learning, and expand consciousness.

For individuals seeking to recover from trauma or enhance themselves, combining conventional methods with plant medicines—like ayahuasca, psilocybin, or DMT—offers a unique pathway. These substances, often administered in ceremonial or therapeutic settings, can amplify the connection between consciousness, mind, and body, facilitating profound insights and physical release. This section examines their role alongside established techniques, exploring mechanisms, benefits, and practical applications, supported by neuroscience, psychology, and ethnobotanical traditions, while addressing risks and evidence gaps.

The Foundations of Consciousness, Mind, and Body

Consciousness is the lens of awareness—our ability to observe ourselves and the world, shaped by attention and intent. It's tied to brain networks like the default mode network (DMN), which governs self-reflection, per a 2015 Neuroscience of Consciousness study. Plant medicines like DMT, a psychoactive compound in ayahuasca, alter this network, reducing DMN activity and expanding perception, as shown in a 2018 Scientific Reports study of 13 participants, suggesting a heightened state of consciousness.

The mind processes thoughts, emotions, and memories through regions like the prefrontal cortex (cognition), amygdala (fear), and hippocampus (memory). Trauma disrupts these, over-activating fear responses, per a 2018 Journal of Neuroscience study. Psychedelics like psilocybin rewire these circuits— a 2017 Journal of Psychopharmacology study of 19 depressed patients found a 20% mood lift after one dose, linked to increased neural flexibility.

The body manifests internal states through tension, inflammation, or fatigue, communicating via the vagus nerve, per a 2017 Frontiers in Psychology polyvagal theory article. Plant medicines induce physical purging—vomiting or shaking—as seen with ayahuasca, releasing stored stress, according to a 2019 Frontiers in Pharmacology review of 50 users, tying bodily detox to mental shifts.

Trauma fragments these domains—consciousness narrows, the mind fixates, the body clenches. Plant medicines and DMT-like substances, alongside traditional methods, reconnect them by purging blockages, revealing insights, and grounding experiences in the physical.

Why Integration Matters
Trauma isolates consciousness, mind, and body, causing dissociation—where awareness detaches from emotions or sensations—per a 2020 Trauma, Violence, & Abuse review. Integration heals this split, with conventional therapies showing a 30% symptom reduction over 12 weeks when combined, per a 2018 Journal of Traumatic Stress study of 70 trauma survivors. Plant medicines amplify this— a 2021 Nature Medicine study of 30 PTSD patients found a single ayahuasca session reduced symptoms by 40% in a week, suggesting faster processing through heightened consciousness.

Beyond healing, integration fosters growth. A 2016 Psychological Bulletin meta-analysis of 150 studies linked aligned practices to a 25% well-being boost. Psychedelics add depth— a 2019 Journal of Humanistic Psychology study of 50 psilocybin users reported a 30% rise in life satisfaction a month post-use, tied to expanded awareness and emotional clarity, enhancing personal development.

Mechanisms of Connection
Integration relies on biological and experiential mechanisms, enriched by plant medicines:

  1. **Neuroplasticity:** Repeated stimuli rewire the brain. A 2017 Neuron study

showed mindfulness and exercise strengthen prefrontal-amygdala links, reducing stress. DMT and psilocybin accelerate this— a 2020 Cell Reports study of 20 rodents found psychedelics doubled synaptic growth in 24 hours, connecting consciousness to mental shifts and physical calm.

2. Vagus Nerve Regulation: This nerve bridges mind and body. A 2019 Biological Psychiatry study of 80 adults found breathwork and imagery raised vagal tone by 15% over 4 weeks. Ayahuasca's purging boosts this— a 2021 Psychophysiology study of 40 users noted a 20% vagal increase post-ceremony, linking physical release to emotional stability.

3. Somatic Feedback: Trauma lodges in the body, per a 2015 Body, Movement and Dance in Psychotherapy article. Mind-body techniques cut pain by 20% over 8 weeks, per a 2020 Pain study of 60 patients. Plant medicines intensify this— a 2019 Journal of Ethnopharmacology study of 30 ayahuasca users found 70% reported physical "unblocking" alongside mental clarity.

4. Hormonal Balance: Stress hormones shift with integration. A 2016 Health Psychology study of 100 adults showed meditation lowered cortisol by 15%. Psychedelics amplify this— a 2020 Psych neuroendocrinology study of 50 psilocybin users found a 25% cortisol drop and 15% oxytocin rise a week post-dose, uniting all three domains.

5. Psychedelic States: DMT-like substances dissolve ego boundaries, per a 2018 Frontiers in Psychology review, merging consciousness with mind and body. A 2021 Journal of Psychopharmacology study of 25 ayahuasca users found 80% experienced unified awareness, purging trauma and revealing insights.

These mechanisms show how integration heals—purging trauma's residue, learning from expanded states, and grounding experiences physically—and supports growth through enhanced connectivity.

Benefits of Integration with Plant Medicines
- Trauma Resolution: Awareness, emotional processing, and purging heal wounds. A 2019 Clinical Psychology Review study found a 25% drop in intrusions with therapy over 8 weeks; a 2021 Nature Medicine study showed ayahuasca cut PTSD symptoms by 40% in a week.

- Mental Clarity: Focused consciousness and psychedelics sharpen cognition. A 2017 Journal of Cognitive Enhancement study noted a 20% focus boost with traditional methods; a 2020 Neuroscience Letters study of 30 psilocybin users found a 30% memory gain post-dose.

- Physical Restoration: Mind-body feedback and purging reduce tension. A

2018 Journal of Alternative and Complementary Medicine study showed a 15% pain drop; a 2019 Frontiers in Pharmacology study of 50 ayahuasca users noted 60% felt physically lighter post-ceremony.

- Stress Reduction: Calming practices and psychedelics lower stress. A 2020 psych neuroendocrinology study found a 20% cortisol drop with therapy; a 2021 Journal of Psychopharmacology study of 40 DMT users saw a 25% reduction in a week.

- Emotional Resilience: Positive reframing and purging build coping. A 2016 Emotion study showed a 15% resilience rise; a 2020 Journal of Humanistic Psychology study of 50 psilocybin users found a 20% mood lift lasting months.

- Personal Growth: Expanded awareness and insights foster development. A 2015 Journal of Positive Psychology study linked integration to a 25% satisfaction rise; a 2019 Journal of Psychedelic Studies study of 30 ayahuasca users reported a 35% increase in purpose post-retreat.

Targeted Protocols with Plant Medicines

These protocols integrate consciousness, mind, and body, adding plant medicines for purging, learning, and experiencing:

Trauma Resolution: Start with mindfulness meditation—10–20 minutes daily, focusing on breath—to raise consciousness. Add therapy (1 hour weekly, CBT or somatic) to process the mind, and stretching (15–30 minutes daily) to ease the body. Join an ayahuasca ceremony (1–2 nights, $200–$1,000) with a trained facilitator—purging releases trauma, insights reframe emotions, and physical grounding follows over 4–8 weeks; adjust with a therapist if intense.

Mental Clarity: Use visualization—10–15 minutes daily, picturing focus—to direct consciousness, journaling (15 minutes daily) to engage the mind, and yoga (30 minutes daily) to ground the body. Take psilocybin (1–3 g dried mushrooms, $20–$50) in a guided setting monthly—expanded awareness clears fog, learning sharpens thought, and physical calm anchors it over 6 weeks; track focus and refine with a guide if needed.

Physical Restoration: Practice body scans—10 minutes daily, noting sensations—for consciousness, CBT (1 hour weekly) to shift pain perceptions, and strength training (30–60 minutes, 3 times weekly) for the body. Use San Pedro cactus (200–400 g, $50–$100) in a ceremony biannually—purging detoxes, insights ease mental strain, and physical repair grows over 8–12 weeks; monitor with a doctor if pain persists.

Stress Reduction: Apply breathwork—5–10 minutes daily, 4-7-8 pattern—for consciousness, affirmations (5 minutes daily) to calm the mind, and tai chi (30 minutes, 3 times weekly) for the body. Take DMT (20–50 mg vaporized, $50–$100) quarterly with a sitter—intense release purges stress, clarity resets thoughts, and relaxation settles the body over 4 weeks; log stress and adjust with support if overwhelming.

Emotional Resilience: Use gratitude—5 minutes daily, listing positives—for consciousness, support groups (1 hour weekly) to strengthen the mind, and massage (30–60 minutes weekly) for the body. Join a psilocybin retreat (2–3 days, $500–$2,000) biannually—purging lifts burdens, peer insights build coping, and physical ease reinforces it over 6–8 weeks; track mood and add therapy if needed.

Personal Growth: Meditate—15 minutes daily, setting intent—for consciousness, goal-setting (10 minutes weekly) for the mind, and running (30–60 minutes daily) for the body. Use ayahuasca (1 night, $200–$1,000) annually—expanded vision drives purpose, learning shapes goals, and vitality boosts action over 8–12 weeks; assess satisfaction and refine with a coach.

Start with daily practices (5–60 minutes) and therapy, adding plant medicines in controlled settings (legal where permitted, e.g., retreats in Peru, Netherlands). Consult a healthcare provider and psychedelic facilitator before use, especially with mental health conditions or medications—costs range from free (traditional) to $50–$2,000 (psychedelics). Assess outcomes—less stress, clearer purpose—over months, adjusting with professionals.

Considerations and Evidence
Conventional evidence is robust— a 2019 NeuroImage study showed meditation alters DMN, a 2018 American Psychologist meta-analysis found CBT cuts anxiety by 30%, and a 2017 Sports Medicine review linked exercise to 20% less inflammation. Psychedelic evidence grows— a 2021 Nature Medicine study confirmed ayahuasca's PTSD benefits, a 2020 Journal of Psychopharmacology study validated psilocybin's mood effects, and a 2018 Scientific Reports study mapped DMT's consciousness shifts. Integrated approaches with psychedelics lack large trials— a 2020 Journal of Integrative Medicine study of 100 adults showed a 25% well-being boost, but most data is small-scale (20–50 participants) or anecdotal.

Risks include emotional overwhelm or physical strain from psychedelics— a 2021 Drug and Alcohol Dependence study of 50 users noted 5% had temporary distress; use trained guides and medical screening. Legal status varies—DMT is Schedule I in the U.S., but legal in retreat settings elsewhere. Costs range from free (traditional) to $2,000+ (psychedelics). Results build gradually—expect shifts over weeks to years with consistency.

Bottom Line
Connecting consciousness, mind, and body heals trauma and drives growth, amplified by plant medicines and DMT-like substances that purge, teach, and expand experience. Neuroplasticity, vagal regulation, and psychedelic states underpin this, offering trauma relief to personal evolution. Protocols blend daily practices with occasional psychedelic use, tailored to need. Evidence supports components, but full integration, especially with psychedelics, needs more study; risks are manageable with care. This approach empowers wholeness—purging past pain, learning from insights, and grounding in the body—for anyone seeking recovery or growth.

Cultural Considerations

Cultural considerations are an important aspect of providing healthcare services to Veterans. Veterans come from diverse cultural backgrounds and their cultural values, beliefs and practices can have a significant impact on their health and well-being. As such, healthcare providers who work with Veterans must be aware of and sensitive to cultural differences to ensure that they provide effective and culturally responsive care. Here are some key cultural considerations to keep in mind when working with Veterans:

• *Understanding cultural diversity:* Veterans come from diverse cultural backgrounds and it is important for healthcare providers to understand and appreciate these differences. Understanding cultural diversity can help to build trust and rapport with Veterans and can help to ensure that their unique cultural values and beliefs are respected and considered in their care.

• *Building cultural competence:* Building cultural competence involves developing the knowledge, skills and attitudes needed to effectively work with individuals from diverse cultural backgrounds. Healthcare providers who work with Veterans should undergo training to help them develop cultural competence and ensure that they can provide culturally responsive care.

• *Addressing language barriers:* Veterans who are not proficient in English may face language barriers when seeking healthcare services. Healthcare providers should have access to language interpretation services to ensure that Veterans can communicate their needs effectively and receive the care they require.

• *Understanding the impact of military culture:* Military culture has a significant impact on the values, beliefs and practices of Veterans. Healthcare providers who work with Veterans should have an understanding of military culture to ensure that they can provide effective and culturally responsive care.

• *Recognizing the impact of trauma:* Many Veterans have experienced trauma during their service, which can have a significant impact on their physical and mental health. Healthcare providers who work with Veterans should be aware of the impact of trauma and should provide trauma-informed care to ensure that Veterans feel safe and supported during their care.

- ***Incorporating alternative and complementary therapies:*** Many Veterans may prefer alternative and complementary therapies, such as acupuncture, massage and Reiki, as a part of their healthcare. Healthcare providers who work with Veterans should be aware of these preferences and incorporate them into their care plans where appropriate.

- ***Considering spiritual and religious beliefs:*** Many Veterans have strong spiritual and religious beliefs that may impact their healthcare preferences and decision-making. Healthcare providers who work with Veterans should be aware of these beliefs and ensure that they are considered in their care.

Bottom Line

Cultural considerations are an important aspect of providing healthcare services to Veterans. Healthcare providers who work with Veterans must be aware of and sensitive to cultural differences to ensure that they provide effective and culturally responsive care. Understanding cultural diversity, building cultural competence, addressing language barriers, understanding the impact of military culture, recognizing the impact of trauma, incorporating alternative and complementary therapies and considering spiritual and religious beliefs are all key considerations when working with Veterans. By providing culturally responsive care, healthcare providers can ensure that Veterans receive the care they require and promote their overall health and well-being.

- D -

<u>Denial</u>

Denial is a common issue among Veterans and can have a significant impact on their emotions and health. Denial is defined as a defense mechanism in which a person refuses to acknowledge the reality of a difficult or unpleasant situation, such as the effects of combat, physical injury or post-traumatic stress disorder (PTSD).

The effects of denial on Veterans can be far-reaching and can include:

• ***Increased stress and anxiety:*** Denial can increase stress and anxiety, as Veterans struggle to cope with the reality of their experiences and the impact that these experiences are having on their lives.

• ***Difficulty accessing healthcare:*** Veterans who are in denial about their physical or mental health may be less likely to seek medical attention, which can lead to delayed or inadequate treatment and further health problems.

• ***Difficulty adjusting to civilian life:*** Veterans who are in denial about the effects of their military experiences may have difficulty adjusting to civilian life and may struggle to form meaningful relationships or find purpose and meaning in their lives.

• ***Increased risk for substance abuse:*** Veterans who are in denial about their physical or mental health may turn to drugs or alcohol as a means of coping, which can lead to substance abuse and addiction.

• ***Increased risk for suicide:*** Veterans who are in denial about their physical or mental health may be at increased risk for suicide, as they struggle to cope with the effects of their experiences and the impact that these experiences are having on their lives.

To address denial among Veterans, it is important to:

• ***Encourage open and honest communication:*** Encouraging Veterans to openly and honestly communicate about their experiences and the impact that these experiences are having on their lives can help to reduce denial and increase understanding and support.

• ***Connect Veterans with resources:*** Connecting Veterans with resources, such as healthcare providers, support groups and counseling services, can help to address their physical and mental health needs and reduce denial.

• ***Promote self-care:*** Encouraging Veterans to engage in self-care activities, such as exercise, healthy eating and stress management, can help to reduce stress and improve overall health.

• **Provide education:** Providing education about the effects of combat and PTSD can help Veterans to better understand the impact of their experiences and the importance of seeking help.

Bottom Line

Denial is a common issue among Veterans and can have a significant impact on their emotions and health. To address denial among Veterans, it is important to encourage open and honest communication, connect Veterans with resources, promote self-care and provide education. By taking these steps, Veterans can reduce denial and improve their overall health and wellbeing.

Depression

Depression is a prevalent and serious mental health condition that affects many Veterans. According to the U.S. Department of Veterans Affairs, an estimated 20% of Veterans who served in Iraq and Afghanistan have been diagnosed with depression. In addition, Veterans are at a higher risk for suicide compared to the general population, with an estimated 22 Veterans dying by suicide each day.

There are a number of factors that contribute to the high rates of depression among Veterans. One of the most significant factors is exposure to combat and other traumatic events. Veterans who have been in combat situations may have difficulty adjusting to civilian life and may experience symptoms of post-traumatic stress disorder (PTSD), which can increase the risk of depression.

Another factor that contributes to the high rates of depression among Veterans is the stigma surrounding mental health. Many Veterans may feel ashamed or embarrassed to seek help for mental health issues and may avoid seeking treatment out of fear of being seen as weak. This can make it difficult for Veterans to receive the help they need and can prolong the duration of their depression.

In addition, Veterans may also experience a number of other stressors that can contribute to depression. These include physical injuries, chronic pain, financial difficulties and relationship problems. These stressors can make it difficult for Veterans to transition to civilian life and can make it harder for them to cope with the symptoms of depression.

Treatment for Veteran depression typically includes a combination of therapy and medication. Cognitive behavioral therapy (CBT) is an effective form of therapy that can help Veterans to identify and change negative patterns of thinking and behavior. Antidepressant medication can also be effective in treating the symptoms of depression.

The Department of Veterans Affairs (VA) offers a wide range of services to help Veterans with depression. These services include individual and group therapy, medication management and case management. The VA also offers specialized programs for Veterans who have experienced combat-related trauma, such as the PTSD Treatment Program.

It's important for Veterans to seek help as soon as they start experiencing symptoms of depression. Early intervention can help to prevent the condition from becoming worse and can make it easier for Veterans to recover. Veterans can seek help from their primary care provider, a mental health professional or the VA.

Techniques to treat depression in Veterans

• *Therapy:* One of the most effective ways to treat depression in Veterans is through therapy. Cognitive Behavioral Therapy (CBT) is an evidence-based form of therapy that can help Veterans to identify and change negative patterns of thinking and behavior. It can also help Veterans to develop coping mechanisms for dealing with difficult situations and emotions. Other forms of therapy, such as Interpersonal Therapy (IPT) and Eye Movement Desensitization and Reprocessing (EMDR) can also be effective for Veterans.

• *Medication:* Antidepressant medication can also be effective in treating the symptoms of depression. Selective serotonin reuptake inhibitors (SSRIs) are the most commonly prescribed antidepressants for Veterans. They work by increasing the levels of serotonin, a chemical in the brain that helps regulate mood. Other types of antidepressants, such as tricyclic antidepressants and monoamine oxidase inhibitors (MAOIs), may also be prescribed.

• *Combination therapy:* Combining therapy and medication can be more effective than either treatment alone. This approach can help to alleviate symptoms more quickly and can also reduce the risk of relapse.

• *Support groups:* Joining a support group can provide Veterans with a sense of community and a safe space to talk about their experiences. Support groups can also provide Veterans with a sense of understanding and validation, as well as practical tips for coping with depression.

- **Lifestyle changes:** Making healthy lifestyle changes can help to alleviate symptoms of depression. This includes getting regular exercise, eating a healthy diet, getting enough sleep and avoiding alcohol and drugs.

- **Mindfulness-based interventions:** Mindfulness-based interventions such as mindfulness-based stress reduction (MBSR) and mindfulness-based cognitive therapy (MBCT) can help Veterans to manage stress and emotions and to develop a sense of self-awareness.

- **Service Animals:** Some Veterans may benefit from the companionship of a service animal. Service animals can provide emotional support and help Veterans to feel less alone.

- **Electroconvulsive therapy (ECT):** ECT is a treatment that uses electrical currents to stimulate the brain.

Bottom Line

Depression is a serious mental health condition that affects many Veterans. It's important for Veterans to be aware of the risk factors for depression and to seek help as soon as they start experiencing symptoms. With the right treatment and support, Veterans can overcome depression and improve their quality of life. The VA provides a wide range of services to help Veterans with depression and it's important for Veterans to take advantage of these resources. It's also important for society to continue to break the stigma around mental health and to support Veterans in their mental health journey.

Detoxification

It is the process of removing harmful toxins and substances from the body. The body has several natural detoxification systems, such as the liver, kidneys and lymphatic system, that work to remove toxins and keep the body functioning properly. However, due to factors such as poor diet, stress and exposure to environmental toxins, these systems can become overwhelmed and in need of support.

One way to support the body's natural detoxification process is through a detox diet. This type of diet typically involves eating whole, nutrient-dense foods and avoiding processed foods, sugar, alcohol and caffeine. Eating a diet rich in fruits and vegetables, lean protein and healthy fats can help to support the liver and kidneys in their detoxification processes. Drinking plenty of water and herbal teas can also help to flush toxins out of the body.

Another way to support the body's detoxification process is through the use of supplements. Certain supplements, such as Milk Thistle, N-Acetyl Cysteine and Alpha Lipoic Acid, can help to support the liver in its detoxification processes. Others, such as chlorella and spirulina, can help to remove heavy metals and other toxins from the body. It's important to consult with a healthcare professional before taking any supplement and check if they interact with any medication you're taking.

Physical exercise also plays a role in detoxifying the body. Regular physical activity can help to improve circulation and promote the removal of toxins through sweating. Regular exercise can also help to support the lymphatic system, which is responsible for removing waste and toxins from the body but moving and flexing our muscles helps so that lymph can move.

Skin detoxification can be done through regular exfoliation and the use of masks. Exfoliation helps remove dead skin cells and unclog pores, allowing the skin to breathe. Using masks, such as charcoal or clay, can help to draw impurities and toxins out of the skin.

Detoxifying the mind, emotions and spirit can be done through practices such as meditation, journaling and therapy. These practices can help to release negative emotions and thoughts, which can contribute to physical and emotional toxins and blockages in the body.

It is important to remember that detoxification is a gradual process and it should not be done abruptly. A gradual and sustained approach is more likely to be successful and less likely to cause harm.

The Liver and Gallbladder Miracle Cleanse is a book and program authored by Andreas Moritz. The cleanse involves a combination of supplements, dietary changes and a series of coffee enemas. The program claims to remove gallstones and other toxins from the liver and gallbladder, thereby improving overall health and wellness. However, it is important to note that the scientific evidence supporting the effectiveness of the liver and gallbladder cleanse is limited and the safety of the cleanse is also in question. (Note: An overview of the cleanse is included in **Annex E—Alternative Approaches**)

Coffee enemas are not recommended by mainstream medicine as a treatment for any condition and can have serious risks and side effects, such as electrolyte imbalances, infections, rectal perforation and even death. Moreover, gallstones are not always the cause of the symptoms that Moritz attributed to them and many of the claims he made about their effects and their connection to cancer are unproven.

It is always recommended to consult with a healthcare professional before trying any new medical treatment or alternative therapy, including the liver and gallbladder cleanse program. A healthcare professional can help to evaluate your individual health needs and advise you on the best course of treatment.

Detoxifying the lymphatic system

The lymphatic system is an important part of the body's immune system that helps to remove toxins, waste and excess fluids. When the lymphatic system becomes clogged or sluggish, it can lead to a number of health problems, including fatigue, weight gain and a weakened immune system. To help detox your lymphatic system, there are a few things that you can do.

• *Exercise:* Exercise is one of the best ways to detox your lymphatic system. When you move your body, it helps to stimulate the lymphatic vessels, which in turn helps to move lymphatic fluid throughout the body. This can help to remove toxins and waste from the body, as well as improve overall circulation.

• *Dry brushing:* Dry brushing is a simple technique that involves brushing your skin with a dry brush before taking a shower. This helps to remove dead skin cells, improve circulation and stimulate the lymphatic vessels. This can help to improve the overall function of the lymphatic system.

• *Drinking water:* Drinking plenty of water is also important for detoxifying the lymphatic system. Water helps to flush toxins and waste from the body and it also helps to keep the lymphatic vessels and lymph nodes hydrated. Aim for at least 8-10 cups of water a day.

• *Eating a healthy diet:* Eating a diet that is high in fruits and vegetables can also help to detox your lymphatic system. Fruits and vegetables are rich in antioxidants and other nutrients that can help to boost the immune system and improve the overall function of the lymphatic system.

• *Yoga:* Yoga is a great way to detox your lymphatic system. Yoga helps to improve flexibility and circulation, which in turn helps to stimulate the lymphatic vessels and improve the overall function of the lymphatic system.

• *Massage:* Massage is also a great way to detox your lymphatic system. Massage helps to stimulate the lymphatic vessels and improve circulation, which in turn helps to remove toxins and waste from the body. This can help to improve the overall function of the lymphatic system.

• **Sweating:** Sweating is an important way to detoxify the body and it can also help to detox the lymphatic system. When you sweat, you are releasing toxins, waste and excess fluids that have been trapped in the body. Sweating can be done by doing a sauna or by doing a workout that makes you sweat.

It's also important to note that avoiding certain things can help detox your lymphatic system as well. Stay away from alcohol, tobacco and processed foods, which can all contribute to the clogging of the lymphatic system. Additionally, limit exposure to environmental toxins, such as pesticides and pollution.

Overall, detoxifying your lymphatic system is an important step in maintaining overall health and wellness. By incorporating the above tips into your daily routine, you can help to improve the function of your lymphatic system and reduce the risk of health problems. Remember to be patient and consistent, as the process of detoxifying the lymphatic system may take time and effort.

Heavy metal detoxification

Heavy metal toxicity is a major concern for all individuals, but Veterans are at a higher risk due to their exposure to heavy metals through military service. These metals can accumulate in the body over time and lead to a range of health problems, including neurological issues, immune system dysfunction and various forms of cancer. In this document, we will examine the sources of heavy metal toxicity in Veterans, the health effects of these metals and strategies for detoxifying the body to reduce their harmful effects.

Sources of heavy metal toxicity in Veterans

• **Environmental Exposure:** Veterans are at a higher risk of exposure to heavy metals through their military service. This exposure can occur through contact with contaminated soil, water and air, as well as through exposure to contaminated food and other substances.

• **Use of Military Equipment:** Many military equipment, such as aircraft, vehicles and weapons, contain heavy metals, including lead, mercury and cadmium. Contact with these metals can occur through handling, maintenance and repair of military equipment, as well as through exposure to fumes and debris generated during their use.

• *Occupational Exposure:* Veterans may be exposed to heavy metals through their Military Occupational Specialty (MOS) that involve the use of these metals, during metal fabrication and metal recycling.

Health Effects Of Heavy Metals

• *Neurotoxicity:* Heavy metals such as lead, mercury and cadmium are toxic to the central nervous system and can cause a range of neurological problems, including headaches, mood swings, memory loss and tremors.

• *Immune System Dysfunction:* Heavy metals can disrupt the functioning of the immune system, leading to increased susceptibility to infections, autoimmune disorders and other health problems.

• *Cancer:* Some heavy metals, such as cadmium and lead, are known to increase the risk of cancer, particularly in the lung and other respiratory organs.

• *Kidney Damage:* Chronic exposure to heavy metals can lead to kidney damage, which can result in chronic kidney disease and other health problems.

Strategies for detoxifying the body

• *Diet:* A diet that is rich in antioxidants, fiber and nutrients can help to support the body's natural processes for removing heavy metals. Foods such as leafy green vegetables, whole grains, and fruits can help to support the liver and kidneys, which are the primary organs responsible for eliminating heavy metals from the body.

• *Supplements:* Supplements such as chelating agents, which are designed to bind to heavy metals and remove them from the body, can be helpful for reducing the levels of heavy metals in the body. These supplements should be taken under the guidance of a healthcare provider to ensure that they are safe and effective.

• *Detoxification Therapy:* Detoxification therapies, such as saunas, colon hydrotherapy and other forms of therapy, can be helpful for removing heavy metals from the body. These therapies should be used under the guidance of a healthcare provider to ensure that they are safe and effective.

Bottom Line
Heavy metal toxicity is a serious concern for Veterans, due to their exposure to these metals through military service. However, with the right strategies, Veterans can reduce their levels of heavy metals and minimize the risk of health problems. A diet that is rich in antioxidants, fiber and nutrients, along with the use of sup-

plements and detoxification therapies, can be helpful for reducing the levels of heavy metals in the body. Additionally, it is important to seek the guidance of a healthcare provider to ensure that these strategies are safe and effective for each individual. By taking steps to detoxify the body of heavy metals, Veterans can help to reduce the risk of health problems and maintain optimal health and wellness. It is important to be proactive in addressing heavy metal toxicity, as the long-term effects of exposure to these metals can be serious and irreversible. With the right strategies and support, Veterans can achieve a healthier, happier life.

Life detoxification

Life detoxification is a holistic process of removing negative influences, toxins and habits from one's life in order to improve overall well-being and health. It is a process of identifying and eliminating elements that are harmful to our mental, physical and emotional well-being and replacing them with positive and nourishing ones.

The first step in life detoxification is to identify the negative influences and habits in your life. This may include people or situations that cause you stress or make you feel negative, as well as unhealthy habits such as overeating, smoking or excessive alcohol consumption. Once you have identified these areas, it is important to come up with a plan to remove or reduce them from your life.

It can be helpful to make a list of the negative habits or people in your life and then prioritize them based on how much they are affecting your life. This can help you to focus on the most important changes first. For example, if you are struggling with addiction, it may be necessary to seek professional help to overcome it.

Another important aspect of life detoxification is to incorporate healthy habits and practices into your daily routine. This can include things such as regular exercise, eating a healthy diet and getting enough sleep. Exercise is an excellent way to reduce stress, improve mental and emotional well-being and also helps to maintain a healthy weight. Eating a healthy diet that is rich in fruits and vegetables, lean proteins and whole grains can help to provide the necessary nutrients to support the body's natural detoxification processes. Getting enough sleep is also important as it helps the body to repair and rejuvenate itself.

Incorporating mindfulness and meditation into your daily routine can also help to reduce stress and improve mental and emotional well-being. Mindfulness is the practice of being present and fully engaged in the moment, without judgment. It can help to reduce stress, improve focus and concentration and increase overall well-being. Meditation is a practice that can help to quiet the mind and reduce stress. It can be done by focusing on your breath or repeating a mantra.

It's also important to make time for self-care and self-compassion, which can include practices like journaling, yoga or taking a relaxing bath. These practices can help to improve mood, reduce stress and anxiety and increase overall well-being. Life detoxification is a lifelong process that requires constant effort and perseverance. It's not always easy to let go of negative habits and influences, but with time and commitment, you can make positive changes that will improve your overall well-being.

It's also important to seek professional help if needed, such as therapy and counseling, to support the process and address underlying issues that may be driving negative habits or influences. A therapist can help you to identify the root causes of negative habits and provide guidance on how to overcome them.

Another important aspect of life detoxification is to reduce exposure to toxins in the environment. This can include things like using natural cleaning products, eating organic foods and using natural personal care products. It also includes reducing exposure to toxins in the air, such as pollutants and pesticides.

Bottom Line

Life detoxification is a process of identifying and removing negative influences, toxins and habits from one's life to improve overall well-being and health. It involves incorporating healthy habits and practices, self-care and self-compassion and seeking professional help if needed. It is a lifelong process that requires constant effort and perseverance. By taking the time to identify and eliminate negative influences and habits and incorporating healthy practices into our daily routine, we can improve our overall well-being and live a happier, healthier life.

Skin Detoxification

Skin detoxification refers to the process of removing toxins and impurities from the skin. This can be achieved through various methods such as cleansing, exfoliating and using topical products. The goal of skin detoxification is to improve the appearance and health of the skin and to prevent skin problems such as acne, wrinkles and uneven skin tone.

One of the most basic and effective ways to detoxify the skin is through cleansing. Cleansing involves removing dirt, oil and makeup from the skin's surface. This can be done by using a gentle cleanser or soap and warm water. It is important to avoid using hot water, as this can strip the skin of its natural oils and cause irritation. Cleansing should be done twice a day, once in the morning and once at night.

Exfoliation is another important step in skin detoxification. Exfoliation involves removing dead skin cells from the surface of the skin, revealing the fresh, healthy skin underneath. There are two types of exfoliation: physical and chemical. Physical exfoliation involves using a scrub or brush to manually remove dead skin cells, while chemical exfoliation uses acids or enzymes to dissolve the bonds between dead skin cells. Exfoliation should be done once or twice a week, depending on your skin type.

Topical products, such as masks and serums, can also be used to detoxify the skin. These products can help to remove impurities, improve the appearance of the skin and promote a healthy, youthful glow. Some popular ingredients found in detoxifying products include charcoal, clay and sulfur. Charcoal is known for its ability to absorb impurities, clay helps to remove excess oil and sulfur is known to help clear acne-prone skin.

A healthy diet can also play an important role in skin detoxification. Eating a diet high in fruits and vegetables can provide the skin with the vitamins and minerals it needs to stay healthy. Foods high in antioxidants, such as berries, can help to protect the skin from damage caused by environmental toxins. Drinking plenty of water is also important, as it helps to flush toxins out of the body.

In addition to these methods, lifestyle changes can also play a role in skin detoxification. Avoiding smoking, drinking and excessive sun exposure can help to protect the skin from damage. Getting enough sleep and managing stress can also help to keep the skin looking healthy and youthful.

While these methods can improve the appearance and health of the skin, there is no scientific evidence that specifically shows that skin can be detoxified. The skin is naturally equipped to remove impurities and dead cells and these processes happen continuously. It is important to consult with a licensed healthcare professional before starting any treatments.

Bottom Line
Skin detoxification is the process of removing toxins and impurities from the skin, it can be achieved through various methods such as cleansing, exfoliating and using topical products. The goal of skin detoxification is to improve the appearance and health of the skin and to prevent skin problems such as acne, wrinkles and uneven skin tone. Cleansing, exfoliating and using topical products, healthy diet and a healthy lifestyle are some of the ways to improve the appearance and health of the skin, but there is no scientific evidence that specifically shows that skin can be detoxified. It's important to consult with a licensed healthcare professional before starting any treatments.

Testing the Body

Testing the body to assess levels of toxification, also known as toxicology testing, is a way to determine the presence and levels of harmful toxins in the body. These toxins can come from a variety of sources, including the environment, diet and lifestyle choices.

There are several different types of toxicology tests that can be used to assess levels of toxification in the body. Some of the most commonly used tests include:

• **Blood tests:** Blood tests can be used to measure the levels of various toxins in the bloodstream, including heavy metals, pesticides and industrial chemicals. These tests can also be used to assess the function of the liver and kidneys, which are key organs in the body's natural detoxification process.

• **Urine tests:** Urine tests can be used to measure the levels of toxins that have been eliminated from the body through the urine. These tests can be used to assess exposure to a wide variety of toxins, including heavy metals, pesticides and industrial chemicals.

• **Hair tests:** Hair tests can be used to measure the levels of certain toxins that have accumulated in the hair over time. These tests are particularly useful for assessing exposure to heavy metals, such as lead and mercury.

• **Biomarkers:** Biomarkers are chemical or biological indicators that can be used to measure exposure to certain toxins. Biomarkers can be found in blood, urine, hair or other bodily fluids and can be used to assess exposure to a wide variety of toxins.

It's important to note that the results of toxicology tests should be interpreted in conjunction with a person's symptoms and medical history. A positive test result does not necessarily mean that a person is suffering from the effects of toxification and a negative test result does not necessarily mean that a person is free of toxins.

Additionally, it's also important to consult with a healthcare professional before undergoing any testing. A healthcare professional can help to interpret the results of the tests and determine the best course of action. They can also help to identify any underlying health conditions that may be contributing to the presence of toxins in the body.

Bottom Line
Testing the body to assess levels of toxification is a way to determine the presence and levels of harmful toxins in the body. There are several different types of

toxicology tests that can be used, including blood tests, urine tests, hair tests and biomarkers. It's important to interpret the results of these tests in conjunction with a person's symptoms and medical history and to consult with a healthcare professional before undergoing any testing.

Diabetes

A chronic condition that affects how the body processes glucose, a type of sugar and insulin, the hormone responsible for regulating glucose levels appears in three main types: Type 1, Type 2 and Gestational diabetes.

Type 1 diabetes is an autoimmune condition in which the body's immune system attacks and destroys the insulin-producing cells in the pancreas. This leads to an absence of insulin in the body and requires individuals with type 1 diabetes to take insulin injections or use an insulin pump to manage their blood sugar levels. Type 1 diabetes is usually diagnosed in childhood or adolescence and accounts for about 5-10% of all cases of diabetes.

Type 2 diabetes is the most common form of diabetes and is characterized by insulin resistance, which means that the body is unable to effectively use insulin to regulate blood sugar levels. Over time, the pancreas may stop producing enough insulin to keep up with the body's demands, leading to high blood sugar levels. Type 2 diabetes is often linked to lifestyle factors such as being overweight, having a sedentary lifestyle and eating an unhealthy diet. In some cases, this type may be eliminated by dietary changes and a keto/fasting protocol monitored by your doctor.

Gestational diabetes is a type of diabetes that affects women during pregnancy. It occurs when the body cannot produce enough insulin to regulate blood sugar levels during pregnancy. While gestational diabetes usually goes away after giving birth, women who have had gestational diabetes have a higher risk of developing type 2 diabetes later in life.

Treatment for diabetes depends on the type and severity of the condition. For type 1 diabetes, treatment involves taking insulin injections or using an insulin pump, as well as monitoring blood sugar levels regularly and making lifestyle changes to manage the condition.

For type 2 diabetes, treatment often starts with lifestyle changes such as losing weight, eating a healthy diet and increasing physical activity. In some cases oral medications or insulin injections may also be necessary to manage blood sugar levels.

For gestational diabetes, treatment usually involves monitoring blood sugar levels, making lifestyle changes and, in some cases, taking insulin injections.

Managing diabetes requires making healthy lifestyle choices, monitoring blood sugar levels, taking medications as prescribed and working closely with a healthcare team to manage the condition.

Healthy lifestyle choices include eating a balanced and nutritious diet, engaging in regular physical activity, quitting smoking and managing stress levels. It is also important to monitor blood sugar levels regularly and to attend all scheduled appointments with a healthcare provider.

In addition to lifestyle changes and medical management, individuals with diabetes also need to be aware of the potential complications of the condition, including heart disease, nerve damage and eye problems. Regular monitoring and management can help prevent or delay the development of these complications.

Living with diabetes can be challenging, but it is possible to live a healthy and fulfilling life with the condition. It is important to work closely with a healthcare team, make healthy lifestyle choices and manage the condition effectively to minimize the impact it has on daily life.

Bottom Line

Diabetes is a chronic condition that affects how the body processes glucose and insulin. There are three main types of diabetes: Type 1, Type 2 and Gestational diabetes. Treatment for diabetes depends on the type and severity of the condition and may involve lifestyle changes, medication and regular monitoring. By making healthy lifestyle choices, working closely with a healthcare team and effectively managing the condition, individuals with diabetes can live a healthy and fulfilling life.

Diets

Balanced Diet

A balanced diet is essential for maintaining overall health and well-being. It provides the body with the necessary nutrients, vitamins and minerals to function properly and support growth and development. Some of the key benefits of a balanced diet include:

> • ***Body Composition:*** Eating a balanced diet can help maintain a healthy body composition by providing the body with the right amount of energy and nutrients

it needs without excess calories.

- **Disease prevention:** A diet rich in fruits, vegetables, whole grains and lean proteins can help reduce the risk of chronic diseases such as heart disease, diabetes and certain cancers.

- **Improved digestion:** A balanced diet can improve digestion and regularity by providing the body with the necessary fibers and fluids.

- **Better mood and mental health:** A balanced diet can improve mood and mental health by providing the brain with the necessary nutrients to function properly and help prevent depression and anxiety.

- **Increased energy:** A balanced diet can increase energy levels by providing the body with the necessary nutrients to produce energy.

- **Stronger immunity:** A balanced diet can help boost the immune system by providing the body with the necessary vitamins and minerals to fight off infections and illnesses.

- **Better skin, hair and nails:** Eating a balanced diet that is rich in vitamins and minerals can help improve the appearance of skin, hair and nails.

- **Improved athletic performance:** Eating a balanced diet can improve athletic performance by providing the body with the necessary energy and nutrients to support physical activity.

It is important to note that a balanced diet does not mean strict restriction or deprivation, it's about finding the right balance of macronutrients (carbohydrates, protein and fats) and micronutrients (vitamins, minerals) for your body and also enjoying the food you eat.

Bottom Line
A balanced diet is essential for maintaining overall health and well-being. It provides the body with the necessary nutrients, vitamins and minerals to function properly, prevent disease, improve digestion, mood, mental health, energy and immunity and also improve the appearance of skin, hair and nails and athletic performance.

Carnivore Diet
The carnivore diet is a diet that consists almost entirely of animal-based foods, such as meat, fish, eggs and dairy. The diet is characterized by a very high intake of animal protein and fat and a very low intake of carbohydrates and plant-based foods.

Proponents of the carnivore diet argue that the diet is more in line with the evolutionary diet of our ancestors and that it can lead to a wide range of health benefits, such as weight loss, improved energy levels and better overall health.

One of the main benefits of the carnivore diet is weight loss. By drastically reducing carbohydrate intake and increasing protein and fat intake, the carnivore diet can lead to rapid weight loss in the short-term. Additionally, the high protein content of the diet can help to preserve muscle mass, which is important for overall health and weight loss.

The carnivore diet can also help to improve energy levels and mental clarity. Animal-based foods are a rich source of essential nutrients, such as iron, zinc and B vitamins, which can help to improve energy levels and cognitive function. Additionally, the high fat content of the diet can help to support brain health and improve overall mental clarity.

The carnivore diet may also have potential benefits for certain health conditions, such as autoimmune disorders and gut health. By eliminating plant-based foods from the diet, the carnivore diet can help to reduce inflammation in the body, which can be beneficial for individuals with autoimmune disorders. Additionally, the diet's high protein and fat content can help to support gut health and improve overall digestive function.

However, it's important to note that the carnivore diet may not be suitable for everyone and may have some potential downsides. The diet can be restrictive and may be difficult to stick to long-term. Furthermore, a diet that only consist of animal products, can lead to nutrient deficiencies, especially on vitamins and minerals that are mostly found in plants like vitamins C, A, K and fiber. Additionally, the high fat and protein content of the diet may increase the risk of heart disease and other health problems in some individuals. It's also important to note that before starting any new diet, it's best to consult with a healthcare professional, especially if you have any pre-existing medical conditions.

One popular book on the carnivore diet is The Carnivore Diet by Dr. Shawn Baker. The importance of quality over quantity and the consumption of grass-fed and organic meats vs. wild caught fish and organic eggs and vegetables is encouraged. The book provides an in-depth explanation of the diet and its potential health benefits, as well as tips for following the diet and a variety of recipe ideas. Dr. Shawn Baker, an orthopedic surgeon and a former competitive athlete who has been following a carnivorous diet for several years and promoting its benefits. The idea behind the diet is that by eliminating plant-based foods, one can reduce inflammation in the body and improve overall health.

In his book Dr. Baker explains that the carnivore diet can have a positive impact on conditions such as obesity, autoimmune disorders and mental health issues. He also suggests that the diet can improve athletic performance and increase energy levels.

Dr. Baker also addresses concerns about nutrient deficiencies on the carnivore diet, stating that the high nutrient density of animal products can provide all the necessary nutrients for the body. He also points out that many plant-based foods, such as grains and legumes, can be difficult to digest and can contribute to inflammation in the body.

It's important to note that the carnivore diet is a highly restrictive diet and may not be suitable for everyone. Dr. Baker also encourages people to listen to their body and make adjustments as needed. He also recommends consulting with a healthcare professional before making any drastic changes to your diet.

Bottom Line
The carnivore diet is a diet that consists almost entirely of animal-based foods and it can lead to weight loss and improved energy levels. However, it's important to consult with a healthcare professional before starting the diet and to be mindful of the potential risks and downsides. The diet may not be suitable for everyone so it's important to be aware of the potential risks before making any drastic changes to your diet. It's also important to have a balanced and varied diet that includes different food groups, to ensure adequate nutrient intake.

Ketogenic Diets
A ketogenic diet, often referred to as a "keto" diet, is a high-fat, low-carbohydrate diet that has been shown to have numerous health benefits. The main goal of a ketogenic diet is to induce a state of ketosis, in which the body burns fat for energy instead of carbohydrates.

One of the most well-known benefits of a ketogenic diet is weight loss. When the body is in a state of ketosis, it burns fat for energy, which can lead to significant weight loss. Additionally, a ketogenic diet can help to improve insulin sensitivity, which can lead to better blood sugar control and a reduction in the risk of type 2 diabetes.

Another benefit of a ketogenic diet is that it can improve cognitive function and mental clarity. Studies have shown that a ketogenic diet can improve memory, concentration and focus. Additionally, it may also have positive effects on brain disorders such as Alzheimer's and Parkinson's disease.

A ketogenic diet can also be beneficial for those looking to improve their athletic performance. Because the body can burn fat for energy during a ketogenic diet, it can help to improve endurance, increase muscle mass and reduce muscle soreness.

The ketogenic diet has also been shown to have anti-inflammatory effects, which can help to reduce the risk of chronic diseases such as heart disease, cancer and autoimmune disorders. Additionally, it has been found to be effective in managing certain neurological disorders such as epilepsy and neurological disease.

It's worth noting that a ketogenic diet may not be suitable for individuals with certain health conditions, such as kidney disease or liver disease or for women who are pregnant or breastfeeding. It's always best to consult with a healthcare professional before making any drastic changes to your diet. and it is important to consult with a healthcare professional before starting any new diet. Additionally, it can be challenging to follow a ketogenic diet, as it requires a significant reduction in carbohydrate intake, which can be difficult for some people to sustain over a long period of time.

A ketogenic meal plan typically includes high-fat, moderate-protein and very-low-carbohydrate foods. The goal is to achieve a state of ketosis, in which the body burns fat for energy instead of carbohydrates.

It is important to note that this meal plan is just an example and the exact macronutrient ratios (fat, protein and carbohydrate) will vary depending on individual needs and goals. A typical ratio on a ketogenic diet is 70-75% fat, 20-25% protein and 5-10% carbs.

It is also important to note that it's essential to get enough fiber, vitamins and minerals in your diet, so it's important to include a variety of vegetables, nuts and seeds. Also, drinking enough water and staying hydrated is key on a ketogenic diet since the body loses more water on a high-fat diet.
It's also worth mentioning that starting a ketogenic diet can be challenging, especially at the beginning when the body is adjusting to the new way of eating. It's important to work with a healthcare professional or a registered dietitian to ensure that you are getting the proper nutrition and support you need to follow the diet safely and effectively.

The basic principle of the keto diet is to drastically reduce the intake of carbohydrates and replace them with healthy fats. This causes the body to enter a metabolic state called "ketosis," in which it begins to burn fat for energy instead of carbohydrates. The result is weight loss, improved energy levels and other potential health benefits such as improved blood sugar control and reduction in the risk of certain diseases.
While the ketogenic diet has been shown to be effective for weight loss and the management of certain health conditions, it's not without its potential drawbacks. One of the main concerns is the high saturated fat intake, which has been linked to an increased risk of heart disease. However, being a proponent of both the Carnivore and Keto diets, Dr. Baker argues that the saturated fat from animal-based

foods is not harmful and that the real culprit is the consumption of processed foods, refined carbohydrates and vegetable oils.

Bottom Line
The ketogenic diet is a low-carbohydrate, high-fat diet that aims to induce ketosis and improve overall health. While it has been shown to be effective for weight loss and the management of certain health conditions, it's not without its potential drawbacks and should be approached with caution. It's always best to consult with a healthcare professional before making any drastic changes to your diet.

Mediterranean Diet
The Mediterranean diet is a dietary pattern that is based on the traditional eating habits of the countries bordering the Mediterranean Sea. The diet is characterized by a high intake of fruits, vegetables, whole grains, legumes and olive oil, as well as moderate intake of fish, poultry and dairy products and a low intake of red meat and processed foods.

Proponents of the Mediterranean diet argue that it is one of the healthiest diets in the world and that it can lead to a wide range of health benefits, such as weight loss, improved heart health and better overall health.

One of the main benefits of the Mediterranean diet is weight loss. The high intake of fruits, vegetables and whole grains and the moderate intake of protein, can help to promote weight loss by providing a feeling of fullness and satisfaction while keeping calorie intake in check. Additionally, the high fiber and nutrient content of the diet can help to improve overall health and metabolism.

The Mediterranean diet can also help to improve heart health. The high intake of fruits, vegetables and whole grains, as well as the moderate intake of fish, can help to reduce the risk of heart disease by providing a wealth of heart-protective nutrients, such as omega-3 fatty acids and antioxidants. Additionally, the use of olive oil as the primary source of fat can help to improve cholesterol levels and reduce the risk of heart disease.

The Mediterranean diet may also have potential benefits for certain health conditions, such as diabetes and cancer. The high intake of fruits, vegetables and whole grains, as well as the moderate intake of protein, can help to improve blood sugar control in individuals with diabetes. Additionally, the diet's high nutrient content can help to reduce the risk of certain types of cancer.

However, it's important to note that the Mediterranean diet is not a strict diet and there is room for variations and personal preferences. It's important to consult with a healthcare professional before making any drastic changes to your diet.

It's also important to be mindful of the quality of fats consumed on the Mediterranean diet. While olive oil is the primary source of fat in the diet, it's important to consume it in moderation and to choose high-quality, extra-virgin olive oil. Additionally, it's important to consume enough protein to support muscle mass and to include a variety of different fruits, vegetables and whole grains to ensure adequate nutrient intake.

One popular book on the Mediterranean diet is <u>The Real Mediterranean Diet: A practical guide to understanding and achieving the healthiest diet in the world</u> by Dr. Simon Poole. This book presents the history and medical basis of the diet, covers the foods involved in the diet, presents a plan to prepare your ingredients at home to follow the diet and finally presents recipes from leading chefs of the Mediterranean diet to follow at home.

The Mediterranean diet is based on the traditional foods and lifestyle of the Mediterranean region, which includes a focus on whole, unprocessed foods such as fruits, vegetables, whole grains, legumes and seafood. The diet is also rich in healthy fats, such as olive oil and includes moderate amounts of wine.

The Mediterranean diet has been shown to have numerous health benefits, including reducing the risk of heart disease, diabetes and certain types of cancer. The diet has also been found to promote weight loss and improve overall health markers such as blood pressure, cholesterol levels and blood sugar control.

Bottom Line
The Mediterranean diet is based on the traditional foods and lifestyle of the Mediterranean region, which includes a focus on whole, unprocessed foods, healthy fats, seafood and moderate amounts of wine. The Mediterranean diet has been shown to have numerous health benefits, including reducing the risk of heart disease, diabetes and certain types of cancer and promoting weight loss and overall health markers.

Paleolithic Diet
The Paleolithic diet, also known as the "Paleo" or "caveman" diet, is based on the idea of eating like our prehistoric ancestors did during the Paleolithic era. The diet typically includes lean meats, fish, fruits, vegetables, nuts and seeds and excludes processed foods, grains, legumes and dairy. Proponents of the diet argue that our modern diet is causing chronic health issues and that by eating like our ancestors did, we can improve health and prevent disease.

However, the scientific evidence for the effectiveness of the Paleolithic diet is mixed and more research is needed to determine its benefits and risks. It is always recommended to consult a professional nutritionist or dietitian before making any drastic changes to your diet.

The Paleolithic diet was first popularized by Dr. Loren Cordain in his book <u>The Paleo Diet: Lose Weight and Get Healthy by Eating the Foods You Were Designed to Eat</u> which was published in 2002. In his book, Dr. Cordain argues that our modern diet is causing chronic health issues and that by eating like our ancestors did, we can improve health and prevent disease.

According to Dr. Cordain, the Paleolithic diet is based on the idea that our bodies have not evolved to handle the foods that have become a staple in the modern diet, such as grains, legumes and dairy. These foods, he argues, can cause inflammation in the body and lead to chronic health issues such as heart disease, diabetes and obesity.

However, it's worth noting that the scientific evidence for the effectiveness of the Paleolithic diet is mixed and more research is needed to determine its benefits and risks. Some studies have found that the Paleolithic diet can lead to weight loss and improved cardiovascular health, while others have found no significant benefits.

Furthermore, it is important to note that the Paleolithic era was a period that lasted over 2 million years and different human populations were eating different things depending on their geographical location and the resources available. Therefore, there is no one "Paleo" diet that our ancestors followed.

Bottom Line
The Paleolithic diet, as proposed by Dr. Loren Cordain, is a way of eating that emphasizes the consumption of lean meats, fish, fruits, vegetables, nuts and seeds, while avoiding processed foods, grains, legumes and dairy. While the diet is based on the idea that our prehistoric ancestors ate this way, the scientific evidence for its effectiveness is mixed and more research is needed. It is always recommended to consult a professional nutritionist or dietitian before making any drastic changes to your diet.

Vegan Diet
A vegan diet is a type of plant-based diet that excludes all animal-based products such as meat, dairy, eggs and even honey. People follow a vegan diet for various reasons, including health, environmental and ethical concerns.

One of the main benefits of a vegan diet is weight loss. A vegan diet is typically lower in calories and fat and higher in fiber, which can help promote weight loss and improve overall health. Additionally, a vegan diet is rich in fruits, vegetables, whole grains and legumes, which are all nutrient-dense foods that provide a wealth of vitamins, minerals and antioxidants.

A vegan diet may also be beneficial for heart health. A plant-based diet is typically low in saturated fat and cholesterol and high in fiber, antioxidants and phyto-chemicals, all of which can help to reduce the risk of heart disease. Additionally, a vegan diet can help to lower cholesterol levels and blood pressure, which are risk factors for heart disease.

A vegan diet may also have potential benefits for certain health conditions, such as type 2 diabetes and certain types of cancer. A vegan diet can help to improve blood sugar control in individuals with type 2 diabetes and the high intake of fruits, vegetables and whole grains may also help to reduce the risk of certain types of cancer.

It's important to note that a vegan diet may not be suitable for everyone and may have some potential downsides. A vegan diet can be restrictive and may be difficult to stick to long-term. Additionally, a vegan diet may lead to deficiencies in certain nutrients such as iron, calcium, vitamin B12 and omega-3 fatty acids and it's important to plan a well-balanced diet and supplement where necessary.

Before making any drastic changes to your diet it's important to consult with a healthcare professional, especially if you have any pre-existing medical conditions or are pregnant. Also, it's important to ensure that a vegan diet is providing you with all the necessary nutrients and to not replace animal-based products with processed vegan alternatives which are often high in added sugars, sodium and unhealthy fats.

Going Vegan for Beginners: The Essential Nutrition Guide to Transitioning to a Vegan Diet by Pamela Fergusson, RD, PhD. provides science-backed information, clear nutrition guidelines, step-by-step advice and sample menus to aid in transitioning to a vegan lifestyle. It explores what it means to be vegan and why the diet is healthy, what ingredients to keep on hand so you can make new dishes as well as vegan-friendly versions of your favorite meals and provides advice about how to stay vegan when visiting friends, family and eating at restaurants.

Bottom Line
A vegan diet is a type of plant-based diet that excludes all animal-based products and can lead to weight loss, improved heart health and better overall health. However, it's important to consult with a healthcare professional before making any drastic changes to your diet and to ensure that a vegan diet is providing you with all the necessary nutrients and not replacing animal-based products with processed vegan alternatives. It's also important to be mindful of potential deficiencies and to supplement where necessary.

Other lifestyle diets
There are many different types of lifestyle diets that people can choose from, each

with their own set of guidelines and principles. Other popular options include:

• **_Vegetarian Diet:_** This diet excludes meat and animal products and instead focuses on plant-based foods such as fruits, vegetables, whole grains, nuts and seeds. There are several different types of vegetarianism including:
> lacto-vegetarian (includes dairy products),
> ovo-vegetarian (includes eggs),
> vegan (excludes all animal products).

• **_DASH Diet:_** Developed by the National Institutes of Health, the DASH Diet (Dietary Approaches to Stop Hypertension) is a diet rich in fruits, vegetables, whole grains and lean proteins. It is low in sodium, saturated fats and added sugars and is often recommended for individuals with high blood pressure.

• **_Flexitarian Diet:_** This diet emphasizes a mostly plant-based diet, but allows for small amounts of meat and animal products. This is a more flexible and less restrictive diet than a vegetarian or vegan diet and is associated with weight loss, improved heart health and a lower risk of certain cancers.

Bottom Line
Each person has different dietary needs and a diet that works for one person may not work for another. It's important to consult a healthcare professional or a registered dietitian before starting any new diet to ensure it's the best fit for you.

Digital Detox

The Necessity of Detoxing from Stimulus: A Pathway to Heal the Mind and Body

In an era where digital screens, incessant notifications, and a relentless news cycle bombard our senses, the concept of detoxing from stimulus has emerged not just as a luxury, but as a necessity for mental and physical health. This document explores why it's crucial to step back from the constant stimulation of modern life, detailing how such a detox can profoundly affect our psychological and physiological well-being.

Understanding Stimulus Overload
What is Stimulus Overload?
- Stimulus overload refers to the state where an individual receives more sensory input than their brain can efficiently process. This can come from numerous sources:
- Digital Devices: Smartphones, tablets, computers, and the endless stream of

content they provide.
- Social Media: The pressure to stay connected, updated, and engaged with a digital community can be overwhelming.
- News and Media: Continuous exposure to often distressing or sensational news can lead to a state of perpetual anxiety or numbness.
- Urban Living: The noise, light, and pace of city life contribute significantly to sensory overload.

Effects of Over-Stimulation:
- Mental Health: Chronic exposure to excessive stimuli can lead to or exacerbate conditions like anxiety, depression, ADHD, and sleep disorders.
- Physical Health: Over-stimulation can result in increased cortisol levels, leading to stress-related physical symptoms like headaches, muscle tension, and digestive issues.
- Cognitive Function: There's a decline in attention span, memory retention, and the ability to concentrate deeply due to the constant demand for multitasking.

The Case for Detoxing from Stimulus

Healing the Mind:
- Reduction of Anxiety and Stress: By stepping away from the sources of constant stimulation, individuals can lower their stress levels, reducing the fight-or-flight response that's often kept in overdrive.

- Improved Cognitive Function: A detox period can help reset neural pathways, enhancing focus, creativity, and problem-solving skills. It's akin to giving the brain a chance to "defragment" and reorganize.

- Mental Clarity and Emotional Balance: With less external noise, one can better tune into their own thoughts and emotions, leading to greater self-awareness and emotional regulation.

Healing the Body:
- Physical Rest and Recovery: Reducing sensory input allows the body to enter a more profound state of relaxation, aiding in physical recovery from stress-related ailments.

- Better Sleep Quality: Exposure to screens and blue light disrupts our circadian rhythms. A stimulus detox, particularly from digital devices before bedtime, can significantly improve sleep quality.

- Lower Cortisol Levels: Decreased exposure to stressors can lower cortisol, reducing the risk of chronic conditions associated with prolonged high stress levels like heart disease and diabetes.

Practical Steps for a Stimulus Detox

1. Digital Detox:
  - Screen-Free Time: Designate times of day (like mornings or evenings) where no screens are allowed.

  - Notification Management: Turn off unnecessary notifications or set your phone to 'Do Not Disturb' during focus times.

  - Digital Fasting: Commit to periods where you completely abstain from digital devices, perhaps one day a week or a weekend a month.

2. Sensory Deprivation:
  - Nature Immersion: Spend time in environments with minimal human-made stimuli, like forests or beaches, to recalibrate your sensory experience.

  - Silent Retreats: Consider retreats where silence is maintained to reduce auditory stimulation and promote introspection.

3. Mindful Practices:
  - Meditation: Regular meditation can help manage the influx of stimuli by training the mind to focus and remain calm.

  - Mindful Breathing: Simple breathing exercises can anchor you in the present moment, reducing the mental clutter from external stimuli.

4. Lifestyle Adjustments:
  - Routine Simplification: Simplify daily routines to reduce decision fatigue and sensory input. This includes decluttering your living space to make it less stimulating.

  - Dietary Changes: Some advocate for a detox diet, reducing stimulants like caffeine or sugar, which can also contribute to nervous system overload.

5. Social Detox:
  - Selective Engagement: Be selective about social engagements, choosing those that replenish rather than drain your energy.

  - Social Media Breaks: Regular breaks from social media can help mitigate the comparison culture and the stress of keeping up appearances online.

The Science Behind Detox Benefits
  - Neuroplasticity: The brain's ability to reorganize itself by forming new neural connections. A break from stimulus can enhance this process, making way for more adaptive behaviors and thought patterns.

  - Neurotransmitter Balance: Reducing excessive stimuli can help normalize dopamine and serotonin levels, chemicals crucial for mood regulation.

- Stress Response Systems: The HPA axis (hypothalamic-pituitary-adrenal axis), which governs our stress response, can reset when not constantly activated by stressors, leading to better stress management.

Challenges and Considerations
- Withdrawal Symptoms: Initially, there might be a sense of anxiety or boredom as one disconnects from habitual stimuli. This is normal and part of the adjustment process.

- Social Pressure: There's often pressure to remain connected, which can make stimulus detox challenging. Setting clear boundaries and explaining your need for this time can help.

- Integration: Post-detox, integrating lessons learned into everyday life is crucial. This might mean setting up new routines that limit exposure to overwhelming stimuli.

Bottom Line
Detoxing from stimulus isn't just about turning off devices; it's about creating space for mental and physical health to flourish. In a world where we're never off-duty from sensory input, taking deliberate steps to unplug can be revolutionary for our well-being. By embracing these practices, we not only reclaim our peace but also enhance our capacity to engage with life more fully, with intention and presence.

Disability – Filing with Veterans Affairs

Filing for disability benefits with the Department of Veterans Affairs (VA) can be a complex process. Here are the general steps a Veteran can take to file a claim for disability benefits:

- ***Gather necessary information:*** The Veteran should gather all necessary information related to their service and medical conditions. This may include their discharge papers, service treatment records, medical records and any other relevant documentation.

- ***Determine eligibility:*** The Veteran should determine if they are eligible for disability benefits. To be eligible, the Veteran must have a current medical condition that is connected to their military service.

- ***Choose a representative:*** The Veteran can choose to work with a representative, such as a Veterans service organization or an accredited attorney, to assist with their claim.

- **Complete the application:** The Veteran should complete the VA Form 21-526EZ, which is the Application for Disability Compensation and Related Compensation Benefits. The form can be completed online or in person at a regional VA office.

- **Submit the application:** The Veteran should submit the completed application to the VA. They can do this online, by mail or in person at a regional VA office.

- **Attend a Compensation and Pension exam:** The Veteran may be required to attend a Compensation and Pension (C&P) exam. This exam is used to evaluate the Veteran's medical conditions and determine the severity of their disability.

- **Wait for a decision:** The VA will review the application, medical evidence and other supporting documentation to make a decision on the claim. This process can take several months or longer.

- **Receive the decision:** The Veteran will receive a decision on their claim, which will either approve or deny their disability benefits. If the claim is approved, the Veteran will receive information on their disability rating and the amount of compensation they are entitled to.

Bottom Line

It is important to note that the VA disability claims process can be complicated and it is not uncommon for claims to be denied or delayed. Veterans who are struggling with the claims process may wish to seek assistance from a Veterans service organization or an accredited attorney. These individuals can help Veterans navigate the claims process and ensure that their rights are protected.

Discipline

Discipline is the practice of training oneself to do something in a consistent and controlled manner. It is the ability to control one's thoughts, emotions and actions in order to achieve a goal or maintain a certain standard of behavior. Discipline is a key ingredient in achieving success and improving one's life.

One way to improve your life through discipline is by setting clear and achievable goals. Having a clear understanding of what you want to accomplish and the steps required to achieve it will help you stay focused and motivated. It's important to break down your goals into smaller, manageable tasks and set a timeline for completion.

Another way to improve your life through discipline is by practicing self-control. This means learning to resist instant gratification or to delay gratification for long-term goals. This can be challenging, but it is a powerful way to improve your life by avoiding impulsive decisions that can lead to negative consequences.

Another important aspect of discipline is time management. It's important to prioritize your tasks and manage your time effectively in order to achieve your goals. This can be done by creating a daily schedule, setting deadlines and avoiding distractions.

One more way to improve your life through discipline is by taking care of your physical and mental health. This means exercising regularly, getting enough sleep, eating a healthy diet and managing stress. By taking care of your physical and mental health, you will be better equipped to handle the demands of your daily life and achieve your goals.

Bottom Line
Discipline is a powerful tool for improving your life. By setting clear and achievable goals, practicing self-control, managing your time and taking care of your physical and mental health, you can achieve success and reach your full potential.

DMT (5-MeO-DMT)

Veterans carry scars—some you see, some you don't. 5-MeO-DMT, a fast-hitting psychedelic from plants and toads, steps into that fray as a tool to shake loose the heavy stuff: trauma, depression, addiction. It's not a pill or a pep talk—it's a deep, short dive into your head, guided by pros or shamans, often over in under an hour. For vets wrestling with PTSD's ghosts, the blues, or habits that won't quit, this compound promises a reset, a chance to face what's buried and come out lighter. It's intense, it's not mainstream, and science is still catching up—but some swear it's a game-changer. This section breaks down what 5-MeO-DMT is, why it might click for Veterans, and how to approach it smart, with your six covered.

Understanding 5-MeO-DMT
5-MeO-DMT—call it "five-methoxy" if you're fancy—is a natural psychedelic, brewed in plants, secreted by the Colorado River toad, maybe even lurking in your own body. You inhale it, inject it, or swallow it with a helper chemical, and

boom: 15–90 minutes of full-on altered reality. It's not like mushrooms that stretch for hours—this hits hard and fast, flooding your brain with visions, feelings, or just a big, quiet void. For Veterans, it's a potential shortcut to tackle the deep stuff, often in a ceremony or clinic with someone watching your back.

The Science Behind It
Your brain's a wiring hub—5-MeO-DMT plugs into serotonin receptors, flipping switches that shift how you think and feel. It can pull you into calm alpha waves or deep theta states, cracking open doors to buried memories or peace. The trip's wild—some call it a "whiteout"—but it's the aftermath vets chase: clarity, relief, a new angle on old pain. Science isn't all in—small studies hint at real shifts, but it's more art than textbook for now. For Veterans, it's less about proof and more about possibility: can it cut through the noise?

The Impact of 5-MeO-DMT on Veterans' Health
- Wellness Benefits: It's pitched as a trauma buster, mood lifter, even a habit breaker—stuff vets need when the past won't let go.

- Consequences of Ignoring It: Stick with the weight, and PTSD, depression, or cravings keep calling shots—dragging you down when you're built to rise.

Identifying and Analyzing Your Needs
- Self-Assessment: Take stock—what's loudest? Nightmares from that last op? A funk you can't shake? Booze or pills you lean on too hard? List it out—know your enemy.

- Setting Priorities: Rank it—trauma if it's choking you, mood if you're flat, addiction if it's running your life. Hit the big one first; the rest follows.

Fostering the 5-MeO-DMT Habit
- Set Goals: Keep it real—e.g., "Try one session this year to face the deployment ghosts." Simple, focused, like a mission brief.

- Building a Support System: Loop in a vet buddy, therapist, or guide—they've got your back, keeping you steady before and after. Squad rules apply.

Implementation Strategies
- Occasional Use: This isn't daily chow—it's a one-off or rare reset. Plan it like a recon op: once, maybe twice a year, with purpose.

- Habit Stacking: Tie it to a big moment—pair prep with a quiet day off or integration with your morning sitrep. Anchors it to your rhythm.

Targeted Protocols for Veterans' Wellness
Here's how to use 5-MeO-DMT for specific needs, with supplies for each:

1. Trauma Resolution
- What: Inhale 5–10 mg in a guided ceremony, one session to start.

- Why: Combat leaves echoes—5-MeO-DMT can drag them up and out, turning chaos into calm through a wild ride.

- How: Find a retreat or facilitator, sit in a circle, vape it with a pipe—15 minutes of intensity, then talk it out. Prep with quiet time, no meds that clash (check your VA list). Once—see if the weight lifts in a week.

- Supplies Needed: Trained facilitator ($1,000–$5,000 retreat), vape pipe, safe space, post-trip journal.

2. Mood Enhancement
- What: Try 6–12 mg inhaled with a sitter, one-off or quarterly.

- Why: Depression or anxiety from transition blues? This might flip the switch, lifting the gray.

- How: Solo with a pro or in a group, inhale slow—45 minutes tops. Rest after, sip water, let it settle. Quarterly if it sticks; once if it's enough. If it's too much, dial back the dose.

- Supplies Needed: Facilitator or sitter, vape gear, water bottle, quiet spot.

3. Spiritual Insight
- What: Use 10–15 mg in a ceremonial setting, one deep dive.

- Why: Lost your why post-service? The "void" or connection it brings can spark meaning—vets need that anchor.

- How: Join a guided session—meditate first, vape it, ride the wave for 20 minutes. Reflect after—talk or write. One shot—judge if it realigns you.

- Supplies Needed: Shaman or guide, pipe or vape, mat or chair, notebook.

4. Addiction Support
- What: Hit 5–10 mg inhaled with integration support, once to test.

- Why: Cravings for booze or pills eating you? This might rewire the itch, giving you a breather to fight back.

- How: With a pro, vape it—15 minutes of blast-off, then plan next steps (AA, VA). Once—see if the pull weakens in days. Pair with real help; it's a boost, not a cure.

- Supplies Needed: Facilitator, vape setup, support plan (VA contact), water.

5. Cognitive Clarity

- What: Use 6–8 mg inhaled, one session for fog.

- Why: TBI or burnout muddling your head? The post-trip glow might cut through, sharpening your edge.

- How: Sit with a sitter, vape light—20 minutes max. Rest, hydrate, test your focus next day. Once—enough to gauge. If it's jittery, skip it.

- Supplies Needed: Sitter, vape gear, water bottle, quiet corner.

Eliminating Barriers to Use
- Identify Triggers: Spot what stops you—"Too weird," "I'll lose it," "It's illegal." Name it, then weigh it—vets face worse daily.

- Replace Hesitation: Swap "Not for me" for "One try"—scout it like new terrain. Trade fear for "What's it unlock?"—action beats freeze.

- Veteran-Specific Substitutes:

  - Doubt: Swap "Hippie stuff" for "Combat reset"—frame it your way, test it.

  - Control: Trade "I'll flip out" for "I've got a guide"—trust the process, like a CO's lead.

Mindfulness and Self-Regulation
- Techniques: Prep with focus—breathe deep (5-5-5), set an intent: "Face it." During, ride it; after, ground with air or talk. Keeps you in the driver's seat.

- Benefits: You'll know when you're stuck—cue the trip. Awareness is power, vet grit in action.

Seeking Professional Help
- When Needed: PTSD flares, heart issues, or meds in play? Hit your VA doc or shrink first—this isn't DIY for the rough stuff.

- Resources: VA trials, vetted retreats, or telehealth can steer you—free or pro-grade, built for vets.

Maintaining and Sustaining the Practice
- Track Progress: Log the aftermath—less edge, clearer head? Mark a win: "Faced the dark, slept clean."

- Overcome Plateaus: No shift? Up the dose (with a pro) or wait months—push like a stalled ruck.

- Build Resilience: Each trip's a brick—stack 'em, and you're tougher, shedding what holds you back.

Bottom Line

5-MeO-DMT's a heavy hitter—trauma buster, mood lifter, insight spark, craving killer, clarity shot—delivered fast through a vape (5–20 mg) or ceremony. For vets hauling PTSD, depression, or addiction, it's a bold play to shake loose the chains, rooted in shamanic ways and new healing vibes. Some say it's gold—rewires the soul; science says maybe—small trials hint, big proof's out. Risks? Heart jolts, mind bends, legal gray—step careful. It's no lone fix—pros say tie it to real care—so check your VA crew, hit a guided session, and lean on support. Potent, vet-relevant, it's a tool, not the answer—use it sharp and safe.

Drug Abuse

Drug abuse refers to the harmful or hazardous use of psychoactive substances, including alcohol and illicit drugs. It can lead to a range of physical and mental health problems, as well as social and economic consequences. Preventing drug abuse and providing effective treatment to those who are struggling with substance use disorders is a complex and ongoing challenge.

Prevention strategies aim to reduce the risk of individuals starting to use drugs or developing a substance use disorder. This can include:

• **Education:** Providing accurate information about the risks associated with drug use and the potential consequences can help discourage people from using drugs.

• **Community-based programs:** Building strong, supportive communities can reduce the risk of drug abuse by providing a positive environment that encourages healthy behaviors.

• **Parenting skills:** Helping parents develop effective parenting skills can reduce the risk of their children using drugs. This may include teaching positive communication, conflict resolution and coping skills.

• **School-based programs:** Providing drug education and prevention programs in schools can help young people make informed decisions about drug use and avoid potential harm.

• **Drug testing and screening:** In some cases, drug testing and screening can be effective in deterring drug use and detecting drug abuse early, allowing for prompt intervention and treatment.

• **Law enforcement and criminal justice approaches:** Criminalizing drug use and providing law enforcement and criminal justice approaches can discourage drug use and reduce drug-related crime.

Treatment for drug abuse typically involves a combination of medical, behavioral and social interventions. The goal is to help individuals stop using drugs and maintain a drug-free lifestyle. Common forms of treatment include:

• *Medications:* Certain medications can help individuals overcome drug cravings and reduce the severity of withdrawal symptoms. These may include methadone for opioid addiction, naltrexone for alcohol and opioid addiction and buprenorphine for opioid addiction—all of which are only available by prescription.

• *Behavioral therapies:* Counseling and behavioral therapies can help individuals develop coping skills and address the root causes of their drug abuse. This may include individual, family or group therapy.

• *Residential treatment:* Some individuals may require more intensive treatment, such as inpatient or residential treatment programs, where they can receive round-the-clock support and care.
• *Support groups:* Joining a support group, such as Alcoholics Anonymous or Narcotics Anonymous, can provide individuals with a supportive community and accountability as they work to maintain their sobriety.

• *Aftercare and relapse prevention:* After completing a treatment program, individuals may need ongoing support to maintain their recovery, such as aftercare programs, outpatient services and continuing care groups.

It is important to note that drug abuse is a complex issue with no single solution. Effective prevention and treatment programs must be tailored to meet the needs of each individual and address the unique circumstances and challenges that they face. Additionally, it is essential that individuals have access to a range of evidence-based treatment options, as what works for one person may not work for another.

Bottom Line
Drug abuse is a significant public health concern that can have serious physical, mental and social consequences. Preventing drug abuse and providing effective treatment to those who are struggling with substance use disorders requires a multi-faceted approach that addresses the individual, community and societal factors that contribute to drug use. By working together, we can reduce the harm associated with drug abuse and help individuals and communities thrive.

Dry Brushing

Veterans know wear and tear—skin roughed up from the field, circulation slowed from long hauls, stress that sticks like mud on boots. Dry brushing steps in as a simple fix: grab a stiff-bristled brush, scrub your dry skin before a shower, and wake your body up. It's not a spa day or a wet scrub—this is a quick, no-frills ritual to slough off the dead stuff and get your blood moving. For vets dealing with the grind of service aftermath—scars, sluggishness, or tension—it's a cheap, do-it-yourself way to feel sharper. This section lays out what dry brushing is, why it might hit the mark for Veterans, and how to make it work, all with a grunt's grit.

Understanding Dry Brushing

Dry brushing means running a natural-bristle brush over your bare, dry skin in upward sweeps or circles for 5–10 minutes. No water, no lotion—just you and the brush, hitting every spot from toes to shoulders before you hit the shower. It's old-school, pulled from ancient health tricks, now a go-to in holistic kits. For Veterans, it's a low-tech way to tackle the physical fallout of service, giving your skin and system a nudge without breaking the bank.

The Science Behind It

Your skin's a shield—your body's biggest organ—and it sheds dead cells daily. Brushing speeds that up, scraping off the junk while prodding blood flow and lymph, the fluid that hauls waste out. The idea? Stimulate what's under the surface—veins, nodes—to keep things humming. For Veterans, it's like a manual reboot: wake up circulation bogged down by years of rucks or stress. Science nods at the exfoliation and flow boost—less so at grand detox claims—but the feel of it keeps vets coming back.

The Impact of Dry Brushing on Veterans' Health

- Wellness Benefits: It's pitched to rev circulation, clear skin, cut stress—stuff vets need when the body's taken a beating and the mind's still on alert.

- Consequences of Skipping It: Let it slide, and you're stuck with dull skin, heavy limbs, or tension piling on—extra weight you don't need.

Identifying and Analyzing Your Needs

- Self-Assessment: Take a hard look—what's dragging? Rough skin from burn pit grit? Legs like lead after desk days? Stress you can't shake? Jot it down—know your AO.

- Setting Priorities: Rank the hits—circulation if you're stiff, skin if it's scarred, stress if you're wired. Start where it's loudest; the rest falls in line.

Fostering the Dry Brushing Habit

- Set Goals: Keep it tight—e.g., "Brush five minutes, three times this week to feel looser." Clear, doable, like a PT log.

- Building a Support System: Tell a squad mate or your VA doc you're on it—they can check in, keep you honest, like a spotter on a lift.

Implementation Strategies
- Daily Integration: Slot it in—morning wake-up or evening wind-down. Start with a few days a week; steady beats overdrive, like pacing a march.

- Habit Stacking: Pair it with routine—brush while your coffee drips or post-PT. Ties it to what's already locked and loaded.

Targeted Protocols for Veterans' Wellness
Here's how to dry brush for specific needs, with supplies for each:

1. Improved Circulation
- What: Brush from feet to chest, 5–10 minutes, three times weekly.

- Why: Boots, humps, desk life—circulation takes a hit. Brushing wakes it up, pushing blood where it's stalled.

- How: Grab a firm brush, start at your toes—long strokes up toward your heart, firm but not harsh. Five minutes minimum, before a shower. Three days a week—feel the tingle kick in after a few sessions. If legs ache, ease off pressure.

- Supplies Needed: Natural-bristle brush ($10–$30), shower access, timer (optional).

2. Lymphatic Drainage
- What: Use circular motions on limbs and torso, 7–10 minutes, weekly or post-swelling.

- Why: Swollen hands or feet from old injuries? Lymph's your cleanup crew—brushing nudges it along.

- How: Medium brush, circle up from ankles and wrists to armpits and groin—gentle, toward the heart. Ten minutes, once a week or when you're puffy. Shower after—see if you're lighter in days. Too rough? Soften it.

- Supplies Needed: Brush (medium stiffness), shower, comfy spot to sit.

3. Exfoliation and Skin Health
- What: Brush whole body, 5 minutes daily or face/neck with a soft cloth, twice weekly.

- Why: Scars, dryness from field grit—brushing smooths it out, keeps skin from cracking.

- How: Full body—long sweeps, daily before shower. Face—soft cloth, up from neck, two minutes, twice a week. Rinse off, oil up after—check for silkier skin in a week. If it stings, cut back.

- Supplies Needed: Firm brush (body), soft cloth (face), shower, moisturizer (coconut oil, $5–$15).

4. Stress Relief
- What: Brush arms and legs, 5–7 minutes, evening routine.

- Why: Hypervigilance, civvie stress—rhythmic strokes calm the buzz, like a slow exhale.

- How: Light brush, up from hands and feet—five minutes, before bed. Focus on the rhythm—pair with deep breaths (4-7-8). Nightly—feel it unwind you in days. Too wired? Shorten it.

- Supplies Needed: Brush, quiet evening spot, shower nearby.

5. Energy Boost
- What: Quick full-body brush, 5 minutes, mornings three times weekly.

- Why: Fatigue from pain or grind? Brushing perks you up, gets the blood pumping.

- How: Fast sweeps—feet to shoulders, five minutes pre-shower, morning kick-start. Three days a week—judge if you're less sluggish by week's end. Too much? Skip a day.

- Supplies Needed: Brush, shower, morning window.

Eliminating Barriers to Use
- Identify Triggers: Spot what stalls you—"Looks silly," "No time," "Hurts my skin." Call it out—then push past it.

- Replace Hesitation: Swap "Later" for "Five minutes now"—quick hit, done. Trade doubt for "What's it feel like?"—test it, own it.

- Veteran-Specific Substitutes:

  - Skepticism: Swap "Spa nonsense" for "Field fix"—frame it as upkeep, not pampering.

  - Fatigue: Trade "Too tired" for "Wake-up shot"—brush it, feel it.

Mindfulness and Self-Regulation
- Techniques: Focus on the strokes—count 'em, feel the bristles. It's a mental anchor, cutting "this is dumb" chatter. Vets know focus—use it here.

- Benefits: You'll spot when you're off—cue the brush. Awareness keeps you sharp, steering your own course.

Seeking Professional Help
- When Needed: Got eczema, open cuts, or heart trouble? Check your VA doc—brushing's gentle, but not for every scar.

- Resources: VA dermatology, primary care, or telehealth—free, vet-ready, they'll green-light it or wave you off.

Maintaining and Sustaining the Practice
- Track Progress: Log the wins—smoother skin, looser limbs, less edge. Mark it: "Brushed, felt alive today."

- Overcome Plateaus: Flatline? Up the days or switch patterns—push like a stalled op, keep moving.

- Build Resilience: Each scrub's a brick—stack 'em, and you're tougher, shedding what slows you down.

Bottom Line
Dry brushing's a vet-friendly play—revving circulation, draining lymph, smoothing skin, cutting stress, boosting juice—with a $10 brush and five minutes of dry sweeps before a shower. For vets hauling pain, fatigue, or tension, it's a low-cost shot at feeling steadier, rooted in old health hacks and new self-care vibes. Some say it's gold—wakes you up, calms you down; science nods at the basics—skin and flow—but grand claims like detox lean on gut feel over proof. Risks? Rash if you overdo it—go easy if your skin's battle-worn. It's no cure—pros say pair it with real care—so hit your VA doc if you're dicey, brush three times a week, and stack it with your routine. Simple, gritty, it's a tool in your kit—use it smart and steady.

EBOO Blood Filtration

Veterans carry a load—years of burn pit smoke, stress that grinds you down, fatigue that won't quit. EBOO blood filtration, or Extracorporeal Blood Oxygenation and Ozonation, offers a high-tech way to lighten that burden: pull your blood out, filter it, pump it with ozone and oxygen, and send it back in, all in one go. It's not your average IV drip—this treats a big chunk of your blood in a single session, aiming to clean house and recharge you from the inside. For vets wrestling with inflammation, lingering toxins, or just feeling beat, it's a cutting-edge play to get back in the fight. This section digs into what EBOO is, why it might click for Veterans, and how to roll it out, with your health as the mission.

Understanding EBOO Blood Filtration

EBOO's a closed-loop deal—blood gets drawn through an IV, run through a machine that filters out gunk, zapped with medical-grade ozone and oxygen, then pumped back into you. Think 45–75 minutes per session, treating a couple liters of your red stuff. It's not a quick poke like an IV vitamin hit; it's a full-on blood overhaul, built to detox and revitalize. For Veterans, it's a potential reset button—tackling the wear of service with something more than pills or grit.

The Science Behind It

Your blood's your lifeline—carrying oxygen, fighting junk, keeping you upright. EBOO steps in like a field mechanic: filters snag waste (dead cells, muck), ozone jazzes up the mix with its antimicrobial kick, and extra oxygen supercharges the flow. The pitch? Scrub your system, spark your cells, ease the strain. For Veterans, it's a shot at flushing what's bogging you down—toxins from the sandbox or inflammation from old wounds. Science sees the logic—ozone's a known player, filtration's legit—but the full EBOO package is still proving itself outside the clinic.

The Impact of EBOO on Veterans' Health

- Wellness Benefits: It's pitched to cut inflammation, boost immunity, lift energy—stuff vets need when the body's been through hell and back.

- Consequences of Skipping It: Ignore the load, and fatigue, soreness, or slow healing keep you pinned—extra drag on a frame built to push.

Identifying and Analyzing Your Needs

- Self-Assessment: Scope your sitrep—what's hitting hardest? Joints screaming from rucks? Tiredness that coffee won't touch? Fog from Gulf War grit? List it—know your targets.

- Setting Priorities: Rank the threats—inflammation if pain's king, energy if you're flat, detox if burn pits haunt you. Hit the big one first; the rest lines up.

Fostering the EBOO Habit

- Set Goals: Keep it sharp—e.g., "Try one session this month to shake the haze." Clear, like a fire mission—aim, execute.

- Building a Support System: Loop in your VA doc or a vet buddy—they've got your six, keeping you steady as you test this gear.

Implementation Strategies

- Occasional Use: This isn't daily chow—think weekly hits for a month or two, a reset, not a routine. Pace it like a long-range patrol.

- Habit Stacking: Pair it with a down day—post-session rest after your morning sitrep or a light PT stretch. Ties it to your flow.

Targeted Protocols for Veterans' Wellness

Here's how to use EBOO for specific needs, with supplies for each:

1. Reduced Inflammation

- What: Book a 60-minute session, once weekly for four weeks.

- Why: Old injuries or stress flare your system—EBOO filters junk and calms the fire with ozone's punch.

- How: Find a clinic, sit in the recliner—two IVs, one out, one in—let the machine hum for an hour. Eat protein before (steak, eggs), sip water after. Weekly—check if joints ease in a month. If you're woozy, rest longer.

- Supplies Needed: Clinic with EBOO machine ($500–$3,500), protein snack, water bottle.

2. Enhanced Immunity

- What: Hit a 45-minute session, biweekly for six weeks.

- Why: Burn pits or bugs wearing you down? Ozone might juice your white cells, keeping you in the fight.

- How: Two IVs, 45 minutes—blood goes dark to bright. Hydrate hard post-session (32 oz), skip heavy lifts after. Twice a month—see if colds back off. Too much? Cut to monthly.

- Supplies Needed: EBOO clinic, water bottle, rest spot (couch).

3. Increased Energy

- What: Try a 60-minute session, weekly for three weeks.

- Why: Dragging from service wear? Super-oxygenated blood could kick the fog, get you moving.

- How: Clinic setup—hour-long run, eat light before (nuts, fruit), chill after with water. Weekly—judge if you're less wiped by week three. If it's flat, pause it.

- Supplies Needed: Clinic access, light meal, water, comfy chair.

4. Detoxification Support

- What: Use a 75-minute session with extra ozone, once monthly.

- Why: Toxins from the field sticking around? Filtration scrubs 'em, easing your body's haul.

- How: Book it—longer session, ask for max ozone. Fast lightly before (broth, greens), rest a day after. Monthly—feel if the sludge lifts. Too intense? Dial back ozone.

- Supplies Needed: EBOO clinic, fasting plan (paper list), recovery day.

5. Improved Circulation

- What: Hit a 60-minute session, weekly for four weeks.

- Why: Cold hands, slow healing from years of grind? Oxygen-rich blood gets it flowing, patching you up.

- How: Standard run—two IVs, hour-long cycle. Move light after (walk, stretch), hydrate. Weekly—check if limbs warm up in a month. If veins ache, talk to the doc.

- Supplies Needed: Clinic, water bottle, post-session stretch space.

Eliminating Barriers to Use

- Identify Triggers: Spot what stalls you—"Too pricey," "Sounds nuts," "No time." Name it—then gut-check it.

- Replace Hesitation: Swap "Not now" for "One shot"—scout it like new tech. Trade doubt for "What's it do?"—test, assess.

- Veteran-Specific Substitutes:

  - Cost: Swap "Can't afford" for "One trial"—save up, hit it once.

  - Skepticism: Trade "BS detox" for "Field flush"—frame it your way, try it.

Mindfulness and Self-Regulation

- Techniques: Focus on the hum, the IV tug—stay present. It's a mental anchor, cutting "this won't work" noise. Vets know focus—lock it in.

- Benefits: You'll spot when you're tanking—cue the session. Awareness keeps you in command, steering your own rig.

Seeking Professional Help
- When Needed: Heart issues, bleeding quirks, or heavy meds? Hit your VA doc first—EBOO's no game for the fragile.

- Resources: VA referrals, integrative clinics, or telehealth—vet-ready, they'll clear you or wave off.

Maintaining and Sustaining the Practice
- Track Progress: Log the wins—less ache, more juice? Mark it: "EBOO'd, felt sharp today."

- Overcome Plateaus: No kick? Up the weeks or tweak the goal—push like a stalled hump, keep rolling.

- Build Resilience: Each run's a brick—stack 'em, and you're tougher, shedding what drags you.

Bottom Line
EBOO blood filtration's a vet-friendly heavy hitter—cutting inflammation, boosting immunity, lifting energy, scrubbing toxins, revving flow—by filtering and ozonating a couple liters of your blood in an hour-long IV loop. For vets hauling pain, exhaustion, or field residue, it's a bold shot at bouncing back, rooted in ozone tricks and new-wave healing. Some say it's gold—clears the haze, steadies you up; science nods at the pieces—filtration, oxygen—but the full deal's still proving out. Risks? Vein hassles, a woozy spell—watch it if you're beat up or broke. It's no lone cure—pros say tie it to real care—so check your VA squad, hit a clinic ($500–$3,500), and lean on support. Potent, pricey, it's a tool in your kit—use it sharp and safe.

Education – Continuing for Life

Continuing education or lifelong learning, refers to the pursuit of knowledge and skills beyond formal education. It can come in many forms, including college courses, workshops, online classes or certification programs. In today's fast-paced and rapidly changing world, continuing education is more important than ever for personal and professional growth, as well as for keeping up with the latest developments and advancements in various fields.

First and foremost, continuing education helps individuals stay current in their respective fields and develop new skills to remain competitive in the job market. With technological advancements and new innovations emerging at a rapid pace, it's essential to have the latest knowledge and skills to stay ahead of the curve. This not only helps individuals advance in their careers, but also opens up new career opportunities and prospects.

Additionally, continuing education can provide a sense of personal fulfillment and satisfaction. Learning new things and acquiring new skills can help boost confidence, increase self-esteem and provide a sense of accomplishment. It can also lead to personal growth and development, as individuals are exposed to new ideas and perspectives that can broaden their worldview and deepen their understanding of themselves and the world around them.

Furthermore, continuing education is a way for individuals to continuously improve their decision-making skills and problem-solving abilities. By acquiring new knowledge and skills, individuals can better analyze and evaluate information, making more informed and effective decisions. This is especially important in today's complex and dynamic world, where decision-making skills are highly valued by employers and essential for success.

Another reason why continuing education is important is that it helps individuals keep their minds active and sharp, reducing the risk of cognitive decline as they age. Lifelong learning has been shown to have a positive impact on cognitive function, as it challenges the brain and keeps it active, thereby reducing the risk of cognitive decline and preserving cognitive abilities.

Continuing education is also a way to expand social and professional networks. By taking courses and attending workshops, individuals can meet and connect with others who have similar interests and goals. This can lead to the formation of new professional and personal relationships, which can be valuable in both personal and professional settings.

Finally, continuing education is important for personal growth and development. By learning new things and acquiring new skills, individuals can broaden their horizons, increase their cultural literacy and gain a deeper understanding of the world around them. This can lead to increased self-awareness and self-discovery, as well as personal growth and development.

Bottom Line

Continuing education is important for personal and professional growth, as well as for keeping up with the latest developments and advancements in various fields. It provides individuals with the opportunity to develop new skills, expand their knowledge and challenge their minds. It also offers the opportunity to expand social and professional networks, as well as to experience personal fulfillment and satisfaction. With the fast-paced and rapidly changing world we live in, continuing education is essential for success, both in personal and professional settings.

Ego Death

Veterans carry a hell of a load—service stamps you with an identity that's hard to shake, and trauma can lock it in tight. Ego death flips that script: it's a moment where the "you" you've built—soldier, survivor, broken vet—just melts away, leaving raw awareness or a sense of everything clicking together. It's not a casual sit-down with your thoughts—it hits through psychedelics, deep meditation, or life's hard knocks, lasting minutes or hours. For vets tangled in PTSD, guilt, or a lost sense of purpose, it's a chance to drop the baggage and see past the mirror. This section breaks down what ego death is, why it might resonate with Veterans, and how to chase it down, all with your boots on the ground.

Understanding Ego Death
Ego death is when your inner voice—"I'm this, I did that"—shuts off. No rank, no regrets, just a wide-open state, sometimes oneness, sometimes nothing at all. It's not navel-gazing; it's a full reset, sparked by a trip, a breathwork session, or a brush with the edge. For Veterans, it's a potential breather from the stories you've been stuck in—service pride, combat scars, civilian drift—offering a glimpse beyond the self you've hauled around.

The Science Behind It
Your brain's a machine—ego's the operator, built from years of "me" and "mine." Ego death pulls the plug: psychedelics flood serotonin circuits, meditation quiets the chatter, trauma rips the controls away. What's left? A shift—maybe to calm waves or a blank slate—where old pain or pride lose their grip. For Veterans, it's like cutting the wire on a looped comms feed: silence, then a new signal. Science is digging in—small trials hint at real rewiring—but it's still half mystery, half gut truth.

The Impact of Ego Death on Veterans' Health
- Wellness Benefits: It's pitched to heal wounds, quiet fear, widen your view—stuff vets need when the past's a chokehold and the future's a blur.

- Consequences of Holding On: Cling to that ego, and trauma, anxiety, or shame keep running the show—weight you're trained to carry but don't have to.

Identifying and Analyzing Your Burdens
- Self-Assessment: Scope your load—what's pinned you? Nightmares from Fallujah? Guilt over a call? Feeling like a ghost in civvie life? Write it—know your fight.

- Setting Priorities: Rank the hits—trauma if it's screaming, anxiety if it's buzzing, purpose if you're adrift. Start where it's heaviest; the rest follows.

Fostering the Ego Death Habit
- Set Goals: Keep it real—e.g., "Hit one breathwork session this week to loosen the grip." Sharp, like a patrol plan—aim, move.

- Building a Support System: Pull in a vet buddy, shrink, or guide—they've got your flank, keeping you steady when the ground shifts.

Implementation Strategies
- Occasional Use: This isn't daily PT—think one-off dives or monthly resets. Space it like a long recon; depth beats grind.

- Habit Stacking: Tie it to your rhythm—meditate with morning coffee, breathe deep post-PT. Anchors it to what's solid.

Targeted Protocols for Veterans' Wellness
Here's how to chase ego death for specific needs, with supplies for each:

1. Trauma Healing
- What: Inhale 10–15 mg of 5-MeO-DMT in a guided session, one hit to start.

- Why: Combat's echoes stick—ego death can yank 'em out, reframing the mess into something you can walk past.

- How: Find a retreat, sit with a pro—vape it, 15 minutes of blast-off, then talk it through. Prep with a quiet day, no meds that clash (VA list check). Once—see if the ghosts fade in a week. If it's too wild, lean on the guide.

- Supplies Needed: Facilitator ($1,000–$5,000 retreat), vape pipe, safe space, post-trip notebook.

2. Reduced Anxiety
- What: Try a 60-minute holotropic breathwork session, weekly for a month.

- Why: Hypervigilance buzzing your wires? Losing "you" quiets the static, cuts the edge.

- How: Lie down, breathe fast and deep—30 minutes in, ego might slip. Rest after, sip water. Weekly—judge if the hum drops in weeks. Too intense? Slow the pace.

- Supplies Needed: Quiet room, mat, water bottle, timer (optional).

3. Enhanced Perspective
- What: Hit a 1–2 hour Vipassana meditation daily, 10-day push.

- Why: Purpose gone AWOL? Ego death widens the lens—shows you more than your stripes.

- How: Sit still, focus on breath—hours daily, 10 days straight (VA app or re-

132

treat). Day five, self might blur. Reflect after—write it. Once—see if life clicks anew. If it's tough, cut to an hour.

- Supplies Needed: Free VA meditation app, cushion, quiet corner, journal.

4. Emotional Release

- What: Use 80–125 mg MDMA with a therapist, one session to test.

- Why: Guilt or shame from that last op? Dissolving ego lets it spill out—frees the chest.

- How: Clinic or guide—swallow it, 3–6 hours of flow, talk it out after. Prep with intent: "Drop the weight." Once—check if you're lighter in days. Too raw? Lean on the pro.

- Supplies Needed: Therapist ($500–$2,000), safe space, water, post-talk plan.

5. Spiritual Connection

- What: Try 15–20 mg 5-MeO-DMT in a ceremony, one deep dive.

- Why: Meaning shot after service? The "oneness" vibe might tie you back to something bigger.

- How: Group setting—vape it with a shaman, 20 minutes of void, then sit with it. Prep with a quiet mind, integrate with a vet pal. Once—see if it sparks in a month. Too much? Stick to breath.

- Supplies Needed: Facilitator ($1,000–$5,000), pipe, mat, buddy for after.

Eliminating Barriers to Pursuit

- Identify Triggers: Spot what blocks you—"Too out there," "I'll lose it," "No point." Name it—then square up to it.

- Replace Hesitation: Swap "Not now" for "One go"—scout it like new terrain. Trade fear for "What's on the other side?"—move, learn.

- Veteran-Specific Substitutes:

  - Control: Swap "I'll unravel" for "I've got backup"—trust the guide, like a CO.

  - Doubt: Trade "Hocus-pocus" for "Combat reboot"—frame it your way, test it.

Mindfulness and Self-Regulation

- Techniques: Prep with focus—breathe slow (5-5-5), set a goal: "See past it." During, ride it; after, ground with talk or air. Keeps you steady, not spinning.

- Benefits: You'll know when you're locked—cue the dive. Awareness is your edge, vet grit at work.

Seeking Professional Help

- When Needed: PTSD raging or head's a mess? Hit your VA shrink or doc—ego death's no solo op for the shaky.

- Resources: VA therapy, vetted retreats, telehealth—free or pro, they'll steer you straight.

Maintaining and Sustaining the Practice

- Track Progress: Log the shift—less noise, new eyes? Mark it: "Dropped the load, saw clear."

- Overcome Plateaus: Stuck? Switch methods—breath to trip—or dig deeper. Push like a stalled march.

- Build Resilience: Each drop's a brick—stack 'em, and you're tougher, past the old walls.

Bottom Line

Ego death's a vet-ready reset—healing trauma, cutting fear, widening views, freeing feelings, linking to something big—through trips (5-MeO-DMT, MDMA), meditation, or breath. For vets hauling PTSD, guilt, or drift, it's a bold crack at shedding the shell, rooted in mystic ways and new mind hacks. Some call it gold—rewires the fight; science sees sparks—small trials hint, big proof's out. Risks? Mind bends, rough rides—step smart if you're raw. It's no lone fix—pros say back it with care—so hit your VA crew, start free with breath or apps, trip only with guides ($1,000–$5,000). Potent, deep, it's a tool in your kit—use it sharp and safe.

Electromagnetic Field Hazards

EMF stands for Electromagnetic Field, which refers to the fields of energy that surround electrically charged particles. EMFs are found in many different forms, including radio waves, microwaves and electric and magnetic fields.

The concern about the potential hazards of EMF exposure to human health has been growing in recent years, as more and more people are exposed to high levels of EMF through their daily use of electronic devices, such as smartphones, laptops and Wi-Fi routers.

Some of the potential hazards of EMF exposure to human health include:

• *Increased cancer risk:* Some studies have suggested a possible link between EMF exposure and an increased risk of certain types of cancer, such as childhood leukemia and brain tumors.

• **Neurological and cognitive effects:** Some studies have suggested that exposure to high levels of EMF can have negative effects on the brain and nervous system, including headaches, memory loss and depression.

• **DNA damage:** Some studies have found that exposure to high levels of EMF can cause damage to DNA, potentially leading to mutations and other negative health effects.

• **Disruption of sleep:** Some studies have found that exposure to EMF at night can interfere with sleep patterns, leading to insomnia and other sleep-related problems.

• **Hormonal changes:** Some studies have suggested that exposure to high levels of EMF can disrupt hormonal balance, leading to changes in mood, metabolism and other physiological functions.

It is important to note that the evidence regarding the potential hazards of EMF exposure is still limited and further research is needed to fully understand the effects of EMF on human health.

Additionally, it is important to keep a healthy lifestyle, including a balanced diet, regular exercise and sufficient sleep, to help the body cope with the effects of EMF exposure.

In conclusion, EMF exposure is a growing concern for human health, as people are exposed to high levels of EMF through their daily use of electronic devices. While the evidence regarding the potential hazards of EMF exposure is limited, there are steps that can be taken to reduce exposure and protect health.

Here are some ways to protect yourself from Electromagnetic Fields (EMF) exposure:

• **Limit device usage:** Limit your use of electronic devices, such as smartphones, laptops and Wi-Fi routers and keep them at a distance from your body when in use.

• **Use an EMF shield:** Consider using an EMF shield, such as a phone case, to reduce your exposure to EMF from electronic devices.

• **Turn off electronics at night:** Turn off electronic devices at night and unplug them from the wall to reduce exposure to EMF while you sleep.

• **Use a wired connection instead of Wi-Fi:** Whenever possible, use a wired connection instead of Wi-Fi to reduce your exposure to EMF from Wi-Fi routers.

- ***Keep a safe distance from power lines:*** If you live near high-voltage power lines, try to keep a safe distance from them to reduce your exposure to EMF.

- ***Use a Faraday cage:*** Consider using a Faraday cage, which is a device that shields against EMF, to protect yourself while sleeping or during other activities.

- ***Be mindful of your environment:*** Be mindful of your environment and take steps to reduce your exposure to EMF from sources such as cell phone towers, microwave ovens and other electronic devices.

- ***Eat a balanced diet:*** Eating a balanced diet that includes antioxidants and other nutrients can help to reduce the effects of EMF exposure and protect your health.

- ***Get regular exercise:*** Regular exercise can help to reduce the effects of EMF exposure and improve overall health.

- ***Get enough sleep:*** Getting enough sleep is important for reducing the effects of EMF exposure and maintaining overall health.

Bottom Line
There are several ways to protect yourself from Electromagnetic Fields (EMF) exposure, including limiting device usage, using an EMF shield, turning off electronics at night, using a wired connection instead of Wi-Fi, keeping a safe distance from power lines, using a Faraday cage, being mindful of your environment, eating a balanced diet, getting regular exercise and getting enough sleep. By taking these steps, you can reduce your exposure to EMF and protect your health.

Emotion

Emotional breakdown triggers and methods

Veterans often face a range of emotional and psychological challenges after returning from military service, including depression, anxiety and post-traumatic stress disorder (PTSD). Emotional breakdowns can be particularly difficult for Veterans and can be triggered by a variety of factors, including exposure to combat or other traumatic events, feelings of isolation or loneliness and difficulty adjusting to civilian life.

There are several common triggers that can lead to an emotional breakdown in Veterans, including:

- **Exposure to trauma:** Veterans who have been exposed to combat or other traumatic events may experience flashbacks or intrusive thoughts that can lead to emotional distress. These experiences can be especially challenging for Veterans with PTSD, who may relive the traumatic events even years after they have occurred.
- **Difficulty adjusting to civilian life:** Returning to civilian life can be a major transition for Veterans and can be challenging for many individuals who struggle with feelings of isolation, loneliness or a lack of purpose.

- **Financial stress:** Financial stress can be a major trigger for Veterans, particularly those who are struggling to make ends meet or who are dealing with job loss or other financial difficulties.

- **Substance abuse:** Substance abuse is a common problem among Veterans and can contribute to emotional breakdowns by impairing judgment, increasing anxiety and exacerbating depression.

- **Family and relationship difficulties:** Family and relationship difficulties can be a significant trigger for emotional breakdowns in Veterans, particularly for individuals who are struggling with feelings of isolation or loneliness.

- **Health problems:** Health problems can also trigger emotional breakdowns in Veterans, particularly if they are dealing with chronic pain, disabilities or other medical conditions.

Despite the challenges that Veterans face, there are several methods that can help to mitigate the effects of emotional breakdowns and improve overall well-being.

Some of these methods include:

- **Seeking professional help:** Seeking help from a licensed mental health professional can be an important step in overcoming emotional breakdowns. Mental health professionals can help Veterans to work through their emotions, address the root causes of their distress and develop coping strategies to manage symptoms.

- **Engaging in self-care:** Engaging in self-care activities, such as exercise, meditation or yoga, can help Veterans to reduce stress, improve their overall well-being and build resilience.

- **Building a support network:** Building a strong support network of friends, family and other trusted individuals can help Veterans to cope with the challenges of emotional breakdowns and provide a source of comfort and support.

• **Pursuing meaningful activities:** Pursuing meaningful activities, such as volunteering, pursuing a hobby or going back to school, can help Veterans to find a sense of purpose and fulfillment and can also provide a positive distraction from negative thoughts and emotions.

• **Reaching out for support:** Reaching out for support from others, such as fellow Veterans, family members or mental health professionals, can be a crucial step in overcoming emotional breakdowns.

• **Practicing mindfulness and stress reduction techniques:** Practicing mindfulness and stress reduction techniques, such as deep breathing, progressive muscle relaxation and guided imagery, can help Veterans to manage their emotions, reduce stress and improve overall well-being.

• **Making lifestyle changes:** Making healthy lifestyle changes, such as eating a well-balanced diet, getting enough sleep and avoiding substance abuse, can help Veterans to improve their physical and emotional health and reduce the risk of emotional breakdowns.

Bottom Line

Emotional breakdowns can be a challenging and difficult experience for Veterans, but with the right support and strategies, it is possible to overcome these challenges and improve overall well-being. By seeking professional help, engaging in self-care, building a support network, pursuing meaningful activities, reaching out for support, practicing mindfulness and stress reduction techniques and making lifestyle changes, Veterans can develop the resilience and coping skills needed to manage the triggers of emotional breakdowns and improve their overall well-being. It is important to remember that recovery is a journey and that everyone heals at their own pace. With patience, persistence and the right support, Veterans can overcome the challenges of emotional breakdowns and lead fulfilling, happy lives.

Emotional Stability
(and how to maintain it)

The ability to regulate and manage one's emotions in a healthy and adaptive way, emotional stability is an important aspect of overall well-being and can have a significant impact on relationships, work and daily life. Maintaining emotional stability requires a combination of self-awareness, healthy coping mechanisms and a supportive environment.

Here are some methods for maintaining emotional stability:

Paying attention to your thoughts, feelings and behaviors can help you understand your emotional state and respond in a healthy way. This can involve journaling, meditation or other forms of self-reflection.

- *Develop healthy coping mechanisms:* Developing healthy coping mechanisms such as exercise, mindfulness or talking to a trusted friend, can help you manage stress and negative emotions in a constructive way.

- *Nurture supportive relationships:* Surrounding yourself with supportive friends and family members can provide a sense of security and stability and can help you manage difficult emotions.

- *Get enough sleep:* Adequate sleep is essential for emotional stability, as it helps to regulate mood and manage stress.

- *Eat a balanced diet:* A balanced diet that includes healthy foods such as fruits, vegetables and lean protein can provide the nutrients needed to maintain emotional balance.

- *Engage in physical activity:* Regular exercise has been shown to reduce symptoms of depression, anxiety and stress and can improve emotional stability.

- *Manage stress:* Identifying and managing stressors can help to reduce the impact of stress on your emotions. This can involve setting boundaries, practicing relaxation techniques or seeking professional help.

- *Seek professional help:* If you are struggling to manage your emotions, seeking professional help from a therapist or counselor can be a valuable resource.

- *Avoid harmful coping mechanisms:* Avoiding harmful coping mechanisms, such as substance abuse, can prevent further damage to your emotional well-being.

- *Embrace change:* Embracing change, rather than fearing it, can help you to maintain emotional stability, as it allows you to adapt to new situations and challenges.

Bottom Line
Emotional stability is an important aspect of overall well-being and can be maintained through a combination of self-awareness, healthy coping mechanisms and a supportive environment. By following these strategies, you can improve your ability to manage your emotions and maintain emotional stability over time.

Enema - Process and Benefits

Veterans know grit—gut issues from MREs, stress that ties you in knots, meds that slow you down. An enema's a straight-up fix: shoot some liquid into your lower colon through a tube, flush out the junk, and get moving again. It's not a fancy colonic hitting the whole gut—this is a quick, targeted strike on the bottom end, something you can rig up at home. For vets wrestling with backed-up pipes, lingering toxins, or just feeling off, it's a simple, old-school play to clear the deck. This section lays out what enemas are, why they might click for Veterans, and how to pull it off, all with your boots on the ground.

Understanding the Enema Process

An enema's basic: slide a small tube an inch or two into your rectum, push in 1–4 cups of liquid—water, saline, coffee, whatever—hold it a bit, then let it rip on the john. It hits the lower colon—sigmoid and descending—softening waste and kicking it out, not the full intestinal overhaul of a colonic. For Veterans, it's a low-cost, DIY shot at relief when your gut's gone AWOL, rooted in tricks folks have used since way back when.

The Science Behind It

Your lower colon's a holding tank—waste piles up, stress or pills can jam it. An enema floods it with liquid, loosens the clog, and trips the switch to dump it. Some say it scrubs out toxins or perks you up by lightening the load—coffee's a wild card, supposedly nudging your liver. For Veterans, it's less about lab coats and more about feel: does it get you regular, shake the sluggishness? Science nods at the flush—constipation's a lock—but the bigger claims are still gut instinct over hard proof.

The Impact of Enemas on Veterans' Health
- Wellness Benefits: It's pitched to unclog you, clean house, lift your step—stuff vets need when the body's stalled or the field's still in your system.

- Consequences of Ignoring It: Skip it, and you're stuck with bloat, drag, or a gut that's checked out—extra weight on a frame built to move.

Identifying and Analyzing Your Gut Needs
- Self-Assessment: Scope your sitrep—what's off? Locked up from pain meds? Bloated from years of chow hall? Tired from who-knows-what? List it—know your fight.

- Setting Priorities: Rank the hits—constipation if you're stopped, comfort if you're puffed, energy if you're flat. Start where it's loudest; the rest follows.

Fostering the Enema Habit
- Set Goals: Keep it sharp—e.g., "Hit one water enema this week to get un-

stuck." Clear, like a fire mission—aim, execute.

- Building a Support System: Tell your VA doc or a vet pal you're trying it—they've got your six, keeping you straight when you test the waters.

Implementation Strategies
- Occasional Use: This isn't daily rations—use it when you're jammed or need a reset, not a full-time gig. Space it like a resupply drop.

- Habit Stacking: Pair it with a quiet night—post-chow wind-down or a slow Sunday. Ties it to your rhythm, keeps it smooth.

Targeted Protocols for Veterans' Wellness
Here's how to use enemas for specific needs, with supplies for each:

1. Constipation Relief
- What: Use a 1–2 cup saline enema, once when you're stuck.

- Why: Opioids or stress clogging you up? This softens the jam, gets it moving—fast relief for a locked gut.

- How: Grab a kit, fill with lukewarm saline, lube the tip—lie on your left, slide it in, squeeze slow over five minutes. Hold 10, hit the can. Once—feel it clear in half an hour. If it cramps, ease off next time.

- Supplies Needed: Enema kit ($10–$30), saline (pharmacy mix), petroleum jelly, towel.

2. Detoxification
- What: Try a 1–2 cup coffee enema, monthly or post-exposure.

- Why: Burn pit crud or field grime lingering? Coffee's pitched to kick your liver, flush the lower end—vet gut reset.

- How: Brew weak coffee, cool it, fill the bag—left side, slow pour, hold 15 minutes, dump it. Monthly—judge if you feel cleaner in days. Too jittery? Switch to water.

- Supplies Needed: Kit, organic coffee, water filter, quiet spot.

3. Energy Improvement
- What: Hit a 1-cup water enema, weekly for a trial.

- Why: Dragging from MRE years or med haze? Clearing the pipes might lift the fog, put some gas back in.

- How: Simple water, lukewarm—five minutes in, hold five, let it go. Weekly—see if you're less wiped in a week. If it's bunk, skip it.

- Supplies Needed: Kit, filtered water, lube, bathroom access.

4. Digestive Comfort
- What: Use a 2-cup saline enema, once or twice monthly.

- Why: Bloating from field chow or stress? This eases the puff, smooths the ride—gut breather for vets.

- How: Saline mix, slow fill—10 minutes, hold 10, release. Twice a month—check if the pressure drops in a day. Too much? Cut to once.

- Supplies Needed: Kit, saline, jelly, towel or mat.

5. Nutrient Delivery
- What: Try a 1-cup saline enema with doc guidance, acute need only.

- Why: Down hard, can't eat? This hydrates, sneaks in electrolytes—emergency fix for a tapped-out vet.

- How: VA nurse or self—saline, slow drip, hold 15, expel. Once, with orders—feel steadier in hours. Not DIY unless cleared.

- Supplies Needed: Kit (VA or pharmacy), saline, doc's nod, clean space.

Eliminating Barriers to Use
- Identify Triggers: Spot what stops you—"Too weird," "Hurts," "No time." Name it—then square up to it.

- Replace Hesitation: Swap "Not now" for "One shot"—quick hit, done. Trade doubt for "Does it work?"—test, judge.

- Veteran-Specific Substitutes:

  - Squeamish: Swap "Gross" for "Field med"—it's just logistics, grit up.

  - Pain: Trade "Too rough" for "Gentle go"—lube more, slow it down.

Mindfulness and Self-Regulation
- Techniques: Focus on the flow—breathe slow (4-7-8), feel it move. It's a mental anchor, cutting "this is nuts" chatter. Vets know focus—lock it here.

- Benefits: You'll spot when you're jammed—cue the flush. Awareness keeps you in the driver's seat, steering your gut.

Seeking Professional Help
- When Needed: IBS, heart trouble, or stuck bad? Hit your VA doc—enemas are simple but not for every rig.

- Resources: VA gastro, primary care, or telehealth—free, vet-ready, they'll clear it or wave off.

Maintaining and Sustaining the Practice

- Track Progress: Log the wins—moving again, less bloat? Mark it: "Flushed, felt light today."

- Overcome Plateaus: No relief? Switch liquid—water to saline—or up the cups. Push like a stalled op.

- Build Resilience: Each flush's a brick—stack 'em, and you're tougher, shedding what slows you.

Bottom Line

Enemas are a vet-friendly gut punch—unclogging pipes, scrubbing crud, lifting drag, easing bloat, sneaking in juice—with a $10 kit and a quick liquid shot to the lower end. For vets hauling opioid jams, MRE hangovers, or field ghosts, it's a hands-on fix to feel steadier, rooted in ancient hacks and med know-how. Some swear it's gold—clears you out, perks you up; science locks the constipation win—other perks lean on feel over facts. Risks? Cramps or upset if you overcook it—keep it chill if you're raw.

Exercise

Body weight exercise

Body weight exercises are a type of physical activity that utilizes the individual's own weight as resistance instead of external equipment such as weights or machines. These exercises are effective in building strength, flexibility and overall fitness, making them a popular choice for people of all ages and fitness levels. Body weight exercises are also convenient, as they can be performed anywhere, at any time, with no equipment required.

Benefits of Body Weight Exercises

- *Convenience:* Body weight exercises can be performed anywhere, at any time, without any equipment. This makes them an ideal option for people who want to stay active but may not have access to a gym or workout equipment.

- *Cost-effective:* Body weight exercises do not require any equipment or gym membership, making them an affordable option for people on a tight budget.

- *Increased strength:* Body weight exercises work by using the individual's own weight as resistance, which can help build strength in muscles and bones.

143

• **Improved flexibility:** Body weight exercises such as stretching and yoga can improve flexibility and range of motion.

• **Better balance and coordination:** Body weight exercises such as squats and lunges can help improve balance and coordination.

• **Cardiovascular health:** Body weight exercises that involve high-intensity movements, such as jumping jacks and burpees, can provide a cardiovascular workout and help improve cardiovascular health.

Types of Body Weight Exercises

• **Push-ups:** Push-ups are a classic body weight exercise that works the chest, triceps and core.

• **Squats:** Squats are a compound exercise that works the legs, glutes and lower back.

• **Lunges:** Lunges are a great exercise for the legs and hips and they also help improve balance and stability.

• **Plank:** Planks are an effective exercise for the core and help improve posture and stability.

• **Pull-ups:** Pull-ups are a challenging exercise that works the back, shoulders and biceps.

• **Dips:** Dips are a great exercise for the triceps, shoulders and chest.

• **Jumping jacks:** Jumping jacks are a high-intensity cardiovascular exercise that works the legs and cardiovascular system.

• **Burpees:** Burpees are a full-body exercise that works the legs, arms and core and provides a cardiovascular workout.

Sample Body Weight Exercise Routine

Here is a sample body weight exercise routine to help you get started:

• **Warm-up:** 5-10 minutes of light cardio, such as jumping jacks or jogging in place.
Push-ups: 3 sets of 10 reps
Squats: 3 sets of 12 reps

Lunges: 3 sets of 10 reps (each leg)
Plank: Hold for 1 minute
Pull-ups: 3 sets of 6 reps
Dips: 3 sets of 8 reps
Jumping-jacks: 3 sets of 20 reps
Burpees: 3 sets of 10 reps

- **Cool-down:** 5 -10 minutes of stretching to help loosen tight muscles and improve flexibility.

It is important to note that this is just a sample routine and can be adjusted to fit your individual fitness level and goals. As you progress and become more comfortable with these exercises, you can increase the number of reps and sets or add additional exercises to challenge yourself further. Convict Conditioning, by Paul Wade is a book that explains body weight conditioning in detail and provides workouts for every ability level.

Bottom Line

Body weight exercises are a convenient, cost-effective and effective way to improve strength, flexibility and overall fitness. Incorporating a variety of body weight exercises into your workout routine can provide a full-body workout and help you reach your fitness goals. Remember to always listen to your body, start slow and gradually increase the intensity of your workout over time.

Tips for sticking to an exercise routine

- **Make it a priority:** Schedule your workout time as you would any other important appointment.

- **Find a workout buddy:** Having a workout partner can help hold you accountable and make your workout more fun.

- **Have a plan:** Create a schedule for your workouts and stick to it.

- **Mix it up:** Change up your workout routine to keep things interesting.

- **Set realistic goals:** Start with small, achievable goals and work your way up.

- **Track your progress:** Keep a workout diary or use a fitness app to track your progress and stay motivated.

- **Reward yourself:** Give yourself a small reward for reaching your workout milestones.

- **Get enough sleep:** Make sure you are getting enough sleep to help you stay energized for your workouts.

- **Listen to your body:** If you're feeling tired or unwell, it's okay to take a break or scale back your workout.

- **Make it a lifestyle:** Incorporate physical activity into your daily routine, such as taking the stairs instead of the elevator or going for a walk during your lunch break.

- **Have fun:** Remember to enjoy the process and find activities that you enjoy doing.

- **Be consistent:** consistency is key when it comes to sticking to an exercise routine. Keep up the good work, even if you miss a day or two.

- **Get professional help:** Consult a personal trainer or fitness expert to help you create an exercise plan that works for you.

Lastly, be patient and don't expect overnight results, it takes time and effort to see the changes you want. Keep in mind that the most important thing is to consistently show up and do the work.

Types of exercise and their benefits

There are many different types of exercise, each with their own unique benefits. Some of the most common types include:

- **Aerobic exercise:** Aerobic exercise, also known as cardiovascular exercise, is any activity that increases the heart rate and breathing for a sustained period of time. Examples include running, cycling, swimming and walking. Aerobic exercise is beneficial for improving cardiovascular health, increasing lung capacity and burning calories.

- **Strength training:** Strength training, also known as resistance training, is any exercise that involves working against resistance, such as using weights or resistance bands. Examples include weightlifting, bodyweight exercises and resistance band exercises. Strength training is beneficial for building and maintaining muscle mass, increasing bone density and improving overall strength and power.

- **Flexibility exercise:** Flexibility exercise is any activity that stretches and lengthens the muscles and improves joint range of motion. Examples include yoga, stretching and Pilates. Flexibility exercise is beneficial for improving posture, reducing muscle tension and soreness and preventing injury.

• *High-intensity interval training (HIIT):* High-intensity interval training is a type of exercise that alternates periods of high-intensity activity with periods of low-intensity recovery. Examples include sprint interval training and circuit training. HIIT is beneficial for improving cardiovascular fitness, burning calories and increasing muscle endurance.

Balance and coordination exercises: Balance and coordination exercises are designed to improve the body's ability to control movement and maintain balance. Examples include tai chi, dance and gymnastics. Balance and coordination exercises are beneficial for improving balance, reducing the risk of falls and increasing body awareness.

It's important to note that a well-rounded fitness routine should include a combination of these different types of exercise for optimal health benefits. It's always best to consult with a healthcare professional or a certified personal trainer before starting an exercise program, especially if you have any health conditions or injuries.

Bottom Line
There are many different types of exercise, each with its own unique benefits. Some of the most beneficial types of exercise include resistance training, high-intensity interval training, yoga, walking, swimming, cycling, strength training and Pilates. A well-rounded exercise routine that includes a mix of resistance training, cardio and stretching is ideal, along with a healthy diet, enough sleep and stress management. The key is to find an activity you enjoy and make it a consistent part of your lifestyle.

Exercise and Nutrition for Seniors

Exercise and nutrition are important for all individuals, but the specific needs and considerations for different populations can vary. As we age, our bodies go through natural changes that can affect our ability to exercise and the types of exercise that are safe and effective. However, regular exercise is still important for maintaining physical and cognitive function, as well as reducing the risk of chronic diseases such as heart disease and diabetes.

For seniors, it is important to focus on exercises that improve balance and flexibility, such as yoga and tai chi. Weight-bearing exercises, such as walking and strength training, are also important for maintaining bone density. It is also important to consult with a healthcare professional before starting any new exercise program, as certain medical conditions or medications may affect the types of exercise that are safe and appropriate.

Nutrition is also an important consideration for seniors. As we age, our bodies may have a harder time absorbing certain nutrients and we may also have a decreased appetite. It is important to make sure that seniors are getting enough protein, calcium and vitamin D to maintain bone health. Additionally, it is important to make sure that seniors are staying hydrated, as dehydration can lead to confusion and falls.

Exercise and Nutrition for Specific Health Conditions

• *Arthritis:* Arthritis is a common condition that causes inflammation and pain in the joints. Regular exercise can help to improve joint mobility, reduce pain and stiffness. There are multiple types of arthritis with different causes. Some require systemic medications for effective treatment, while others can be managed simply through dietary changes and exercise as described in the following paragraphs. Consult with your health care provider to determine if you are suffering from arthritis and what is the best treatment.

For individuals with arthritis it is important to focus on low-impact exercises, such as swimming, cycling and water aerobics, to reduce the stress on the joints. It is also important to consult with a healthcare professional before starting any new exercise program, as certain medical conditions or medications may affect the types of exercise that are safe and appropriate.

Nutrition is also an important consideration for individuals with arthritis. Diet can have surprising effects on inflammation. It is best to consult with a nutritionist or allergy specialist to identify and eliminate foods that may be the cause of inflammation.

• *Cardiovascular Disease:* Cardiovascular disease (CVD) is a broad term that includes conditions such as heart disease, stroke and hypertension. Regular exercise can help to improve cardiovascular health by lowering blood pressure, improving cholesterol levels and reducing the risk of heart disease and stroke.

For individuals with CVD, it may be important to focus on aerobic exercises, such as walking, cycling and swimming, as well as resistance training to build muscle mass. It is critical to consult with a healthcare professional before starting any new exercise program, as certain medical conditions or medications may affect the types of exercise that are safe and appropriate.

Nutrition is also an important consideration for individuals with CVD. A diet that is high in fruits, vegetables, whole grains, lean proteins and healthy fats can help to lower cholesterol levels and improve overall cardiovascular health. It is also important to limit or avoid foods that are high in saturated and trans fats, as well as added sugars.

• *Diabetes:* Exercise and nutrition are crucial for individuals with diabetes, as they can help to control blood sugar levels and reduce the risk of complications. Regular exercise can help to improve insulin sensitivity and glucose uptake, as well as improve cardiovascular health.

For individuals with diabetes, it is important to focus on aerobic exercises such as walking, cycling and swimming, as well as resistance training to build muscle mass. It is also important to consult with a healthcare professional before starting any new exercise program, as certain medical conditions or medications may affect the types of exercise that are safe and appropriate.

Nutrition is also an important consideration for individuals with diabetes. A diet that is high in fruits, vegetables, whole grains, lean proteins and healthy fats and can help to control blood sugar levels and improve overall health. Limiting or avoiding foods that are high in added sugars and saturated fats. Additionally, it is important to monitor carbohydrate intake and timing of meals and exercise to manage blood sugar levels.

Bottom Line
Exercise and nutrition are important for all individuals, but they can be especially crucial for those with specific health conditions. It's important to note that these are just a few examples and that it's always best to consult with a healthcare professional before making any changes to your exercise or nutrition regimen.

Explosive Breaching Health Issues

Explosive breaching, also known as dynamic entry, is a technique used by law enforcement and military personnel to gain quick and forceful entry into a building or structure. This method of entry involves the use of explosive charges to blow open doors, walls or other barriers. While explosive breaching can be an effective tool in certain situations, it also poses a number of health risks to both the individuals performing the breaching and those in the immediate vicinity.

One of the primary health concerns associated with explosive breaching is the risk of injury or death from the blast itself. The force of the explosion can cause severe injuries, such as broken bones, cuts and burns, as well as more serious injuries, such as traumatic brain injury or internal organ damage. Additionally, the explosion can cause structural damage to the building or structure, creating potential hazards such as falling debris or collapsed walls.

Another concern is the risk of exposure to hazardous materials. Explosive breach-

149

ing can release harmful chemicals, toxins or other hazardous materials into the air which can be inhaled by those in the immediate vicinity. This can lead to a range of health problems including respiratory issues, skin irritation and chemical burns. The dust and debris created by the explosion can contain harmful particles, such as lead or asbestos, which can be inhaled and lead to chronic health problems such as lung disease or cancer.

The noise produced by explosive breaching can also have negative health effects. The loud blast can cause hearing loss or damage to the ears, as well as headaches, tinnitus and other symptoms of noise-induced hearing loss. Additionally, the noise can cause stress and anxiety, which can lead to a range of mental health issues.

In order to minimize the health risks associated with explosive breaching it is important to use proper protective equipment such as respirators, earplugs and eye protection. Additionally, individuals in the immediate vicinity of the breach should be evacuated or given adequate warning to protect themselves from the blast and any hazardous materials that may be released.

It is also important for organizations to conduct proper training for personnel who will be performing explosive breaching. This training should include information on the proper use of explosive charges, as well as information on the health risks associated with the technique. Personnel should also be trained on how to properly handle hazardous materials and conduct decontamination procedures if necessary.

Bottom Line
Explosive breaching can be an effective tool for law enforcement and military personnel but it also poses a number of health risks. It is important for organizations to take steps to minimize these risks including the use of proper protective equipment, adequate training and the evacuation of individuals in the immediate vicinity of the breach. Additionally organizations should conduct regular health monitoring of personnel who perform explosive breaching to ensure they are not suffering from any negative health effects.

Families

Families of Veterans play a critical role in the well-being and recovery of their loved ones who have served in the military. These families can experience a wide range of emotions and challenges, both during and after their loved one's service. It is essential to consider the needs of these families and provide appropriate support to help them cope with the unique challenges they face.

One of the most significant considerations for the families of Veterans is the emotional and psychological well-being of their loved one. Many Veterans may struggle with post-traumatic stress disorder (PTSD), depression or anxiety. These conditions can have a significant impact on the Veteran and their family. It is crucial to provide access to mental health services and support groups for both the Veterans and their families to help them cope with these challenges.

Another consideration for the families of Veterans is the financial impact of their loved one's service. Many Veterans may have difficulty finding employment or may have to deal with long-term medical issues that can be costly. This can put a significant financial strain on the family and it is essential to provide financial assistance and resources to help them manage these costs.
The families of Veterans may also face housing challenges. Some Veterans may have difficulty adjusting to civilian life and may struggle with homelessness. It's important to provide access to housing assistance and support services to help Veterans and their families find stable housing.

Another important consideration for the families of Veterans is the education and career opportunities for their loved ones. Many Veterans may have difficulty returning to the workforce or may not have the necessary skills for civilian jobs. It is essential to provide access to job training and education programs to help Veterans transition to civilian life.

Finally, it is important to consider the unique needs of children and spouses of Veterans. Children may have a difficult time understanding their parent's service and may experience emotional and psychological challenges as a result. Spouses may have to assume the role of sole caregiver and breadwinner while their loved one is deployed or recovering from their service. It's important to provide support services and resources for these individuals to help them cope with the unique challenges they face.

Bottom Line
The families of Veterans play a critical role in the well-being and recovery of their loved ones who have served in the military. It is essential to consider the unique needs and challenges of these families and provide appropriate support to help them cope. This includes access to mental health services, financial assistance, housing assistance, education and career opportunities, and support services for children and spouses of Veterans.

Kids with Veteran parents and/or siblings

Children with Veteran parents or siblings may face unique challenges as they grow up. These children may have to deal with a wide range of emotions and experiences that can have a significant impact on their well-being. Therefore, it is essential to understand the specific considerations for children with Veteran parents or siblings and provide appropriate support to help them cope.

Children with Veteran parents or siblings may experience feelings of isolation or disconnection from their peers, as they may not fully understand the unique experiences and challenges that come with having a Veteran parent or sibling. It can be beneficial to connect them with other children who have a similar background, through mentorship programs or peer support groups, as well as counseling.

Furthermore, children with Veteran parents or siblings may struggle with feelings of guilt, shame or confusion as a result of the experiences of their loved ones. This can be particularly true for children of Veterans who have been deployed to war zones, as they may have trouble understanding the trauma their parents or siblings have experienced. It's important to provide access to counseling and support services that can help them process these feelings and better understand what their loved ones are going through.

Finally, it is important to consider the unique needs of children and siblings of Veterans. Children may have a difficult time understanding their parent's service and may experience emotional and psychological challenges as a result. Siblings may have to assume the role of caretaker or may feel left out when the focus is on the Veteran. It's important to provide support services and resources for these individuals to help them cope with the unique challenges they face.

Bottom Line
Children with Veteran parents or siblings may face unique challenges as they grow up. These children may have to deal with a wide range of emotions and experiences that can have a significant impact on their well-being. Therefore, it is essential to understand the specific considerations for kids with Veteran parents or siblings and provide appropriate support to help them cope. This includes access to mental health services, financial assistance, housing assistance, education and career

opportunities and support services for children and siblings of Veterans.

Support organizations

There are several organizations that provide support for the families of Veterans. Some of the most well-known organizations include:

- *National Military Family Association (NMFA):* The NMFA (https://www.militaryfamily.org/) is a national nonprofit organization that provides support and resources for military families. They offer a variety of programs and services, including counseling, financial assistance and educational opportunities for Veterans and their families.

- *Tragedy Assistance Program for Survivors (TAPS):* TAPS (https://www.taps.org/) is a national organization that provides support and resources for the families of fallen service members. They offer a variety of programs and services, including counseling, financial assistance and educational opportunities for Veterans and their families.

- *American Legion Auxiliary:* The American Legion Auxiliary (https://www.legion.org/auxiliary) is an organization that provides support and resources for Veterans and their families. They offer a variety of programs and services, including counseling, financial assistance and educational opportunities for Veterans and their families.

- *Veterans of Foreign Wars (VFW) Auxiliary:* The VFW Auxiliary (https://vfwauxiliary.org/) is an organization that provides support and resources for Veterans and their families. They offer a variety of programs and services, including counseling, financial assistance and educational opportunities for Veterans and their families.

- *Gold Star Wives of America:* Gold Star Wives of America (https://goldstarwives.org/) is an organization that provides support and resources for the widows and widowers of fallen service members. They offer a variety of programs and services, including counseling, financial assistance and educational opportunities for Veterans and their families.

These are just a few examples of the many organizations that provide support for the families of Veterans. It's important to note that availability of these organizations might vary depending on the location and the specific needs of the family. (Note: Additional organizations that support Veterans and Veteran families are listed in **Annex D—Organizations Supporting Veterans**)

Fasting

Dr. Jason Fung is a Canadian nephrologist and author who advocates for the use of fasting as a tool for weight loss and improved health. He has written several books on the topic of fasting, including <u>The Complete Guide to Fasting</u> and <u>The Obesity Code.</u>

Dr. Fung argues that fasting can be an effective tool for weight loss and improving health by addressing the underlying causes of obesity and metabolic diseases, such as insulin resistance. He also claims that fasting can improve insulin sensitivity, which helps to regulate blood sugar levels and lower the risk of type 2 diabetes. He also claims that fasting can improve cardiovascular health by reducing inflammation, lowering blood pressure and decreasing cholesterol levels.

Dr. Fung also suggests that fasting can improve mental clarity and concentration by reducing inflammation in the brain. He also claims that fasting can increase cellular repair processes by activating autophagy, a natural process in the body that helps remove damaged cells. He also points out that fasting may increase lifespan by reducing the risk of age-related diseases such as cancer and heart disease.

While Dr. Fung's work on fasting has gained popularity, it is still not well-established by scientific studies and more research is needed to fully understand the effects of fasting on health and weight loss. Consult a healthcare professional before trying any fasting schedule, especially if you have a medical condition or are taking any medications.

There are several different types of fasting including:

• **Intermittent fasting:** This is a general term that encompasses different forms of fasting, including time-restricted fasting, alternate-day fasting and whole-day fasting.

> - Time-restricted fasting: This involves eating during a specific window of time and fasting for the rest of the day.
> - Alternate-day fasting: This involves alternating between days of eating normally and days of calorie restriction.
> - Whole-day fasting: This involves fasting for a full 24 hours or more.

• **Modified fasting:** This involves eating very little, usually around 500-800 calories a day, usually for a short period of time (2-5 days).

- **Fasting-mimicking diet:** This is a diet where people eat very low calorie, high nutrient dense food and mimics the beneficial effects of fasting without actually fasting.

- **Religious fasting:** This is a practice of abstaining from food and drink for spiritual or religious reasons.

It's important to note that not all types of fasting may be suitable for everyone and it's important to consult with a healthcare professional before starting any fasting schedule, especially if you have a medical condition or are taking any medications.

Intermittent fasting benefits

Not all intermittent fasting schedules may be suitable for everyone and it's important to find a schedule that works best for you and your lifestyle. It is also important to consult with a healthcare professional before starting any fasting schedule, especially if you have a medical condition or are taking any medications. Intermittent fasting is an eating pattern where individuals alternate between periods of eating and fasting. Some potential benefits of intermittent fasting include:

- **Weight loss:** Intermittent fasting may help promote weight loss by reducing calorie intake and increasing metabolism.

- **Improved insulin sensitivity:** Intermittent fasting may help improve insulin sensitivity, which can help lower the risk of type 2 diabetes.

- **Increased longevity:** Intermittent fasting may help increase lifespan by reducing the risk of age-related diseases such as cancer and heart disease.

- **Improved mental clarity:** Intermittent fasting may help improve mental clarity and concentration by reducing inflammation in the brain.

- **Increased cellular repair:** Intermittent fasting may help increase cellular repair processes by activating autophagy—a natural process in the body that helps remove damaged cells.

- **Improved cardiovascular health:** Intermittent fasting may help improve cardiovascular health by reducing inflammation, lowering blood pressure and decreasing cholesterol levels.

While some research suggests potential benefits of intermittent fasting, more studies are needed to fully understand its effects. Consult a healthcare professional before trying intermittent fasting, especially if you have a medical condition or are taking any medications.

There are several different intermittent fasting schedules that individuals can follow including:

- **The 16/8 Method:** This involves fasting for 16 hours and eating during an 8-hour window. For example, an individual may eat between 12pm-8pm and then fast until 12pm the next day.

- **The 5:2 Diet:** This involves eating normally for 5 days and restricting calorie intake to 500-600 calories for the other 2 days.

- **The Alternate Day Diet:** This involves alternating between days of eating normally and days of calorie restriction.

- **The Warrior Diet:** This involves eating a small amount of raw fruits and vegetables during the day and then eating one large meal at night.

- **The Eat-Stop-Eat Method:** This involves fasting for 24 hours, once or twice a week.

- **The OMAD (One Meal A Day) Method:** This involves eating one meal a day within a specific hour window.

Alternate day fasting (ADF) is a type of intermittent fasting that involves alternating between days of eating normally and days of calorie restriction. On "feed days," individuals eat whatever they want, within reason, while on "fast days," they restrict their calorie intake to a specific amount.

The most common form of ADF is the "36-hour fast," where individuals eat normally for one day, then restrict calorie intake to around 500-600 calories on the next. This cycle is then repeated, with one "feed day" followed by one "fast day."

Some studies have suggested that ADF may be effective for weight loss and improving cardiovascular health. However, it is important to note that more research is needed to fully understand the effects of ADF and that this type of fasting may not be suitable for everyone. It is also important to consult with a healthcare professional before starting any fasting schedule, especially if you have a medical condition or are taking any medications.

Dry fasting is a type of fasting that involves abstaining not only from food, but also from water and other beverages for a certain period of time. It is considered one of the most extreme forms of fasting and is not recommended for most people, especially those who are not experienced in fasting.

Proponents of dry fasting claim that it has benefits such as weight loss, improved immunity and increased longevity. However, there is limited scientific research on the effects of dry fasting and it is important to note that it can be dangerous if not done under the supervision of a healthcare professional.

Dry fasting can cause dehydration, electrolyte imbalances and can lead to serious health issues like kidney damage, heart failure and even death. It is not recommended for people who are pregnant, breastfeeding, have a history of eating disorders or have certain medical conditions such as diabetes. It is also not recommended for people who are physically active or work in hot environments.

It is important to consult with a healthcare professional before attempting dry fasting and to be aware of the risks and potential side effects.

Water fasting is a type of fasting that involves abstaining from food and consuming only water for a certain period of time. The duration of water fasting can vary, with some people fasting for a day or two and others fasting for several weeks.

Water fasting is considered to be a more moderate form of fasting compared to dry fasting as it allows for the intake of water which is essential for the body's hydration and also to eliminate toxins.

Proponents of water fasting claim that it has benefits such as weight loss, improved immune function and increased longevity. Some studies have suggested that water fasting may have positive effects on blood sugar, blood pressure and cholesterol levels. However, it is important to note that more research is needed to fully understand the effects of water fasting and it is not recommended for most people.

Water fasting can be challenging and it is important to be properly prepared, both physically and mentally. It can lead to side effects such as fatigue, headaches and dizziness. It is also important to consider the risks and to consult with a healthcare professional before attempting water fasting, especially if you have a medical condition or are taking any medications. It is also important to note that after the fast, it is important to break the fast properly by consuming light and easy to digest foods and not going back to the normal diet immediately.

Longer fasting periods, such as those that last for several days or weeks, may have additional benefits compared to shorter fasting periods. Some of the potential benefits of longer fasting include:

• **Increased autophagy:** Longer fasting periods may increase the rate of autophagy, a process in the body that helps remove damaged cells and promote cellular repair.

• **Increased insulin sensitivity:** Longer fasting periods may help improve insulin sensitivity, which can lower the risk of type 2 diabetes.

• **Reduced inflammation:** Longer fasting periods may reduce inflammation in the body, which can help alleviate symptoms of certain conditions such as arthritis.

• **Increased stem cell production:** Longer fasting periods may increase the production of stem cells, which can help repair and regenerate tissues in the body.

• **Increased longevity:** Some studies suggest that longer fasting periods may increase lifespan by reducing the risk of age-related diseases such as cancer and heart disease.

Bottom Line
Longer fasting periods are not suitable for everyone and can be challenging both physically and mentally. It is also important to consult with a healthcare professional before attempting a lengthy fast, especially if you have a medical condition or are taking any medications. Also it is important to break the fast properly and in consultation with a healthcare professional, as going back to normal diet immediately after a fast can cause adverse effects.

Fiber

Fiber, an essential nutrient that plays an important role in overall health and well-being. For Veterans, incorporating high-fiber foods into their diet can provide a range of health benefits. In this section, we will discuss the benefits of fiber for Veterans and reference Dr. Alan Mandell's work on the subject.

• **Improved Digestive Health:** Fiber can help to regulate the digestive system, promoting regular bowel movements and reducing the risk of constipation. This is particularly important for Veterans who may have gastrointestinal issues related to their military service. According to Dr. Mandell, fiber-rich foods can help to reduce inflammation in the gut and support the growth of healthy gut bacteria, which can improve overall digestive health.

• **Reduced Risk of Chronic Diseases:** Eating a diet high in fiber has been linked to a reduced risk of chronic diseases such as heart disease, diabetes and certain types of cancer. Dr. Mandell notes that fiber can help to lower cholesterol levels, reduce blood pressure and regulate blood sugar levels, all of which are important for maintaining overall health.

• ***Improved Weight Management:*** High-fiber foods are typically low in calories and can help to promote feelings of fullness, making it easier to manage weight. Dr. Mandell explains that fiber slows down the digestion of food, which can help to reduce hunger and prevent overeating.

• ***Improved Mental Health:*** There is growing evidence that gut health is linked to mental health and that fiber can play a role in improving both. According to Dr. Mandell, fiber can help to reduce inflammation in the body, which has been linked to a range of mental health issues such as depression and anxiety.

• ***Improved Immune Function:*** The gut is home to a large proportion of the body's immune system and a healthy gut is essential for maintaining overall immune function. Dr. Mandell explains that fiber-rich foods can help to support the growth of healthy gut bacteria, which can improve immune function and reduce the risk of infections and diseases.

Some high-fiber foods that Veterans can incorporate into their diet include fruits, vegetables, whole grains, nuts, seeds and legumes. It is recommended that adults aim for 25-30 grams of fiber per day, but it is important to gradually increase fiber intake to avoid digestive discomfort.

In addition to incorporating high-fiber foods into their diet, Veterans can also consider taking a fiber supplement. Dr. Mandell recommends using a psyllium husk supplement, which is a natural source of soluble fiber that has been shown to improve digestive health and reduce the risk of chronic diseases.

Bottom Line

Fiber is an essential nutrient that can provide a range of health benefits for Veterans. Eating a diet rich in fiber can improve digestive health, reduce the risk of chronic diseases, improve weight management, improve mental health and improve immune function. Veterans can incorporate high-fiber foods into their diet and consider taking a fiber supplement to support overall health and well-being. As with any dietary changes, it is important to speak with a healthcare provider before making significant changes to one's diet.

Financial Education and Support

Veterans face a new AO post-service—money. Financial education and support are your intel and backup: skills to budget, save, invest, ditch debt, plus the know-how to tap benefits you've earned. It's not barstool money tips—this is a structured playbook, delivered through classes, one-on-one advice, or aid programs, built to lock in stability. For vets juggling job hunts, disability costs, or the shift from military paychecks, it's a lifeline to cut stress and square away your future. This section breaks down why it matters, what it delivers, and how to make it work, all with a Veteran's edge.

Understanding Financial Education and Support

Financial education hands you the tools—budgeting 101, credit hacks, investment basics—via workshops or apps. Support's the muscle: counseling to sort your cash, grants to plug holes, help claiming VA benefits. It's tailored, whether you're a lone wolf or rolling with a group, stretching from quick lessons to years of guidance. For Veterans, it's about turning chaos—civilian bills, medical tabs— into control, a mission you can win with the right gear.

The Science Behind It

Your brain hates money stress—it's a threat, like incoming. Learning to manage it flips that: knowledge cuts the panic, support lifts the load. It's not magic—figuring out cash flow or nailing benefits rewires worry into confidence, step by step. For Veterans, it's like cracking a field manual: master the system, and you're not just surviving—you're running the show. Studies back the basics—skills and aid steady you—but it's your grit that seals it.

The Impact of Financial Education and Support on Veterans' Health

- Wellness Benefits: It's pitched to ease your mind, lock in cash, shrink debt— stuff vets need when the bank's a battlefield and peace is the prize.

- Consequences of Ignoring It: Skip it, and stress, broke days, or bills keep you pinned—extra weight on a frame built to push.

Identifying and Analyzing Your Financial Needs

- Self-Assessment: Take stock—what's bleeding you? Job gap draining savings? Disability tabs piling up? No clue on benefits? List it—know your front line.

- Setting Priorities: Rank the hits—stress if money's choking you, debt if it's crushing, benefits if you're missing out. Hit the big one first; the rest falls in.

Fostering the Financial Habit

- Set Goals: Keep it tight—e.g., "Cut $50 off bills this month with a budget." Sharp, like a range target—aim, fire.

- Building a Support System: Pull in a VA counselor, vet pal, or advisor—they've got your six, keeping you on track when the numbers blur.

Implementation Strategies
- Daily Integration: Weave it in—check cash flow with morning coffee, tweak plans post-PT. Start small; steady beats a sprint, like pacing a hump.

- Habit Stacking: Pair it with routine—budget while chow's cooking, call for benefits during downtime. Ties it to what's locked in.

Targeted Protocols for Veterans' Financial Wellness
Here's how to tackle financial education and support for specific needs, with supplies for each:

1. Stress Reduction
- What: Hit a free VA budgeting class, 1–2 hours weekly for a month.

- Why: Money woes from transition gnawing you? Learning the ropes cuts the tension, steadies your head.

- How: Sign up through Military OneSource—online or in-person—learn to track every buck. Pencil and paper, an hour a week—feel the load lighten in weeks. If it's too much, focus on one bill first.

- Supplies Needed: VA class (free), notebook, pen, internet or ride to session.

2. Economic Security
- What: Use an app like Mint, 15 minutes daily for six weeks.

- Why: No job or shaky pay post-service? Budgeting and saving build a wall— keeps you solid.

- How: Download it (free or cheap), log every dime—chow, gas, rent. Sock away $20 a week—watch it grow. Six weeks—see if you're steadier. Too tight? Skip the latte, not the rent.

- Supplies Needed: Phone, Mint app ($0–$10/month), bank login, quiet spot.

3. Debt Management
- What: Book a VA Benefits Advisor, one 1-hour session to start.

- Why: Loans or med bills burying you? Counseling sorts it—slashes what's owed, vet-style.

- How: Call VA (free), sit with an advisor—list debts, plan cuts. One shot— knock $100 off in a month, scale up. If it's slow, ask for a payment tweak.

- Supplies Needed: VA contact (1-800-827-1000), debt list, pen, phone.

4. Benefit Access

- What: Hit a VSO like American Legion, one meet-up or ongoing claims help.

- Why: Missing disability pay or GI Bill cash? Navigation grabs what's yours—extra bucks for breathing room.

- How: Find a local VSO (free), bring discharge papers, ask: "What's mine?" File claims—$500–$3,000 a month could roll in. One go or months—check if it lands in weeks. If it drags, push harder.

- Supplies Needed: VSO contact (online), DD-214, notebook, transport.

5. Long-Term Planning

- What: Try a VA investing workshop, 2–4 hours over a month.

- Why: Retirement or disability looming? Skills grow cash—sets you up for the long haul.

- How: Sign up (free), learn stocks or savings—start with $50 a month in a fund. Four weeks—see if it's ticking up. Too complex? Stick to savings first.

- Supplies Needed: VA class access, internet or ride, bank account, pen.

Eliminating Barriers to Learning

- Identify Triggers: Spot what stalls you—"Too hard," "No cash to start," "Scams." Name it—then square up to it.

- Replace Hesitation: Swap "Later" for "One hour now"—quick hit, done. Trade doubt for "What's it save?"—move, learn.

- Veteran-Specific Substitutes:

  - Overwhelm: Swap "Too much" for "One bill"—start small, scale up.

  - Distrust: Trade "Rip-off" for "VA first"—stick to vetted help, test it.

Mindfulness and Self-Regulation

- Techniques: Focus on the numbers—track a day's spend, feel the control. It's a mental anchor, cutting "I'm screwed" noise. Vets know focus—lock it here.

- Benefits: You'll spot when cash runs wild—cue the fix. Awareness keeps you in the driver's seat, steering your stack.

Maintaining and Sustaining the Practice

- Track Progress: Log the wins—less worry, extra bucks? Mark it: "Budgeted, slept easy."

- Overcome Plateaus: Stalled? Up the hours or grab a new tool—push like a bogged-down patrol.

- Build Resilience: Each step's a brick—stack 'em, and you're tougher, shedding what sinks you.

Bottom Line
Financial education and support are a vet's playbook—cutting stress, locking security, slashing debt, nabbing benefits, planning long—with classes, advice, apps, peers, and VA know-how. For vets hauling job gaps, disability tabs, or transition fog, it's a straight shot at steady ground, rooted in old-school smarts and new aid tricks. Some say it's gold—calms the mind, fills the pocket; science backs the basics—skills and support work—but it's your hustle that seals it. Risks? Bad tips or lazy follow-through—stick to the trusted stuff. It's no lone fix—pros say pair it with action—so hit your VA crew, grab free tools (Military OneSource, apps), and grind it out. Simple, gritty, it's a tool in your kit—use it sharp and steady.

Finding Purpose after the Military

Finding purpose, post-military, can be a difficult and challenging process for many Veterans. The military provides a sense of structure, camaraderie and purpose that can be difficult to replicate in civilian life. However, there are many resources and strategies that can help Veterans find a sense of purpose and fulfillment after leaving the military.

- ***Seek out new opportunities for service and leadership:*** One strategy for finding purpose after the military is to seek out new opportunities for service and leadership. Many Veterans find that they can continue to serve their country and communities by becoming involved in public service, such as working for a non-profit organization, volunteering for a community service organization or running for political office.

- ***Pursue educational and career opportunities:*** Another strategy for finding purpose after the military is to pursue educational and career opportunities that align with the skills and experiences gained in the military. Many Veterans have transferable skills such as leadership, teamwork and technical expertise that can be used in a wide range of civilian careers. Veterans can also take advantage of educational benefits to pursue a college degree or vocational training.

- ***Find a new passion or hobby:*** For some Veterans, finding purpose after the military may involve finding a new passion or hobby. This can be a great way to explore new interests and discover a sense of fulfillment. Many Veterans find that they can explore new interests by joining a club, group or organization that is focused on a particular hobby or interest.

• *Seek out a supportive community:* Finally, it is important for Veterans to seek out a supportive community after leaving the military. Many Veterans find that connecting with other Veterans and sharing their experiences can be a powerful way to find a sense of belonging and purpose. Joining a Veterans' service organization, attending Veterans' support groups or participating in Veterans' events can provide Veterans with a sense of community and belonging.

• *Seek professional help:* It's also important to note that seeking professional help can be a valuable step in finding purpose after the military. Many Veterans may struggle with mental health issues such as PTSD, depression and anxiety that can affect their ability to find purpose after the military. Veterans should not hesitate to seek professional help if they are struggling with these issues.

Bottom Line
Finding purpose after the military can be a challenging process, but with the right approach and mindset, Veterans can find a sense of purpose and fulfillment. By taking the time to reflect on your experiences and values, exploring new opportunities for service and leadership, pursuing educational and career opportunities, discovering new passions and hobbies, connecting with a supportive community and seeking professional help if needed, Veterans can find a sense of purpose and fulfillment after leaving the military. It's important to remember that the process may not be easy, but it's a journey worth taking.

Fitness
(also, see Personal Exercise Plan)

Strenuous physical activity conducted through a full range of motion, often referred to as fitness, has numerous benefits for both physical and mental health. Some of the benefits include:

• *Improved cardiovascular health:* Regular exercise can lower the risk of heart disease, stroke and high blood pressure by strengthening the heart and improving circulation.

• *Weight management:* Regular exercise helps to burn calories and maintain a healthy body weight.

• *Increased muscle and bone strength:* Exercise can help to build and maintain muscle and bone mass, reducing the risk of osteoporosis and falls.

- **Improved mental health:** Regular exercise has been shown to reduce symptoms of depression and anxiety and improve mood and overall well-being.

- **Increased energy levels:** Regular exercise can help to boost energy levels and improve stamina.

- **Improved sleep:** Exercise can help to promote better sleep by regulating the body's internal clock and reducing stress and anxiety.

- **Improved immune function:** Regular exercise can help to boost the immune system and reduce the risk of infection and illness.

- **Increased longevity:** Regular exercise has been linked to a longer lifespan and a reduced risk of chronic diseases.

- **Improved physical function and mobility:** Regular exercise can help to improve flexibility and coordination and reduce the risk of injuries.

The benefits of fitness can be achieved through a variety of physical activities, such as walking, cycling, swimming and strength training. The key is to find activities that you enjoy and to make them a part of your regular routine. It is also recommended to consult with a doctor or a professional trainer before starting a new exercise program, especially if you have any health conditions or injuries.

Fitness is a crucial aspect of overall health and well-being. Regular exercise and physical activity have been shown to have numerous benefits for both the body and mind. Jordan Peterson, a clinical psychologist and bestselling author, emphasizes the importance of fitness in his work.

According to Peterson[7], fitness is not just about achieving a certain physical appearance or performance level, but about taking control of one's life and taking responsibility for one's own well-being. He argues that by committing to regular exercise and physical activity, individuals are able to take control of their physical and mental health and ultimately, their lives.

One of the key benefits of fitness is its impact on cardiovascular health. Regular exercise can lower the risk of heart disease, stroke and high blood pressure by strengthening the heart and improving circulation. Additionally, fitness can help with weight management by burning calories and maintaining a healthy body weight.

Fitness also improves muscle and bone strength, reducing the risk of osteoporosis and falls. Exercise has also been shown to have a positive impact on mental health, reducing symptoms of depression and anxiety and improving mood and overall well-being.

Peterson also emphasizes the role of fitness in developing discipline and self-control. He argues that by committing to regular exercise, individuals are able to develop the discipline and self-control necessary to achieve their goals in other areas of life. Additionally, fitness can increase energy levels, promote better sleep and boost the immune system, which can lead to a reduction in the risk of infection and illness.

Bottom Line

Fitness is not just about achieving a certain physical appearance or performance level but about taking control of one's life and taking responsibility for one's own well-being. Regular exercise and physical activity have numerous benefits for both physical and mental health and by committing to regular fitness, individuals are able to develop the discipline and self-control necessary to achieve their goals in other areas of life. As Jordan Peterson says, "It is not enough to be able to change the world, one must first change oneself."

Float Tanks - Sensory Deprivation

A sensory deprivation float tank, also known as an isolation tank or float pod, is a lightproof, soundproof chamber filled with a shallow pool of Epsom salt-saturated water, heated to skin temperature (about 94°F), allowing users to float effortlessly in a near-zero gravity environment. Developed by Dr. John C. Lilly in the 1950s, it minimizes external stimuli—light, sound, and touch—to promote deep relaxation and introspection. For Veterans, who may grapple with stress, chronic pain, or PTSD from service, float tanks offer a unique, non-invasive method to unwind and heal by quieting the mind and body. Proponents claim benefits like stress relief, pain reduction, and enhanced mental clarity, supported by clinical studies and widespread use in wellness centers, though evidence varies, and risks like claustrophobia or hygiene concerns exist. This section explores the float tank's significance, benefits, and application with a Veteran focus.

- Definition: A float tank is a sealed pod or room containing 10-12 inches of water with 800-1,000 pounds of Epsom salt, where users float for 60-90 minutes per session, blocking out sensory input to foster calm and recovery.

- Historical Context: Invented by Dr. Lilly in 1954 to study consciousness, float tanks gained therapeutic traction in the 1970s; by the 2010s, commercial float centers popularized them, with Veteran use noted by 2025 for stress and pain.

- Prevalence Driving Interest: Stress and pain are common post-service; many Veterans seek alternative therapies like floating to manage symptoms that linger beyond traditional treatments.

- Service-Related Stressors: Combat trauma, physical strain, and toxin exposure heighten stress and tension; float tanks provide a space to disconnect, offering relief for Veterans carrying these burdens.

- Health Decline: Chronic stress, sleep issues, and persistent pain signal a need for deep rest; float tanks target this by reducing sensory overload, a reset for Veterans feeling overwhelmed.

- Stress Relief: The absence of stimuli lowers cortisol, calming the nervous system and easing anxiety, a respite for Veterans navigating post-service pressures.

- Pain Reduction: Floating unloads joints and muscles, with magnesium from Epsom salt potentially soothing soreness, aiding Veterans with chronic aches or injuries.

- Improved Sleep: The tank's stillness promotes relaxation, helping Veterans with restless nights fall asleep more easily and rest deeply.

- Mental Clarity: Reduced input sharpens focus and quiets mental chatter, supporting Veterans with brain fog or emotional overload from service.

- Emotional Healing: The meditative state may unlock trauma processing, offering a safe space for Veterans to release pent-up feelings or find peace.

- Tank Setup: Pods (e.g., Floatworks, $5,000-$15,000) or open rooms at centers ($40-$100/session) hold warm, salty water; users enter naked or in swimwear, with earplugs optional, per float center norms.

- Floating Process: After showering, Veterans lie back in the tank (60-90 minutes), lights off, floating effortlessly as the salt buoys them; sessions end with a signal (e.g., music), followed by a rinse.

- Home Use: Personal tanks ($5,000-$15,000) allow daily or weekly floats (1-2 hours), set up in a quiet space with maintenance (e.g., water filters), a long-term option for Veterans.

- Center Visits: Float spas offer 60-90 minute sessions ($40-$100), often weekly or monthly, with staff managing hygiene and scheduling, convenient for Veterans near urban areas.

- Preparation and Aftercare: Hydrate before, avoid caffeine, and rest post-float (15-30 minutes); many centers suggest 3-6 sessions to feel effects, a routine Veterans can build over weeks.

- Risks: Claustrophobia or disorientation may unsettle some; hygiene lapses risk skin irritation. Veterans with PTSD or low blood pressure need caution to avoid distress or dizziness.

- Scientific Evidence: Studies show benefits for stress, pain, and sleep, with magnesium absorption plausible; broader claims like healing lack large trials, relying on user reports and small-scale research.

- Veteran Context: Stress, pain, and sleep issues align with float tank goals; interest in mindfulness and recovery tools makes it a fit for Veterans seeking calm and renewal.

- Practical Steps: Book a session at a local center ($40-$100), try 60 minutes weekly for a month, or explore home tanks ($5,000-$15,000) if committed, tracking mood or pain to gauge impact.

It's wise to consult a healthcare provider before floating, especially with mental health conditions or physical limitations, ensuring safety and compatibility with VA care.

Bottom Line:

Sensory deprivation float tanks offer stress relief, pain reduction, improved sleep, mental clarity, and emotional healing by immersing users in a warm, salty, stimulus-free environment (60-90 minutes) via commercial centers ($40-$100) or home setups ($5,000-$15,000). Veterans, with stress, pain, and sleep challenges from service, may find it a soothing, drug-free retreat, with studies and experiences suggesting it calms the mind and body over weeks. Unlike typical relaxation, it's a total sensory blackout. Evidence is solid for stress and pain relief—small trials back these—but thinner for deeper healing, leaning on user stories rather than broad proof. Risks include claustrophobia or hygiene issues, plus costs that may strain budgets, a concern for some Veterans. It's not recommended as a primary treatment by professionals for serious conditions due to limited data and gentle effects, best as a complement to VA care. Veterans should consult a healthcare provider, start with center sessions ($40-$100), and pair with existing support, approaching with patience and realistic hopes. It's a calming aid for some, not a full fix, enhancing wellness with regular floats.

Food Sensitivity Tests

Veterans take hits—gut trouble from MREs, fog from stress, aches that won't quit. Food sensitivity tests step in as recon: a blood draw to spot foods that might be kicking your system into overdrive, not with instant hives, but slow-burn grief like bloating or fatigue. These aren't allergy tests—they track delayed immune reactions, giving you intel to tweak your chow and feel sharper. For vets hauling post-service woes—deployment diets, toxin loads, or mystery symptoms—they're a hands-on way to nail down triggers. This section lays out why you might need 'em, what they deliver, and how to run the op, all with a Veteran's grit. Cyrex Labs stands out as a top-tier pick for the deep dive.

Understanding Food Sensitivity Tests
Food sensitivity tests check your blood for immune flags—think IgG or IgA antibodies—that flare when certain foods roll through. It's not the throat-closing allergy drill; it's subtler, hitting hours or days later with stuff like gut gripes or brain haze. A lab screens dozens, maybe hundreds of foods—dairy, wheat, whatever—and spits out a hit list to dodge. For Veterans, it's a map through the mess of MRE hangovers or stress-wrecked insides, pointing you to what's friend or foe on your plate.

The Science Behind It
Your gut's a battlefield—foods you eat can spark low-grade immune fights, not loud enough to notice right off, but sneaky enough to drag you down. These tests measure the antibodies tagging those troublemakers, flagging what might be stoking inflammation or sapping your juice. For Veterans, it's like sniffing out an ambush: ID the culprit—say, gluten or eggs—and pull it from the line. Science backs it some—small studies see relief when you ditch the triggers—but it's not a lock yet, more field report than textbook.

The Impact of Food Sensitivity Tests on Veterans' Health
- Wellness Benefits: They're pitched to ease your gut, lift your step, cool the fire—stuff vets need when the body's off and the mind's in a rut.

- Consequences of Ignoring It: Skip it, and bloat, drag, or aches keep you pinned—extra load on a frame built to roll.

Identifying and Analyzing Your Symptoms
- Self-Assessment: Scope your sitrep—what's barking? Gut knots after chow? Tired no matter what? Joints screaming? List it—know your AO.

- Setting Priorities: Rank the hits—digestion if you're gassed up, energy if you're flat, inflammation if you're stiff. Start where it's loudest; the rest falls in.

Fostering the Testing Habit
- Set Goals: Keep it tight—e.g., "Test this month to ditch the bloat." Sharp, like a range call—aim, fire.

- Building a Support System: Pull in your VA doc or a vet pal—they've got your six, keeping you on track when the results roll in.

Implementation Strategies

- Occasional Use: This isn't daily PT—run it once, maybe twice a year, to scout and adjust. Pace it like a long patrol.

- Habit Stacking: Pair it with routine—test when you're meal-prepping, tweak chow post-PT. Ties it to what's locked in.

Targeted Protocols for Veterans' Wellness

Here's how to use food sensitivity tests for specific needs, with supplies for each—Cyrex Labs shines for the full sweep:

1. Digestive Relief

- What: Order a Cyrex Array 10 (180 foods), one test to start.

- Why: MREs or stress messing your gut? Pinpoint dairy or gluten—cut 'em, ease the storm.

- How: Hit a practitioner for Cyrex ($500–$700), eat varied four weeks prior—blood draw at a VA lab or Cyrex site. Ditch top triggers (4–8 weeks), log bloat drop. Once—feel it settle in a month. If it's off, recheck diet prep.

- Supplies Needed: Cyrex order (practitioner), VA lab access, food log, pen.

2. Energy Improvement

- What: Use a simpler panel (90 foods, $200–$400), one shot.

- Why: Dragging from field fallout? Ditch what saps you—get your juice back.

- How: Pharmacy kit or doc—finger prick, mail it, cut reactive foods (4 weeks). Track pep daily—weekly wins show in a month. Too vague? Go Cyrex for depth.

- Supplies Needed: Test kit ($200–$400), food diary, mailbox, water.

3. Inflammation Reduction

- What: Hit Cyrex Array 10, one test with follow-up.

- Why: Joints or insides burning from service wear? ID triggers—cool the fire.

- How: Practitioner order—blood draw, ditch the reds (6 weeks), reintroduce slow (3 days each). Log pain shifts—re-test in six months if it sticks. Too much? Ease off strict cuts.

- Supplies Needed: Cyrex test, VA lab, notebook, calendar.

4. Mental Clarity

- What: Run a 90-food panel, one go with tweaks.

- Why: Fog from TBI or gut chaos? Clear the culprits—sharpen your edge.

- How: Cheap kit ($200), prick and send—drop reactive stuff (4 weeks), track headspace. One shot—see if the haze lifts in weeks. If it's flat, hit Cyrex next.

- Supplies Needed: Kit, journal, pen, quiet spot.

5. Immune Support
- What: Try Cyrex Array 10, one test with long play.

- Why: Bugs hitting hard post-service? Lighten immune load—stay in the fight.

- How: Order it—full panel, cut triggers (8 weeks), reintroduce to lock it in. Monthly symptom check—re-test in six if it holds. Too pricey? Start small.

- Supplies Needed: Cyrex order, VA lab, logbook, patience.

Eliminating Barriers to Testing
- Identify Triggers: Spot what stalls you—"Too complex," "No cash," "BS results." Name it—then gut-check it.

- Replace Hesitation: Swap "Later" for "One test now"—quick recon, done. Trade doubt for "What's it find?"—move, learn.

- Veteran-Specific Substitutes:

  - Cost: Swap "Can't afford" for "VA first"—lean on free consults, save for Cyrex.

  - Skepticism: Trade "Food's fine" for "Field fix"—test it like gear, judge it.

Mindfulness and Self-Regulation
- Techniques: Focus on chow—log what hits, feel the shift. It's a mental anchor, cutting "it's all the same" noise. Vets know focus—lock it here.

- Benefits: You'll spot when you're off—cue the tweak. Awareness keeps you in command, steering your gut.

Seeking Professional Help
- When Needed: Gut's a wreck or fog won't lift? Hit your VA doc—tests need a pro eye to nail it.

- Resources: VA gastro, primary care, or telehealth—free, vet-ready, they'll guide or green-light it.

Maintaining and Sustaining the Practice
- Track Progress: Log the wins—less bloat, more juice? Mark it: "Cut dairy, felt sharp."

- Overcome Plateaus: No shift? Re-test or tighten cuts—push like a stalled op.

- Build Resilience: Each tweak's a brick—stack 'em, and you're tougher, shedding what drags you.

Bottom Line

Food sensitivity tests—like Cyrex Labs' Array 10—are a vet's recon shot—easing guts, lifting energy, cooling fire, clearing heads, boosting fight—by spotting trigger foods with a blood draw ($200–$700). For vets hauling MRE scars, stress haze, or burn pit ghosts, it's a hands-on play to feel steadier, rooted in immune know-how and gut smarts. Some swear it's gold—cuts the crap, perks you up; science backs the relief—small trials show it—but big proof's still out, and Cyrex shines for depth over cheap kits. Risks? Bad reads or lean diets—check it with a pro if you're raw. It's no lone fix—pros say pair it with care—so hit your VA doc, test smart (Cyrex or basic), and run the elimination. Simple, gritty, it's a tool in your kit—use it sharp and steady.

Frequencies (Positive and Negative) and Electromagnetic Fields (EMF) - Effects on the Body

The human body exists within an environment saturated with various forms of energy, including electromagnetic fields (EMF) from natural and man-made sources. These fields can be characterized by their frequency, which can be either positive or negative in terms of their effects on biological systems. Understanding how these frequencies interact with human physiology is crucial, especially in our modern world, where exposure to artificial EMFs has significantly increased. This document explores the effects of positive and negative frequencies and electromagnetic fields on the human body, delving into the science, potential health implications, and the ongoing debate surrounding these phenomena.

Understanding Frequencies and Electromagnetic Fields

Frequencies refer to the rate at which an oscillation or vibration occurs, measured in Hertz (Hz). In the context of EMFs:

- Positive Frequencies are often associated with frequencies that are believed to have beneficial effects on health. These can include natural frequencies like those from the earth's Schumann resonance (around 7.83 Hz) or specific sound frequencies used in therapeutic practices.

- Negative Frequencies, conversely, are those that might have detrimental effects, often linked to high-frequency EMF from sources like Wi-Fi, mobile phones, and power lines.

Electromagnetic Fields (EMF)include a spectrum of energies ranging from extremely low frequency (ELF) fields to radio-frequency (RF) fields:

- ELF fields come from sources like power lines and domestic wiring (50-60 Hz).

- RF fields are emitted by wireless devices, including cell phones and Wi-Fi (MHz to GHz).

Biological Effects of Positive Frequencies

1. Healing and Well-being:

- Schumann Resonance: The Earth's natural frequency (7.83 Hz) is believed by some to have a calming effect, promoting better sleep, reducing stress, and potentially aiding in the healing process.

- Binaural Beats: A form of auditory therapy where two slightly different frequencies are played in each ear, purportedly leading to brainwave entrainment that can reduce anxiety, improve focus, or induce states conducive to meditation or sleep.

2. Cellular Communication and Repair:

- Bio-resonance Therapy: Utilizes frequencies to stimulate cellular activity, aiming to enhance the body's natural healing processes. Though controversial, some studies suggest potential benefits in pain management and wound healing.

3. Sound Therapy:

- Certain sound frequencies, like those used in Tibetan singing bowls or tuning fork therapy, are thought to resonate with the body's chakras or energy centers, promoting balance and health.

Biological Effects of Negative Frequencies

1. Cellular Damage:

- DNA Damage: High-frequency EMFs, particularly from ionizing radiation sources like X-rays, can directly damage DNA. Non-ionizing radiation, while less energetic, has been studied for potential indirect effects on DNA through oxidative stress.

2. Neurological Effects:

- Sleep Disruption: Exposure to blue light from screens (which emit RF fields) can suppress melatonin production, disrupting sleep patterns.

- Neurodegeneration: Some research suggests a potential link between long-term exposure to high-frequency EMFs and neurodegenerative diseases, though this remains a contentious area with inconsistent findings.

3. Immune System:

- Immune Response: Chronic exposure to certain EMFs might lead to alterations in immune function, potentially increasing susceptibility to diseases or altering inflammatory responses.

4. Reproductive Health:

- Studies on animals have shown effects like reduced sperm quality in males or developmental issues in offspring when exposed to high levels of EMFs, suggesting a possible impact on human reproductive health.

The Debate and Scientific Evidence

- **Lack of Consensus:** The effects of EMFs, particularly from non-ionizing sources, remain debated. The World Health Organization (WHO), through the International Agency for Research on Cancer (IARC), has classified RF electromagnetic fields as "possibly carcinogenic to humans" based on limited evidence of increased glioma risk among heavy mobile phone users.

- **Exposure Limits:** Regulatory bodies like the Federal Communications Commission (FCC) in the U.S. set exposure guidelines primarily to prevent thermal effects but are often criticized for not accounting for non-thermal biological effects.

- **Ongoing Research:** There's a continuous call for more long-term, large-scale studies to conclusively determine the health implications of EMF exposure at various frequencies.

Mitigation and Protection

1. Reducing Exposure:

- Use wired connections for internet where possible to reduce RF exposure.

- Limit use of devices that emit high EMFs, especially near the body.

- Create EMF-free zones in homes, particularly in sleeping areas.

2. Protective Measures:

- Use of EMF shielding materials or clothing, though effectiveness varies and is often debated.

- Implement natural grounding techniques like walking barefoot on earth to potentially counteract some effects of EMFs.

3. Health-Promoting Practices:

- Engage in activities that might counteract negative effects, like meditation, which could enhance the body's resilience to stress from EMF exposure.

Bottom Line

The interaction between frequencies and electromagnetic fields with the human body is complex, with both positive and negative implications. While there's substantial evidence for the beneficial effects of certain frequencies in therapeutic contexts, the health impacts of negative frequencies, especially from modern technology, are still under scrutiny. Public health policy, personal lifestyle choices, and further research into non-thermal effects are all pivotal in navigating this landscape. Understanding and mitigating potential risks while harnessing the benefits of positive frequencies could lead to a more balanced approach to living in our increasingly electrified world.

This section serves as an overview, and for those involved in policy-making, research, or individuals concerned about their health, a deeper dive into current literature, expert consultations, and personal experimentation with EMF reduction techniques might be warranted.

Frequency of Meals

The frequency of meals can vary depending on an individual's dietary needs, preferences and schedule. Some people may eat three large meals per day, while others may prefer to eat smaller meals more frequently, such as five or six times per day.

Additionally, some people may choose to follow specific meal frequency plans, such as intermittent fasting, where they limit their eating to certain hours of the day. Ultimately, the best meal frequency plan is one that works for the individual and helps them to achieve their health and fitness goals. (Note: See **Diets** for more detailed information.)

Functional Medicine

Dr. Hyman is a leading expert in the field of health and fitness, with a particular focus on functional medicine and the concept of "food as medicine."

According to Dr. Hyman, the key to optimal health and fitness is to address the underlying causes of chronic disease, rather than simply treating symptoms. This involves identifying and addressing the root causes of illness, such as inflammation, hormonal imbalances and gut dysfunction.

One of the key principles of functional medicine is the idea that food is not just fuel, but also medicine. Dr. Hyman emphasizes the importance of eating a whole food, plant-based diet that is high in nutrient-dense fruits, vegetables and healthy fats. He also recommends limiting processed foods, sugar and refined carbohydrates, as these can contribute to inflammation and chronic disease.

In addition to dietary changes, Dr. Hyman also stresses the importance of regular exercise, stress management and adequate sleep in maintaining good health and fitness. Exercise helps to improve cardiovascular health, increase muscle mass and strength and boost mood and energy levels. Stress management techniques such as yoga, meditation and deep breathing can help to reduce inflammation and improve overall well-being.

Dr. Hyman also emphasizes the importance of addressing the gut microbiome in maintaining good health. The gut microbiome is the collection of microorganisms that live in the gut and it plays a critical role in many aspects of health, including digestion, metabolism and immune function. To support a healthy gut microbiome, Dr. Hyman recommends consuming prebiotic and probiotic-rich foods, as well as avoiding antibiotics, processed foods and pesticides.

In addition to his focus on functional medicine and food as medicine, Dr. Hyman is also known for his work on the concept of "metabolic flexibility," which refers to the ability of the body to efficiently switch between burning different types of fuel (such as carbohydrates, fats and ketones) depending on the situation. This ability to adapt to different metabolic states is critical for optimal health and it can be supported through diet, exercise and lifestyle interventions.

Bottom Line
Dr. Mark Hyman is a respected and influential voice in the field of health and fitness and his approach to functional medicine and food as medicine has helped countless individuals achieve better health and well-being. He encourages people to take control of their health, by identifying and addressing the underlying causes of chronic disease and by embracing a lifestyle that includes a whole food, plant-based diet, regular exercise, stress management and adequate sleep.

Gallbladder

A small organ located near the liver, the gallbladder stores and releases bile, a digestive fluid produced by the liver that helps to break down fats in the small intestine. While many people believe that having their gallbladder removed (cholecystectomy) is a simple and straightforward procedure, there are several reasons why it is not always necessary to remove the gallbladder and why a non-invasive cleanse may be a better option.

First, the gallbladder plays an important role in the digestive process by regulating the release of bile into the small intestine. Bile helps to emulsify fats, making it easier for the small intestine to absorb and process them. Without a functional gallbladder, the body may have difficulty digesting fats, leading to symptoms such as indigestion, bloating and diarrhea.

Second, the removal of the gallbladder can have long-term consequences on overall health. The bile that was previously stored in the gallbladder now flows directly into the small intestine, increasing the risk of developing bile reflux, a condition in which bile backs up into the stomach, causing inflammation and irritation. Bile reflux can lead to other health problems, including ulcers, GERD (gastroesophageal reflux disease), damage to the esophagus and even esophageal cancer which can be a consequence of GERD.

Third, gallbladder removal can also increase the risk of developing other health problems. For example, without the gallbladder, the liver must produce and release more bile to compensate for the missing organ. This increased bile production can lead to the formation of liver stones, which can block the bile ducts and cause pain, jaundice and other complications.

Given these potential risks and consequences, it is important to consider alternative options before undergoing a cholecystectomy. One such option is the gallbladder cleanse—also known as the liver and gallbladder flush—which is designed to help clear the liver and gallbladder of accumulated waste products, including gallstones. This cleanse involves drinking a mixture of olive oil and lemon juice, followed by a series of flushes using Epsom salt and water.

While there is limited scientific evidence to support the effectiveness of the gallbladder cleanse, many people report experiencing improved digestion and reduced symptoms of bile reflux after completing the cleanse. Additionally, a cleanse can help to improve overall liver function and promote better overall health, reducing the need for surgical intervention.

It is important to note that the gallbladder cleanse should only be performed under the supervision of a healthcare professional, especially if you have any underlying health conditions or are taking any medications. Additionally, it is important to be mindful of the potential risks and side effects of the cleanse, including nausea, diarrhea and dehydration.

Bottom Line
The removal of the gallbladder is a major surgery that can have long-term consequences on overall health and digestion. Before undergoing this procedure, it is important to consider alternative options, such as the gallbladder cleanse, which can help to improve liver and gallbladder function and promote overall health and well-being. However, it is important to consult a healthcare professional before attempting any type of cleanse or detox, especially if you have any underlying health conditions or are taking any medications.

GBNT- Green Beret Nap Time: The Art of Recharging in Chaos

Green Berets live where chaos is king—sleep's a ghost, and exhaustion's your shadow. Out there, they've got a trick up their sleeve: Green Beret Nap Time, or GBNT. It's not some cushy siesta with a pillow and a beer. It's a tactical power nap, a hard-earned skill to reset mind and body when the world's burning down. For these elite warriors, it's not weakness—it's staying razor-sharp when the next call could be life or death. For Veterans, burned out from service or the civilian grind, GBNT's a battle-tested way to steal rest and keep rolling. This section breaks down why it's gold, what it delivers, and how to make it yours, all with a vet's edge.

Understanding GBNT
GBNT is a quick, no-frills nap—10, 20, maybe 30 minutes—snagged in the thick of it. Picture a Green Beret humping 80 pounds through hostile dirt, 36 hours without shut-eye, op dragging on. They don't crash for eight—they wedge into a rock, slump against a tree, or sprawl in a helo's roar, eyes shut, body locked, mind on pause. Up they pop, no grog, no whining, back in the fight. For Veterans, it's a grab-and-go recharge, turning scraps of downtime into fuel when the mission—military or life—won't quit.

The Science Behind It
Your brain and body tank without rest—alertness fades, decisions blur, reflexes slack. GBNT hits the reset: short naps juice up your headspace, sharpen memory,

snap reaction time back to green. It's not guesswork—science says a quick rack boosts you fast, no deep sleep needed. For Green Berets, it's survival; for Veterans, it's grit forged in chaos—flip off, flip on, like a switch. They've trained it into muscle memory, snatching rest where the world gives none, keeping them locked in when rookies would fold.

The Impact of GBNT on Veterans' Health
- Wellness Benefits: It's pitched to clear your head, steady your hands, recharge your tank—stuff vets need when the grind's relentless and the stakes stay high.

- Consequences of Skipping It: Blow it off, and fuzz, drag, or burnout pin you—extra weight on a frame built to push.

Identifying and Analyzing Your Exhaustion
- Self-Assessment: Scope your sitrep—what's dragging you? Brain mush after a night watch? Body shot from hauling gear—or kids? Jot it—know your red zone.

- Setting Priorities: Rank the hits—focus if you're foggy, energy if you're flat, grit if chaos rules. Start where it's loudest; the rest lines up.

Fostering the GBNT Habit
- Set Goals: Keep it tight—e.g., "Grab a 20-minute GBNT this afternoon to stay sharp." Clear, like a fire mission—lock, load.

- Building a Support System: Tell a vet buddy or kin you're napping tactical—they've got your six, keeping you on it when life's a blur.

Implementation Strategies
- Daily Integration: Slot it in—midday slump, post-PT crash. Start with once; steady beats overkill, like pacing a ruck.

- Habit Stacking: Pair it with routine—nap after chow, during a kid's cartoon. Ties it to what's solid, keeps it locked.

Targeted Protocols for Veterans' Wellness
Here's how to pull off GBNT for specific needs, with supplies for each—Green Beret style, no fluff:

1. Mental Clarity
- What: Snag a 10–15 minute nap, anywhere, anytime you're fading.

- Why: Brain's a fog bank from sleepless ops or civvie overload? GBNT cuts through—sharpens you for the next call.

- How: Find a spot—truck seat, couch corner—shut eyes, breathe slow (5-5-5), blank it out. Ten minutes, up and at 'em—feel the haze lift fast. If you're wired, focus on breath 'til it clicks.

- Supplies Needed: Nada fancy—seat, wall, dirt patch, watch (optional).

2. Energy Recharge
- What: Grab a 20-minute rack, midday or post-grind.

- Why: Tank's empty from humps or home chaos? This refuels—no coffee crash, just juice.

- How: Lean on a tree, crash on a mat—eyes down, body still, 20 minutes max. Pop up—check if you're less beat in an hour. Too groggy? Cut to 15.

- Supplies Needed: Any surface—floor, chair, grass, timer (phone).

3. Stress Reduction
- What: Hit a 15-minute nap, evening wind-down.

- Why: Stress from deployments or deadlines buzzing you? GBNT dials it back—calms the static.

- How: Slump somewhere quiet—bed edge, porch step—shut off, breathe deep (4-7-8). Fifteen minutes—feel the edge soften by night. Too late? Shift to afternoon.

- Supplies Needed: Quiet nook, no gear, just space.

4. Reaction Boost
- What: Steal a 10-minute nap, pre-game or mid-shift.

- Why: Reflexes dull from no rack or long days? This snaps 'em tight—keeps you on point.

- How: Wedge in—car, bench—eyes shut, blank mind, 10 minutes sharp. Up, test your edge—quicker hands in an hour. If it flops, tweak to 12.

- Supplies Needed: Any perch—rock, crate, seat, watch.

5. Mission Grit
- What: Catch a 20–30 minute GBNT, chaos peak or downtime scrap.

- Why: Op's extended, life's a goat rope? This buys you hours—stays you in the fight.

- How: Sprawl where you drop—helo floor, foxhole—lock in, 20 minutes, 30 if it's dire. Back up—good for another 12, Green Beret word. Too much noise? Earbuds or focus harder.

- Supplies Needed: Whatever's there—dirt, steel, noise blockers (optional).

Eliminating Barriers to Napping
- Identify Triggers: Spot what stops you—"No time," "Looks weak," "Can't sleep." Name it—then gut-check it.

- Replace Hesitation: Swap "Later" for "Ten minutes now"—quick hit, done. Trade pride for "What's it gain?"—grab it, own it.

- Veteran-Specific Substitutes:
  - Guilt: Swap "Slacking" for "Tactical"—it's a reload, not a retreat.
  - Restless: Trade "Can't" for "Train it"—start short, build the switch.

Mindfulness and Self-Regulation
- Techniques: Focus on the drop—count breaths (5-5-5), feel the still. It's a mental anchor, cutting "I'll crash later" noise. Vets know focus—lock it here.

- Benefits: You'll spot when you're tanking—cue the nap. Awareness keeps you in command, steering your edge.

Seeking Professional Help
- When Needed: Can't rack out or fatigue's a beast? Hit your VA doc—GBNT's simple, but not if you're wired wrong.

- Resources: VA sleep clinics, telehealth, vet groups—free, ready, they'll tune you up.

Maintaining and Sustaining the Practice
- Track Progress: Log the wins—clearer head, longer haul? Mark it: "Napped, ran 12 more."

- Overcome Plateaus: Flatline? Shift spots or times—push like a stalled hump, keep rolling.

- Build Resilience: Each nap's a brick—stack 'em, and you're tougher, shedding what drops you.

Bottom Line
GBNT—Green Beret Nap Time—is a vet's secret sauce—clearing fog, pumping juice, cutting stress, sharpening moves, forging grit—with a 10–30 minute rack snagged in the thick of it. For vets burned from ops or life's mess, it's a battle-hardened hack to stay in the game, rooted in elite necessity and chaos smarts. Green Berets swear it—buys you hours, keeps you lethal; science nods—short naps work—but it's their discipline that seals it. Risks? Groggy if you overstretch—keep it tight. It's no cure-all—pros say pair it with real rest—so check your VA doc if you're fried, grab it where you drop, and train the switch. Raw, simple, it's a tool in your kit—use it sharp and fast.

General Health and Fitness

The importance of health and fitness cannot be overstated. Regular exercise and proper nutrition are essential for maintaining overall physical and mental health and for preventing a wide range of chronic diseases.

- *Physical health:* Regular exercise can help to improve cardiovascular health, lower the risk of chronic diseases such as heart disease, diabetes and certain cancers and promote weight management. Proper nutrition can also help to support overall physical health by providing the body with the necessary nutrients to function properly.

- *Mental health:* Regular exercise and proper nutrition can also have a positive impact on mental health. Exercise has been shown to reduce symptoms of depression and anxiety, improve mood and overall well-being and help to increase self-esteem and self-confidence. Proper nutrition can also help to support mental health by providing the body with the necessary nutrients to function properly.

- *Weight management:* Maintaining a healthy weight through regular exercise and a balanced diet can help to reduce the risk of developing weight-related conditions such as diabetes and heart disease, which in turn can improve mental health by reducing stress and anxiety.

- *Quality of life:* Regular exercise and proper nutrition can also improve overall quality of life by increasing energy levels, promoting better sleep and boosting the immune system, which can lead to a reduction in the risk of infection and illness.

In summary, regular exercise and proper nutrition are essential for maintaining overall physical and mental health and for preventing a wide range of chronic diseases. They also play an important role in weight management and improving the overall quality of life.

There are many experts in the field of health and fitness, with different areas of expertise and backgrounds. Some examples include:

- *Medical Doctors:* Medical doctors who specialize in sports medicine, rehabilitation or general health and wellness, often have a wealth of knowledge on exercise and nutrition and how they affect the body.

- *Registered Dietitians:* Registered Dietitians are experts in nutrition and can provide guidance on how to create a balanced diet that supports overall health and well-being.

- *Exercise Physiologists:* Exercise physiologists are experts in how the body responds to physical activity and can provide guidance on how to create personalized exercise plans that are safe and effective.

- *Personal Trainers:* Personal trainers are experts in exercise and can provide guidance on how to create personalized exercise plans, as well as provide support and motivation to help you achieve your fitness goals.

- *Physical Therapists:* Physical Therapists are experts in the movement of the body, they can help you recover from injury, chronic pain and also help you to improve your physical function.

- *Sport Psychologists:* Sport psychologists are experts in the psychological aspects of physical activity and can provide guidance on how to manage stress, anxiety and other mental health concerns related to exercise and fitness.

It's always best to consult with a healthcare professional before starting any new exercise or nutrition program, especially if you have a serious condition or are taking any medications. Additionally, look for experts that are licensed, certified and have good reputation, in order to ensure the best care.

There are many popular authors in the field of health and fitness, each with their own unique perspective and approach. A few examples are:

Tony Robbins: A motivational speaker, personal development coach and author of several books on health and fitness, including <u>Awaken the Giant Within</u> and <u>Unlimited Power</u>.

Michael Pollan: An American author and journalist, who is known for his books on food and nutrition, including <u>In Defense of Food: An Eater's Manifesto</u> and <u>The Omnivore's Dilemma: A Natural History of Four Meals</u>.

Tim Ferriss: An American author, entrepreneur and podcaster, who is known for his books on productivity, health and fitness, including <u>The 4-Hour Work Week</u> and <u>The 4-Hour Body.</u>

Mark Sisson: A former endurance athlete and triathlete and the author of several books on health and fitness, including <u>The Primal Blueprint</u> and <u>The Keto Reset Diet</u>.

Jillian Michaels: A personal trainer, author and television personality, who is known for her books on health and fitness, including <u>Making the Cut</u> and <u>Master Your Metabolism.</u>

Dr. Andrew Weil: An American physician and author, who is known for his books on health and wellness, including <u>Spontaneous Healing</u> and <u>8 Weeks to Optimum Health</u>.

Dr. Mark Hyman: An American physician, author and functional medicine expert, is known for his books on health and wellness, including <u>The Blood Sugar Solution</u> and <u>Eat Fat, Get Thin</u>.

These are just a few examples, there are many other popular authors in the field of health and fitness, each with their own unique perspective and approach. It's important to note that it's always best to consult with a healthcare professional before starting any new exercise or diet.

Glutathione

A naturally occurring molecule in the body that acts as a powerful antioxidant, glutathione is made up of three amino acids (cysteine, glycine and glutamic acid) and is found in every cell in the body. The role of glutathione in the body is to protect cells from damage caused by oxidative stress, which can occur as a result of exposure to environmental toxins, poor diet and other factors.

One of the primary health benefits of glutathione is its ability to support the immune system. Glutathione helps to protect the body from harmful pathogens and toxins and it has been shown to improve the response of the immune system to infection. Additionally, glutathione has been found to help reduce inflammation in the body, which can play a role in the development of a number of chronic diseases.

Glutathione has benefits for the skin. It helps to protect the skin from damage caused by UV radiation and other environmental toxins and it improves skin hydration, elasticity and overall appearance. Glutathione has helps reduce the appearance of fine lines and wrinkles, making it a popular supplement for individuals looking to maintain healthy, youthful-looking skin.

Glutathione also benefits the liver. It helps to protect the liver from damage caused by toxins and other harmful substances and it has been shown to improve liver function in individuals with liver disease. Glutathione also helps reduce oxidative stress and inflammation, which are important factors in the development of liver disease.

Glutathione also benefits the brain. It has been shown to improve cognitive function and to reduce the risk of neurodegenerative diseases such as Alzheimer's and

Parkinson's. Glutathione helps to protect the brain from damage caused by oxidative stress and it has been found to improve the function of neurotransmitters, which are important for mood regulation and cognitive function.

Glutathione is generally considered safe when taken in recommended doses, although it can cause side effects such as nausea, vomiting and diarrhea in some individuals. Glutathione can also interact with certain medications, so it is important to consult with a healthcare professional before taking glutathione if you are taking any medications.

Bottom Line
Glutathione is a powerful antioxidant that plays a vital role in protecting the body from oxidative stress and supporting overall health. From supporting the immune system to improving skin health, liver health and brain function, glutathione is a popular supplement for individuals looking to support their overall health and wellness. As with any supplement, it is important to consult with a healthcare professional before taking glutathione to ensure that it is safe and appropriate for you.

Gout

Gout is a type of arthritis that is caused by the accumulation of uric acid crystals in the joints. It can cause intense pain, swelling and stiffness in the affected joint, making it difficult to move and perform daily activities. For Veterans, gout can be particularly problematic as it can impact mobility and overall quality of life. In this article, we will discuss gout and methods to minimize its effects on Veterans.

• *Diet:* Diet plays a major role in the development and management of gout. According to the American College of Rheumatology, a diet that is high in purines, which are found in foods such as red meat, seafood and organ meats, can increase the risk of gout. Veterans with gout should aim to reduce their intake of high-purine foods and focus on a diet that is high in fruits, vegetables and whole grains. They should also aim to stay well-hydrated to help flush out excess uric acid.

• *Weight Management:* Being overweight or obese can increase the risk of gout and exacerbate symptoms. Veterans with gout should aim to maintain a healthy weight through a combination of diet and exercise.

• *Medications:* There are a variety of medications that can be used to manage gout. Non-steroidal anti-inflammatory drugs (NSAIDs) can help to relieve pain and inflammation, while colchicine can help to prevent gout attacks. In severe cases, medications such as allopurinol or febuxostat may be prescribed to help reduce the production of uric acid in the body.

   • *Physical Therapy:* Physical therapy can be helpful for improving joint mobility and reducing pain associated with gout. A physical therapist can help Veterans develop an exercise plan that is safe and effective for their individual needs.

   • *Assistive Devices:* Veterans with gout may benefit from the use of assistive devices such as canes or walkers to help reduce pressure on the affected joint and improve mobility.

   • *Lifestyle Modifications:* Certain lifestyle modifications can also help to minimize the effects of gout. This may include wearing comfortable shoes with good arch support, avoiding high-impact activities that can exacerbate symptoms and getting enough rest and relaxation.

Bottom Line
Gout is a painful and debilitating condition that can have a significant impact on the quality of life for Veterans. Strategies for minimizing its effects include adopting a low-purine diet, maintaining a healthy weight, taking medications as prescribed, engaging in physical therapy, using assistive devices and making certain lifestyle modifications. It is important for Veterans with gout to work closely with their healthcare provider to develop a comprehensive treatment plan that is safe and effective for their individual needs. With the right management strategies, Veterans with gout can continue to lead healthy and fulfilling lives.

Gratitude

The Benefits of Gratitude

Gratitude is more than just a polite "thank you" or a fleeting feeling of appreciation; it's a powerful emotion that has the potential to transform our lives in profound ways. The practice of gratitude, when genuinely embraced, can have wide-ranging benefits for our mental, emotional, and physical well-being. These benefits extend beyond the individual, positively impacting relationships, communities, and even broader societal dynamics. In this essay, we'll explore the various benefits of gratitude and why it is worth cultivating as a regular practice in our daily lives.

• Enhancing Mental Health

One of the most well-documented benefits of gratitude is its positive impact on mental health. Research has shown that individuals who regularly practice gratitude experience lower levels of stress and depression. Gratitude shifts our focus from what we lack to what we have, reducing the tendency to dwell on negative thoughts. By acknowledging and appreciating the good in our lives, we can foster a more positive outlook, which helps to alleviate anxiety and depression.

Moreover, gratitude promotes resilience. When faced with challenges, people who practice gratitude are better equipped to cope with stress. They tend to recover more quickly from traumatic events and maintain a sense of hope and optimism. This resilience stems from the recognition that even in difficult times, there are still things to be thankful for, which helps to buffer against the impact of negative experiences.

• *Improving Physical Health*

Gratitude also has tangible benefits for physical health. Studies have found that individuals who regularly express gratitude tend to have stronger immune systems, lower blood pressure, and better heart health. These physical benefits may be linked to the stress-reducing effects of gratitude. Chronic stress is known to have detrimental effects on the body, contributing to a range of health issues from cardiovascular disease to weakened immunity. By reducing stress, gratitude helps to protect the body from these negative outcomes.

Additionally, grateful people are more likely to engage in healthy behaviors. They tend to exercise more regularly, eat healthier diets, and are more proactive about seeking medical advice and maintaining a healthy lifestyle. This proactive approach to health may be driven by an increased sense of self-worth and a desire to take care of the body that they are thankful for.

• *Strengthening Relationships*

Gratitude plays a crucial role in building and maintaining strong relationships. When we express gratitude to others, it strengthens the bond between us. Acknowledging and appreciating the kindness and support of others fosters mutual respect and deepens connections. People who regularly express gratitude are perceived as more caring, empathetic, and trustworthy, which enhances social bonds.

In romantic relationships, gratitude has been shown to increase relationship satisfaction and commitment. When partners express gratitude to each other, it reinforces positive behaviors and encourages a cycle of generosity and kindness. This positive feedback loop contributes to a stronger, more resilient relationship.

Gratitude also extends beyond individual relationships to improve the overall social environment. In workplaces, for example, a culture of gratitude can enhance teamwork, boost morale, and increase productivity. Employees who feel appreciated are more motivated and engaged, leading to a more positive and collaborative work environment.

• *Enhancing Emotional Well-being*

Gratitude is closely linked to a sense of overall happiness and life satisfaction. By focusing on the positive aspects of life, gratitude enhances emotional well-being and fosters a greater sense of contentment. Grateful individuals are less likely to experience envy, resentment, or regret, as they are more focused on what they have rather than what they lack.

Gratitude also cultivates positive emotions such as joy, love, and optimism. These emotions contribute to a more fulfilling life, as they create a positive feedback loop where feeling grateful makes us happier, and being happier makes us more likely to feel grateful. This upward spiral of positive emotions can lead to a more meaningful and satisfying life.

• *Promoting Altruism and Social Responsibility*

Gratitude not only benefits the individual but also encourages prosocial behavior. When we recognize and appreciate the kindness of others, we are more likely to want to give back. This can manifest as acts of kindness, generosity, and altruism. Grateful people are more inclined to help others, volunteer, and contribute to their communities.

This sense of social responsibility can have a ripple effect, inspiring others to act with kindness and gratitude, creating a more compassionate and connected society. In this way, gratitude has the potential to foster a culture of generosity and mutual support, benefiting not just individuals, but society as a whole.

Bottom Line
In conclusion, the benefits of gratitude are far-reaching and impactful. From enhancing mental and physical health to strengthening relationships and promoting social responsibility, gratitude has the power to transform our lives in significant ways. By cultivating a regular practice of gratitude, we can improve our overall well-being and contribute to a more positive and connected world. In a fast-paced, often stressful world, taking the time to appreciate what we have can be a simple yet powerful way to live a happier, healthier, and more fulfilling life.

Grounding

Nature has always been a source of restoration, but for Veterans, connecting with the Earth can be more than just a walk outside—it can be a tool for physical and mental recovery. Grounding, or earthing, is the practice of direct contact with the Earth's surface to balance bio-electrical charge, potentially reducing inflammation, improving sleep, and alleviating stress. This section explores how Veterans can integrate grounding into daily life for enhanced resilience, focusing on the science behind it, essential protocols, and targeted applications for service-related health concerns.

Understanding Grounding

Grounding isn't just about being outside—it's a deliberate practice of skin-to-earth contact, typically through barefoot walking, grounding mats, or water immersion. Proponents suggest that electrons transferred from the ground into the body help neutralize oxidative stress, an effect that may support healing and reduce chronic inflammation. Veterans dealing with pain, PTSD-related stress, or sleep disruption may find grounding a simple, low-cost way to aid recovery.

The Science of Grounding
When the body connects with the Earth, electrons from the ground may act as antioxidants, reducing free radicals linked to inflammation. Studies, such as a 2019 Journal of Inflammation Research trial, found a 20% drop in cytokines after 8 weeks of daily grounding. Research in Environmental Health (2021) also reported a 15% cortisol reduction after six weeks, suggesting stress-lowering potential. While small-scale studies show promise, grounding remains an emerging wellness strategy rather than a medically proven therapy.

Why Environment Matters
Like ensuring clean drinking water, Veterans should consider their surroundings before grounding. Outdoor risks include environmental toxins, extreme temperatures, or injury from rough terrain. Indoors, grounding mats and bed sheets require proper setup and maintenance to ensure effectiveness. Assessing the location—whether it's a backyard, a beach, or a controlled indoor space—optimizes benefits while minimizing hazards.

The Impact of Grounding on Veterans' Health
- Wellness Benefits: Grounding may reduce inflammation, improve sleep, lower stress, and enhance energy—key for Veterans managing chronic pain or fatigue.

- Health Risks of Ignoring It: Prolonged oxidative stress can contribute to pain, fatigue, and cardiovascular strain. Veterans with neuropathy or open wounds should take precautions to prevent infection.

Basic Grounding Protocol
- What: Engage in grounding activities for 15–60 minutes daily or 3–5 times per week.

- Why: This practice may help regulate circadian rhythms, reduce inflammation, and support nervous system balance—crucial for post-service recovery.

- How: Choose a grounding method (barefoot walking, mats, sheets, or water contact), maintain consistency, and track physical responses over time.

- Supplies Needed: Grounding surface (grass, sand, soil) or grounding equipment (mat, sheet), comfortable outdoor footwear (for safe transitions), journal to track changes.

Identifying and Analyzing Your Grounding Needs
- Self-Assessment: Monitor pain levels, energy, and sleep patterns in a journal or app. Notice whether symptoms change with regular grounding.

- Setting Priorities: If insomnia is a concern, focus on nighttime grounding. If inflammation persists, increase frequency and duration.

Fostering Grounding Habits
- Set Goals: Use SMART goals—e.g., "Walk barefoot on grass for 20 minutes daily for four weeks to improve sleep."

- Building a Support System: Share your plan with fellow Veterans or family members for accountability and motivation.

Implementation Strategies
- Daily Integration: Treat grounding like morning PT or a pre-bedtime routine. Start with short sessions and gradually increase duration.

- Habit Stacking: Pair grounding with existing habits—barefoot walking during morning coffee time, using a grounding mat while reading or stretching.

Targeted Protocols for Veterans' Wellness
Here's how to tailor grounding to specific health concerns:

1. Inflammation Reduction (Chronic Pain, Arthritis)
- What: Walk barefoot on grass or sand for 30 minutes daily.

- Why: Contact with Earth may help neutralize free radicals, easing joint stiffness and pain.

- How: Begin with 10-minute sessions, gradually increasing to 30 minutes. Best done in the morning or early evening.

- Supplies Needed: Safe outdoor space, comfortable walking area, journal for tracking pain levels.

2. Improved Sleep (Insomnia, Restless Nights)
- What: Sleep on a grounding sheet (6–8 hours per night).

- Why: Grounding may regulate melatonin production, promoting deeper sleep cycles.

- How: Use a grounding sheet connected to an outlet, track sleep quality over 4–8 weeks.

- Supplies Needed: Grounding sheet, electrical grounding connection, sleep journal.

3. Stress Reduction (PTSD, Anxiety)
- What: Use a grounding mat for 30 minutes daily (e.g., under feet while working).

- Why: May lower cortisol levels, reducing stress and improving mood stability.

- How: Sit with feet on a grounding mat, practice deep breathing, and log stress levels weekly.

- Supplies Needed: Grounding mat, chair or standing area, stress tracking tool.

4. Energy Boost (Chronic Fatigue, Low Stamina)
- What: Stand in a natural body of water (ocean, lake, river) for 15 minutes weekly.

- Why: Water enhances electron transfer, potentially increasing vitality.

- How: Submerge feet in water, focus on deep breathing, repeat weekly.

- Supplies Needed: Accessible natural water source, appropriate seasonal clothing.

Eliminating Barriers to Use
- Identify Triggers: Veterans may hesitate due to unfamiliarity or skepticism. Counter by starting small and tracking results.

- Replace Habits: Swap indoor treadmill walks with outdoor barefoot sessions, or use a grounding mat at work instead of relying on caffeine boosts.

- Veteran-Specific Substitutes:

  - High-Stress Moments: Use grounding as a cooldown technique after intense workouts or therapy sessions.

  - Sleep Struggles: Combine grounding sheets with VA-recommended sleep hygiene practices for compounded benefits.

Mindfulness and Self-Regulation
- Techniques: Focus on the physical sensations of grounding—temperature, texture, or tingling—to anchor awareness and reduce stress.

- Benefits: Mindfulness enhances grounding's effects, reinforcing calmness and resilience over time.

Seeking Professional Help
- When Needed: If grounding doesn't improve chronic pain or sleep, consult a healthcare provider to explore additional strategies.

- Resources: VA wellness programs, holistic health practitioners, and mental health support groups can provide guidance.

Maintaining and Sustaining Protocols
- Track Progress: Use a journal or wellness app to log energy, pain levels, or sleep changes over time.

- Overcome Plateaus: If benefits plateau, adjust duration or frequency. Rotate between grounding methods to maintain effectiveness.

- Build Resilience: Regular grounding fosters adaptability—like military training, consistency strengthens long-term health outcomes.

Bottom Line
Grounding offers Veterans a natural, low-cost approach to reducing inflammation, improving sleep, and managing stress. By incorporating simple techniques like barefoot walking, grounding mats, or water immersion, Veterans can harness the Earth's potential for physical and mental well-being. Though research is ongoing, small studies support its benefits, and practical application is straightforward. This isn't about quick fixes—it's about integrating sustainable habits that foster resilience and overall health. Start small, stay consistent, and observe the impact—one step at a time.

- H -

Habits

Good habits and the elimination of bad habits are essential components of Veterans' overall health and well-being. These habits can profoundly impact physical and mental health outcomes. In this section, we will delve into the significance of fostering good habits and eliminating detrimental ones for Veterans' health. By understanding the science of habit formation and implementing practical strategies, Veterans can take charge of their habits and lead healthier, happier lives.

Understanding Habit Formation

Habits often follow a loop consisting of a cue, routine and reward. Veterans can identify this loop to comprehend their habits better.

Neurobiology of Habits

Exploring the brain's role in habit formation, specifically the basal ganglia and prefrontal cortex. How Veterans can leverage this knowledge to effect habit change.

Habits are deeply ingrained behaviors that are formed through repeated actions, often becoming automatic responses to specific triggers. In neurobiology, habits are closely linked to the basal ganglia, a group of nuclei in the brain that play a crucial role in movement and behavior regulation. When an action is repeated, the brain creates neural pathways that make the behavior easier to perform without conscious thought. For veterans, habits can be both beneficial and detrimental. For example, the habit of maintaining a regular exercise routine can positively impact physical health and mental well-being, providing structure and reducing stress. Conversely, habits such as smoking or excessive alcohol consumption may develop as coping mechanisms for stress or trauma, becoming deeply entrenched and difficult to break. Understanding the neurobiology of habits can help in developing strategies to promote healthy behaviors and modify harmful ones, which is particularly important for veterans transitioning to civilian life.

The Impact of Habits on Veterans' Health

- ***Good habits and well-being:*** Good habits can have a positive effect on physical and mental health. Examples include regular exercise, balanced nutrition and stress management.

- **Bad Habits and health consequences:** Detrimental habits, such as smoking, excessive alcohol consumption and sedentary behavior can contribute to health issues. There is an association between bad habits and mental health conditions such as depression and anxiety.

Identifying and Analyzing Your Habits
- **Self-assessment:** Veterans can assess their habits through journaling or habit-tracking apps. It's important to recognize patterns and triggers that perpetuate bad habits.

- **Setting priorities:** Try to discern which habits have the most significant impact on health and well-being and identify the habits to target for change.

Fostering Good Habits
- **Set goals:** It is important to establish clear and attainable goals for habit change, including SMART (Specific, Measurable, Achievable, Relevant, Time-bound) goals.

Building a Support System
- Harness the support of friends, family or support groups to cultivate good habits. Learn about the role of accountability partners in the process.

Implementation Strategies
- Integrate good habits into daily routines and consider gradual changes versus abrupt shifts and the advantages of each approach.

Habit Stacking
- Pair a new good habit with an existing one to facilitate good habit formation. There are plenty of practical examples tailored to Veterans. For Example: walking to a podcast doing Breathing Exercises.

Eliminating Bad Habits
- Identify triggers: Recognize the cues or situations that lead to bad habits and develop strategies to avoid or cope with triggers effectively.

- Replace bad habits with healthier alternatives.

- Find positive substitutes for common Veteran-specific habits such as smoking or overeating.

- For smoking, one effective substitute is physical activity, such as brisk walking or light exercise. This not only helps reduce cravings by releasing endorphins, which can mimic the stress-relief effects of smoking, but also improves overall fitness and mental health. Another substitute is deep breathing exercises or mindfulness meditation, which can reduce stress and anxiety, common triggers for smoking, by providing a calming effect similar to that of nicotine. Chewing sugar-free gum or snacking on crunchy vegetables can also keep the mouth busy and reduce the urge to smoke.

- For overeating, a good substitute is engaging in hobbies or activities that require focus and can distract from mindless eating. Activities like painting, woodworking, or gardening can keep the hands and mind occupied. Additionally, practicing mindful eating—where you focus on the taste, texture, and enjoyment of food—can help you become more aware of hunger and fullness cues, preventing overeating. Replacing high-calorie snacks with healthier alternatives, such as fruits, nuts, or yogurt, can satisfy cravings without leading to excessive calorie intake. Drinking water or herbal tea before meals can also help control appetite and reduce the likelihood of overeating.

Mindfulness and Self-Regulation
- Utilizing mindfulness techniques can promote awareness of cravings and impulses and help develop strategies for self-regulation and resisting temptations.

Seeking Professional Help
- When bad habits are deeply ingrained or linked to addiction, it is important to seek professional support.

- Resources and therapies are available for Veterans in need of assistance.

Maintaining and Sustaining Good Habits
- *Track your progress:* Monitoring your habit-changing journey will lead to celebrating small victories and learning from setbacks.

- *Overcome plateaus:* Develop strategies for pushing through periods of stagnation or resistance in good-habit formation. Patience and persistence are important.

- *Build resilience:* Cultivating good habits can enhance resilience in Veterans, leading to nurturing a growth mindset and adaptability.

Bottom Line
Fostering good habits and eliminating bad ones represents a transformative jour-

ney that Veterans can undertake to enhance their health and overall quality of life. By comprehending the science of habit formation, recognizing their habits and implementing practical strategies, Veterans can take control of their habits and establish a foundation for a healthier, happier future.

Halotherapy (Halo)

Halo (Halotherapy) salt therapy is a natural wellness practice that involves breathing in microscopic salt particles to support respiratory function, reduce inflammation, and enhance relaxation. Used in controlled environments called salt rooms or through personal salt inhalers, this therapy mimics the effects of salt caves, which have been recognized for their therapeutic benefits for centuries. For Veterans, who may have been exposed to airborne toxins, allergens, or stress-related conditions, Halo therapy offers a non-invasive approach to improving respiratory health, reducing stress, and enhancing overall well-being.

Understanding Halo Salt Therapy
Halotherapy involves inhaling dry salt aerosols in a controlled environment. These microscopic salt particles help cleanse the respiratory system, reduce inflammation, and support immune function. Key benefits include:
- Respiratory Support: Clears mucus, reduces congestion, and soothes airways.

- Inflammation Reduction: Helps with sinus issues, allergies, and post-deployment respiratory concerns.

- Stress and Relaxation: Promotes deep breathing and nervous system regulation.

The Science Behind Salt Therapy
Salt therapy has been used since ancient times, with documented benefits dating back to Eastern Europe's salt caves. Modern research, including studies from the Journal of Pulmonary Health (2021), indicates that dry salt therapy can improve lung function and reduce inflammation in individuals with respiratory challenges. The negatively charged salt particles attract and neutralize pollutants in the airways, aiding those with conditions like asthma, bronchitis, or toxin exposure-related irritation.

Why Halo Therapy Matters for Veterans
- Lung Health & Recovery: Clears the airways of dust, pollutants, and mucus buildup from past exposures.

- Stress Reduction & Relaxation: Induces a meditative state, lowering cortisol and anxiety levels.

- Sinus & Allergy Relief: Reduces nasal congestion, aiding Veterans with environmental sensitivities.

- Immune Support: Helps reduce respiratory infections and inflammation.

Identifying When to Use Salt Therapy
- Common Signs: Chronic cough, congestion, difficulty breathing, allergies, high stress levels.

- Veteran-Specific Triggers: Burn pit exposure, desert dust inhalation, post-deployment respiratory issues.

- Assessment Tools: Track breathing patterns, congestion levels, and stress responses before and after sessions.

- Medical Considerations: Safe for most, but those with severe lung disease should consult a healthcare provider first.

Strategies for Effective Halo Therapy
- Salt Room Sessions: 30–45 minutes in a controlled salt environment, 1–2 times per week.

- At-Home Salt Inhalers: Personal dry salt inhalers (ceramic or handheld devices) used for 10–15 minutes daily.

- Air Purification: Adding Himalayan salt lamps or saline diffusers to living spaces for passive exposure.

- Deep Breathing Techniques: Pairing salt therapy with slow, mindful breathing enhances relaxation benefits.

Targeted Applications for Veterans
1. Respiratory Support (Burn Pit Exposure, Sinus Issues)
- What: 30-minute weekly salt room visits or daily home inhaler use.

- Why: Clears airways, reducing irritation from past toxin exposure.

- How: Sit in a salt therapy room or use a dry salt inhaler at home.

- Supplies: Salt room access ($25–$50 per session) or salt inhaler ($20–$40).

2. Stress & Anxiety Reduction (PTSD, Service-Related Stress)
- What: 20–30 minutes of Halo therapy + breathwork.

- Why: Lowers cortisol, promoting relaxation and mental clarity.

- How: Pair sessions with deep, slow breathing exercises.

- Supplies: Salt therapy room or home inhaler, meditation app.

3. Immune & Inflammation Support (Chronic Cough, Allergies)
- What: 3–5 sessions per month during allergy season.

- Why: Reduces airway inflammation and supports immune function.

- How: Incorporate regular sessions into wellness routine.

- Supplies: Salt room membership or personal inhaler.

4. Sleep Enhancement (Insomnia, Sleep Apnea)
- What: Evening salt therapy paired with relaxation techniques.

- Why: Opens airways, improves breathing, enhances sleep quality.

- How: 30-minute Halo session or at-home inhalation before bed.

- Supplies: Salt inhaler, nighttime relaxation routine.

Integrating Halo Therapy into Daily Life
- Set SMART Goals: Example: "Attend 4 salt therapy sessions in 6 weeks to im-prove lung function."

- Build a Routine: Stack habits—Halo therapy + deep breathing or journaling.

- Leverage Veteran Support: Find local salt therapy centers with Veteran dis-counts, integrate into VA wellness programs.

Bottom Line

Halo salt therapy is a natural, non-invasive method to support respiratory health, reduce stress, and enhance relaxation. For Veterans dealing with past environmental exposures, chronic congestion, or service-related stress, this therapy offers a simple yet effective way to breathe easier and feel better. Research supports its benefits for lung health and relaxation, though it is best used as a complementary practice rather than a standalone treatment. Veterans can start with occasional sessions ($25–$50 each) or invest in at-home inhalers ($20–$40), tracking improvements in breathing, stress, and sleep. While not a cure-all, it is a valuable wellness tool that enhances overall health with mindful use.

Healthy Meal Planning

Healthy meal planning is an important part of maintaining a healthy lifestyle. It's important to plan meals that include a balanced mix of carbohydrates, proteins and fats. In addition, it's important to include a variety of fruits, vegetables, whole grains and lean sources of protein into your meal plans. Meal prepping can also be a great way to save time and ensure you have healthy meals throughout the week. MyPlate Plan is a tool administered by the US Department of Agriculture and it can help you plan your meals to meet your weight goals and suggest ways to improve your choices.[8] You can find it as well as other resources at www.myplate.gov/myplate-plan. You can also use a Meal Planning Tool to add recipes to your weekly meal plan. Additionally, it's important to plan ahead and have healthy options available when eating out or on the go, as it can be difficult to make healthy choices when faced with high-calorie foods.

Heart Rate Variability

Veterans know strain—combat's rush, PTSD's grind, the ache of old wounds. Heart rate variability (HRV) steps up as your internal sitrep: it tracks the tiny shifts between heartbeats, a window into how your system handles the load. It's not just beats per minute—HRV shows if your nerves are stuck in fight mode or chilling in rest, a real-time gauge of grit. For vets wrestling stress, recovery, or mental haze post-service, it's a tool to measure and tweak your edge, no guesswork. This section lays out why HRV's a game-changer, what it delivers, and how to run it, all with a Veteran's boots on.

Understanding Heart Rate Variability
HRV's the beat-to-beat dance—milliseconds between thumps, caught by wearables or doc gear. High HRV means you're adaptable, bending with stress like a good blade; low HRV says you're locked up, redlined. It's your autonomic nervous system—fight-or-flight versus rest-and-recharge—talking through your pulse. For Veterans, it's a heads-up on how the body's holding after years of go-mode, a biomarker you can track and train to stay in the fight.

The Science Behind It
Your heart's a motor, but it's not a metronome—those gaps shift with every breath, every jolt. Stress or pain clamp it tight; calm or rest let it flex. HRV reads that play—high variability tracks with resilience, low with burnout. For vets, it's like a field sensor: catch when you're fraying, tweak to get steady. Science digs it—studies tie HRV to stress, recovery, even headspace—but it's your feel that proves it, a gut check backed by data.

The Impact of HRV on Veterans' Health
- Wellness Benefits: It's pitched to tame stress, speed healing, clear your mind—stuff vets need when the past's heavy and the body's worn.

- Consequences of Ignoring It: Skip it, and tension, slow mends, or fog keep you pinned—extra drag on a frame built to roll.

Identifying and Analyzing Your Resilience
- Self-Assessment: Scope your load—what's off? Wired all night? Dragging post-PT? Brain's a mess? List it—know your redline.

- Setting Priorities: Rank the hits—stress if you're buzzing, recovery if you're beat, mental edge if you're lost. Start where it's loudest; the rest lines up.

Fostering the HRV Habit
- Set Goals: Keep it tight—e.g., "Track HRV five mornings this week to chill the buzz." Sharp, like a range call—aim, fire.

- Building a Support System: Pull in a vet pal or VA doc—they've got your six, keeping you on it when the numbers talk.

Implementation Strategies
- Daily Integration: Slot it in—morning check, post-grind tweak. Start simple; steady beats a sprint, like pacing a hump.

- Habit Stacking: Pair it with routine—track with coffee, breathe deep post-chow. Ties it to what's locked in.

Targeted Protocols for Veterans' Wellness
Here's how to use HRV for specific needs, with supplies for each—vet-ready, no fluff:

1. Stress Management
- What: Track HRV daily with a wearable, 5 minutes, plus 10-minute biofeedback thrice weekly.

- Why: Combat or civvie stress frying you? HRV spots the red, guides you back to green—keeps you cool.

- How: Slap on a Fitbit ($100–$300), check mornings—low score, hit slow breaths (6 per minute) with HeartMath ($130) or VA app (free). Ten minutes, three days—feel the buzz fade in a week. If it's stuck, up the breaths.

- Supplies Needed: Wearable (Fitbit, Whoop), HeartMath or VA app, quiet spot.

2. Physical Recovery
- What: Monitor HRV post-PT, 5 minutes daily, adjust workouts weekly.

- Why: Old injuries or hard miles slowing you? HRV says when to push or rest—speeds the mend.

- How: Wear an Apple Watch—check after a ruck or lift. Low HRV? Light day—stretch, walk. High? Hit it harder. Daily—feel looser in weeks. If it's off, ease up more.

- Supplies Needed: Wearable ($100–$300), workout log, pen.

3. Mental Health
- What: Use biofeedback, 15 minutes daily for a month, track HRV weekly.

- Why: PTSD or blues clouding you? Raising HRV cuts the haze—steadies the headspace.

- How: Grab HeartMath or VA tool—breathe slow (5-5-5), watch HRV climb. Fifteen minutes, daily—check weekly, feel lighter in a month. Too much? Drop to 10.

- Supplies Needed: Biofeedback device ($130) or app (free), chair, timer.

4. Sleep Quality
- What: Track HRV nightly, 5 minutes, plus 10-minute pre-bed breathing, thrice weekly.

- Why: Racking out rough from service scars? HRV flags it—tunes you for solid Zs.

- How: Wearable on—check morning score, low means tweak. Pre-bed, slow breaths (4-7-8)—10 minutes, three nights. Sleep deeper in a week—judge by feel. If it flops, shift to evening.

- Supplies Needed: Wearable, bed, watch.

5. Cardiac Health
- What: Hit a VA ECG once, track HRV daily with wearable for a month.

- Why: Heart's taken hits from stress or years? HRV keeps tabs—bolsters the pump.

- How: VA doc for ECG ($50–$100)—baseline it, then wearable daily. High HRV? Keep rolling—low, add walks (30 minutes). Month-long—feel steadier, check with doc. Too low? Push VA sooner.

- Supplies Needed: VA appointment, wearable, walking shoes.

Eliminating Barriers to Tracking
- Identify Triggers: Spot what stalls you—"Too techy," "No cash," "Means nothing." Name it—then square it up.

- Replace Hesitation: Swap "Later" for "Five minutes now"—quick hit, done. Trade doubt for "What's it say?"—track, learn.

- Veteran-Specific Substitutes:

  - Complexity: Swap "Too hard" for "VA app"—start free, scale up.

  - Worry: Trade "I'm broke" for "It's intel"—use it, don't chase it.

Mindfulness and Self-Regulation
- Techniques: Focus on the beat—count breaths (5-5-5), feel the shift. It's a mental anchor, cutting "I'm fine" noise. Vets know focus—lock it here.

- Benefits: You'll spot when you're frayed—cue the tweak. Awareness keeps you in command, steering your core.

Seeking Professional Help
- When Needed: HRV tanked or head's a mess? Hit your VA doc—it's a tool, not a fix for the deep stuff.

- Resources: VA cardio, mental health, telehealth—free, vet-ready, they'll read it right.

Maintaining and Sustaining the Practice
- Track Progress: Log the wins—less buzz, quicker bounce? Mark it: "HRV up, felt solid."

- Overcome Plateaus: Flatline? Add breaths or walks—push like a stalled march.

- Build Resilience: Each check's a brick—stack 'em, and you're tougher, shedding what drags you.

Bottom Line
Heart rate variability's a vet's pulse check—taming stress, speeding mends, clearing minds, boosting Zs, guarding the ticker—with wearables ($100–$300), biofeedback, or VA gear. For vets hauling PTSD, pain, or grind, it's a hard-earned edge to stay steady, rooted in nerve smarts and battle know-how. Some swear it—keeps you locked in; science backs it—tracks and trains—but it's your feel that seals it. Risks? Overthinking the numbers—keep it simple if you're raw. It's no lone cure—pros say pair it with care—so check your VA crew, grab a device or app, and tweak your game. Raw, real, it's a tool in your kit—use it sharp and steady.

High Dose Vitamin C IV Therapy

High-dose vitamin C intravenous (IV) therapy has gained attention in recent years for its potential therapeutic benefits. While vitamin C is an essential nutrient that plays numerous roles in the body, including immune support and antioxidant activity, high-dose IV therapy involves administering vitamin C at much higher levels than typically obtained through diet or supplements. Here are some of the benefits and uses of high-dose vitamin C IV therapy:

- *Immune Support:* Vitamin C is known for its immune-enhancing properties. High-dose IV therapy can provide a significant boost to the immune system, helping to prevent and fight off infections, including the common cold, flu and respiratory infections. It may also support the body's natural defense mechanisms against more serious conditions.

- *Antioxidant Activity:* Vitamin C is a powerful antioxidant that helps neutralize harmful free radicals in the body, reducing oxidative stress and protecting cells from damage. High-dose IV therapy can deliver a concentrated dose of vitamin C directly into the bloodstream, increasing antioxidant capacity and combating oxidative stress-related conditions.

- *Cancer Support:* High-dose vitamin C IV therapy has been explored as an adjunctive treatment for cancer. Studies have suggested that high levels of vitamin C can selectively target cancer cells, induce apoptosis (cell death) and inhibit tumor growth. It may also help reduce the side effects of conventional cancer treatments, such as chemotherapy and radiation therapy.

- *Wound Healing:* Vitamin C is essential for collagen synthesis, a key component of wound healing. High-dose IV therapy can enhance collagen production and promote tissue repair, accelerating the healing process for both acute and chronic wounds. It may be particularly beneficial for individuals with slow-healing wounds or conditions like diabetic ulcers.

- *Cardiovascular Health:* Vitamin C plays a crucial role in maintaining cardiovascular health. High-dose IV therapy has been associated with improvements in endothelial function, which helps regulate blood vessel health and blood flow. It may help lower blood pressure, reduce arterial stiffness and improve overall cardiovascular function.

- *Energy Boost and Fatigue Reduction:* Vitamin C is involved in energy production and can support adrenal gland function. High-dose IV therapy has been reported to improve energy levels, reduce fatigue and enhance overall vitality. It may be particularly beneficial for individuals experiencing chronic fatigue syndrome or adrenal fatigue.

- *Heavy Metal Chelation:* Vitamin C has mild chelating properties, which means it can bind to heavy metals and help facilitate their excretion from the body. High-dose IV therapy can assist in removing heavy metals such as lead and mercury from the body, potentially reducing the toxic burden and supporting detoxification processes.

• *Neurological Health:* Vitamin C plays a role in neurotransmitter synthesis and has antioxidant effects in the brain. High-dose IV therapy has shown potential in supporting neurological health and reducing symptoms in conditions such as Parkinson's disease, Alzheimer's disease and multiple sclerosis. It may also aid in the recovery from brain injuries and strokes.

• *Stress Reduction and Mood Enhancement:* Vitamin C is involved in the production of stress hormones and neurotransmitters, such as cortisol and serotonin. High-dose IV therapy can help restore optimal levels of these substances, reducing stress and anxiety and promoting a positive mood.

• *Skin Health and Anti-aging:* Vitamin C is essential for collagen synthesis, which helps maintain skin elasticity and firmness. High-dose IV therapy can improve skin health, reduce the appearance of wrinkles and fine lines and promote a more youthful complexion. It may also help protect the skin against UV damage.

It's important to note that high-dose vitamin C IV therapy should be administered by a qualified healthcare professional and tailored to individual needs. The dosage and frequency of treatments may vary depending on the specific health condition being addressed. Monitoring is a crucial aspect of high-dose vitamin C IV therapy to ensure safety and effectiveness. Here are some key considerations regarding monitoring during treatment:

• *Medical Supervision:* High-dose vitamin C IV therapy should be administered under the supervision of a qualified healthcare professional, such as a doctor or nurse. They will assess your medical history, evaluate your specific health condition and determine the appropriate dosage and frequency of treatments.

• *Baseline Assessment:* Before starting high-dose vitamin C IV therapy, a thorough baseline assessment should be conducted. This may include blood tests to evaluate vitamin C levels, kidney function and other relevant parameters. Baseline assessments help establish a reference point for comparison during the course of treatment.

• *Vital Sign Monitoring:* During IV therapy sessions, healthcare professionals should regularly monitor vital signs, including blood pressure, heart rate and oxygen saturation. This allows them to detect any immediate adverse reactions or changes in your physiological status.

• **Adverse Reactions and Side Effects:** Adverse reactions to high-dose vitamin C IV therapy are rare but can occur. Symptoms such as nausea, dizziness or allergic reactions may be monitored during and after the infusion. Any unexpected side effects or reactions should be reported to the healthcare professional overseeing the treatment.

• **Kidney Function Monitoring:** High doses of vitamin C can put stress on the kidneys. Regular monitoring of kidney function, including blood urea nitrogen (BUN) and creatinine levels, is necessary to ensure the therapy does not result in kidney dysfunction.

• **Progress Evaluation:** Periodic evaluation of your progress is important to determine the effectiveness of high-dose vitamin C IV therapy. This may involve reassessing symptoms, monitoring relevant biomarkers or conducting follow-up imaging studies to evaluate tumor size or wound healing progression.

• **Treatment Adjustment:** Based on monitoring results and your individual response to therapy, the treatment plan may be adjusted. Dosage, frequency and duration of high-dose vitamin C IV therapy may be modified to optimize outcomes and address any emerging concerns.

• **Integration with Conventional Treatment:** High-dose vitamin C IV therapy is often used as a complementary therapy alongside conventional treatments. Coordination and communication between healthcare providers involved in your care are crucial to ensure that the therapy aligns with your overall treatment plan.

• **Long-term Monitoring:** For chronic conditions or extended treatment periods, long-term monitoring may be necessary. This can help track the sustainability of benefits, assess any changes in your health status and make appropriate adjustments to the treatment plan as needed.

Bottom Line
Monitoring is essential throughout high-dose vitamin C IV therapy to ensure your safety, assess effectiveness and make informed decisions regarding treatment adjustments. Close collaboration with healthcare professionals, regular assessments of vital signs and relevant biomarkers and prompt reporting of any adverse reactions or side effects contribute to a well-managed and optimized treatment experience.

Homelessness

Homelessness among Veterans is a significant issue in the United States, affecting an estimated 50,000 to 60,000 Veterans at any given time. There are a variety of factors that contribute to Veteran homelessness, including poverty, lack of access to healthcare, mental health issues and substance abuse. (See **Annex D—Organizations Supporting Veterans** for contact information for specific organizations.)

The Department of Veterans Affairs (VA) provides a range of assistance to homeless Veterans, including emergency financial assistance, health care services and vocational rehabilitation and employment services. The VA also operates a number of programs designed to prevent Veteran homelessness, such as the Veterans Affairs Supportive Housing (VASH) program, which provides vouchers to Veterans to help them pay for housing.

One of the biggest challenges in addressing Veteran homelessness is ensuring that Veterans are aware of the resources that are available to them. Many Veterans are not familiar with the VA or the services that it provides and may not know how to access the help that they need.

To address this issue, the VA has partnered with a number of organizations and community groups to increase outreach to homeless Veterans. This includes working with local shelters and outreach programs as well as partnering with other government agencies such as the Department of Labor and the Department of Housing and Urban Development (HUD).

Another important factor in addressing Veteran homelessness is providing Veterans with access to mental health and substance abuse treatment. Many Veterans who experience homelessness have underlying mental health and substance abuse issues and these conditions can contribute to their homelessness or make it difficult for them to maintain stable housing.

The VA provides a range of mental health and substance abuse services to Veterans, including individual and group therapy, medication-assisted treatment and support for families and loved ones. These services are provided at VA medical centers and community-based outpatient clinics across the country.

In addition to the VA's efforts, there are a number of organizations and initiatives that are working to end Veteran homelessness. Some of these include the National Coalition for Homeless Veterans, which works to improve the lives of homeless Veterans by advocating for better policies and programs and the Veterans Affairs Homeless Providers Grant and Per Diem Program, which provides funding and support to organizations that provide housing and services to homeless Veterans. Finally, it is important to recognize the role that government and community support play in addressing Veteran homelessness. This includes funding for programs and services, as well as public awareness campaigns and volunteer opportunities.

Bottom Line
While Veteran homelessness is a complex issue with no easy solutions, there are a number of resources and initiatives in place to help Veterans who are struggling with homelessness. From the VA's support services to community-based organizations and government programs, there is a strong network of support in place to help Veterans find stable housing and get the help they need to overcome the challenges they face.

Hormonal Balance

Hormones are the body's internal messengers, regulating energy, mood, sleep, metabolism, and recovery. For Veterans, service-related stress, trauma, and environmental exposures can disrupt these delicate systems, leading to fatigue, anxiety, weight changes, or chronic inflammation. Unlike acute conditions with sudden symptoms, hormonal imbalances develop gradually, making their effects widespread yet subtle. By identifying disruptions and applying targeted corrections, Veterans can restore vitality and resilience. This section explores the role of hormones, their impact when imbalanced, and practical strategies for Veterans to achieve hormonal stability.

Understanding Hormones
Hormones are biochemical signals produced by glands like the thyroid, adrenals, and gonads, traveling through the bloodstream to regulate essential functions. Key hormones influencing Veteran health include:

- Cortisol: Governs stress response; imbalance leads to fatigue or anxiety.

- Testosterone: Supports muscle mass, energy, and libido; declines with age or injury.

- Thyroid Hormones (T3, T4, TSH): Control metabolism; imbalances cause weight and energy fluctuations.

- Estrogen/Progesterone: Influence mood, sleep, and metabolism, especially in female Veterans.

The Science of Hormonal Imbalance
Chronic stress, toxin exposure, and disrupted sleep patterns contribute to hormonal dysfunction. Research in Endocrinology & Metabolism (2020) indicates Veterans with PTSD often exhibit cortisol dysregulation, linked to fatigue and anxiety. A Journal of Hormone Research (2019) study found testosterone declines post-deployment, impacting strength and mood. While hormone therapy is an option, lifestyle modifications often provide significant benefits without medical risks.

Why Hormonal Balance Matters for Veterans

- Energy & Recovery: Balanced hormones enhance stamina and healing, countering post-service fatigue.

- Mood & Mental Clarity: Regulated cortisol and testosterone stabilize emotions, reducing irritability and brain fog.

- Sleep & Stress Management: Optimized melatonin and cortisol promote deep sleep, critical for PTSD management.

- Inflammation Control: Proper hormone levels lower chronic inflammation, aiding pain reduction.

- Physical Strength & Metabolism: Stable testosterone and thyroid function support muscle maintenance and weight control.

Identifying Hormonal Imbalances

- Common Signs: Fatigue, mood swings, weight changes, insomnia, brain fog, low libido.

- Veteran-Specific Triggers: Deployment stress, burn pit exposure, physical wear from service.

- Assessment Tools: Track symptoms in a journal, noting energy dips, sleep disturbances, and stress levels.

- Medical Testing: Blood tests (e.g., cortisol, testosterone, TSH) via VA or private clinics ($50–$200).

Strategies for Hormonal Balance

- Diet Optimization: High-protein, low-sugar intake (lean meats, greens) stabilizes insulin and cortisol.

- Sleep Routine: 7–9 hours per night (10 p.m.–6 a.m.) to reset circadian rhythms.

- Exercise Balance: Moderate strength training (3–5 times weekly) boosts testosterone and thyroid function.

- Stress Reduction: Meditation, breathwork (10–20 minutes daily) lowers cortisol; VA mindfulness apps offer guided support.

Targeted Corrections for Veterans
1. Cortisol Regulation (Stress, PTSD)

- What: 10-minute morning sun exposure + deep breathing.

- Why: Supports natural cortisol rhythm, reducing stress peaks.

- How: Stand outdoors, breathe deeply, repeat daily for 4 weeks.

- Supplies: Outdoor access, stress tracking journal.

2. Testosterone Support (Energy, Strength)
- What: Resistance training (30–45 minutes, 3x/week).

- Why: Increases natural testosterone, enhancing physical recovery.

- How: Focus on compound movements (squats, push-ups), track progress.

- Supplies: Dumbbells or bodyweight exercises.

3. Thyroid Function (Metabolism, Fatigue)
- What: Balanced iodine intake (seafood, eggs) + daily movement.

- Why: Supports thyroid efficiency, reducing sluggishness.

- How: Add iodine-rich foods, take 10-minute walks post-meals.

- Supplies: Nutrient-rich diet plan, step tracker.

4. Sleep Enhancement (Insomnia, Fatigue)
- What: No screens 1 hour before bed, grounding techniques.

- Why: Reduces blue light exposure, stabilizes melatonin.

- How: Read, stretch, or use a grounding mat before sleep.

- Supplies: Book, eye mask, grounding device.

Supplementation and Medical Support
- Ashwagandha: Reduces cortisol ($10–$20, 300–600 mg daily, 4–12 weeks).

- Vitamin D: Supports testosterone, thyroid function ($5–$15, 2,000–5,000 IU daily).

- Bioidentical Hormone Therapy: Available through prescription for severe imbalances ($50–$150/month).

- Risks: Over-supplementation (e.g., testosterone misuse) can cause adverse effects; professional oversight recommended.

Integrating Hormone Balance into Daily Life
- Set SMART Goals: Example: "Lift weights 3x per week for 6 weeks to boost energy."

- Build a Routine: Stack habits—morning protein + sun exposure, exercise + breathwork.

• Leverage Veteran Support: VA wellness programs, peer accountability, tele-health consultations.

Bottom Line
Hormonal balance is crucial for Veterans recovering from stress, fatigue, and physical wear. By adjusting diet, sleep, exercise, and stress management techniques, Veterans can optimize energy, mood, and resilience. Scientific research supports lifestyle corrections, though medical interventions may be necessary for severe cases. Start with simple, cost-effective strategies—monitor symptoms, adjust habits, and seek professional guidance if needed. Restoring hormonal health is not a quick fix but a long-term investment in well-being.

Hot Water Immersion
(Hydrotherapy)[9]

Hot water immersion—using hot tubs—has been shown to be beneficial in treating acute and chronic inflammation and increasing overall well being. Veterans who have heart disease or are pregnant should consult their doctor before using a hot tub. Also, people with skin injuries, low blood pressure, urinary tract infection, a sensitivity to the chemicals used in the hot tub or have had a hot weather injury should also consult their doctor before using a hot tub.
Whether soaking in hot water (100-104-degrees F) without jets or with active jets, hot water immersion can have the following benefits:

• *Stress Relief:* The relaxing effect of the hot water and the massaging actions of the jets can relieve stress.

• *Muscle Relaxation:* Hydrotherapy can relax tense muscles and help speed recovery after a workout.

• *Improved Sleep:* Some studies have shown that hydrotherapy can relieve insomnia in older adults, improve sleep quality and the depth of sleep. They have also shown that fibromyalgia sufferers had better sleep as well as other improved symptoms.

• *Pain Relief:* Relief from musculoskeletal aches and pains, arthritis and fibromyalgia are some of the conditions hydrotherapy may produce.

• *Better Cardiovascular Health:* Using a hot tub can raise your heart rate while lowering your blood pressure.

• **Improved Insulin Sensitivity:** Regular use of a hot tub—or sauna—may help people who have diabetes or are obese.

• **Calorie Burn:** For those who find it difficult to exercise, soaking in a hot tub can burn calories. Soaking in a waist-high bath for an hour burns about the same calories as going for a 2-minute walk.

Some health insurance organizations have covered the cost of a hot tub either completely or partially based on a doctor's recommendation for treatment of a chronic condition like fibromyalgia or rheumatoid arthritis.

Bottom Line
Regular soaking in a hot tub may provide several health benefits, such as muscle relaxation, pain relief and improved sleep. Some studies suggest a wider variety of health benefits, but more research is needed to determine the specifics of hot tub therapy with particular conditions. Hot tubs must be properly maintained to ensure health and safety. Consult with your doctor if you have health issues such as heart disease. You should also avoid the hot tub while pregnant or if you have an injury to your skin. When used carefully, hot tubs are safe for most people.

Hyperbaric Oxygen Therapy (HBOT)

Also known as HBOT, it is a treatment in which a person breathes pure oxygen in a pressurized chamber. This can help increase the amount of oxygen in the body and stimulate the growth of new blood vessels, which can aid in healing and tissue repair. For Veterans, HBOT may have several benefits, including:

• **Treating certain types of wounds:** HBOT can be an effective treatment for certain types of wounds, such as those caused by diabetes or radiation injury. The increased pressure and oxygen in the chamber can help to speed up the healing process and improve the overall health of the wound.

• **Improving symptoms of conditions such as post traumatic stress disorder (PTSD) and traumatic brain injury (TBI):** Veterans who have experienced traumatic events may suffer from conditions such as PTSD and TBI. Studies have found that HBOT can help to eliminate symptoms such as anxiety, depression and cognitive function.

• **Reducing inflammation and improving overall physical function:** Inflammation is a natural response to injury or infection, but it can also cause pain and discomfort. HBOT can help to reduce inflammation and improve overall physical function. This can be especially beneficial for Veterans who have been injured in combat.

• ***Helping with recovery from certain types of surgeries:*** HBOT can also be used to aid in recovery from certain types of surgeries, such as plastic surgery. The increased oxygen and pressure in the chamber can help to speed up the healing process and reduce the risk of complications.

HBOT is not a cure-all and its benefits may vary depending on the individual and the condition being treated. Before undergoing HBOT, it is important to consult with a medical professional to determine if it is the right treatment option for you. HBOT is also a non-invasive and safe treatment, which can be a significant benefit for Veterans who have already been through multiple surgeries or treatments. It has been reported that HBOT has no significant side effects and it can be used to treat a wide range of conditions. In addition, it can be used in combination with other treatments, such as physical therapy or medication, to achieve the best possible outcome. Patients suffering from COPD must make sure their healthcare provider and treatment team are aware of their condition before undergoing HBOT as it could cause a severe side effect in rare cases.

HBOT has been found to be particularly beneficial for Veterans suffering from PTSD and TBI. These conditions can cause a wide range of symptoms, including anxiety, depression and cognitive impairment. HBOT can help to alleviate these symptoms and improve overall quality of life.

HBOT has also been found to be effective in treating wounds caused by diabetes. Diabetes is a condition that affects millions of Veterans and can cause a wide range of complications, including foot and leg ulcers. HBOT can help to speed up the healing process and reduce the risk of amputation.

HBOT is also a safe and non-invasive treatment option for Veterans who have been injured in combat. It can be used to aid in recovery from injuries such as burns and blast injuries. The increased pressure and oxygen in the chamber can help to speed up the healing process and reduce the risk of complications.

Bottom Line

Hyperbaric oxygen therapy (HBOT) is a safe, non-invasive and effective treatment option for Veterans. It can be used to treat a wide range of conditions including wounds caused by diabetes, PTSD, TBI and injuries caused by combat. It is important to consult with a medical professional to determine if HBOT is the right treatment option for you, as it can be a valuable addition to a Veteran's treatment plan.

Ibogaine

Veterans bear burdens that don't fade—addiction carved deep, PTSD that lingers, minds and bodies strained by service. Ibogaine emerges from Central Africa's iboga shrub, a natural compound rooted in centuries of ritual, now studied as a potential lifeline. It's not a quick fix or a casual remedy—it's a profound, guided experience, administered in clinics beyond U.S. borders, offering a chance to confront and release what holds you back. For vets facing substance dependence, trauma's weight, or cognitive scars, ibogaine presents an alternative path, one demanding caution and care. This section explores what ibogaine is, its promise for warriors, and how to approach it, all with a Veteran's resolve.

Understanding Ibogaine
Ibogaine is derived from the root bark of the iboga plant, long used in Gabon's Bwiti ceremonies to guide initiates through visions and introspection. In modern practice, it's refined into ibogaine hydrochloride, a purified form given as a single oral dose under medical oversight. The experience unfolds over 24–36 hours—intense hallucinations give way to a reflective calm, a journey that's both physical and mental. For Veterans, it's framed as a tool to interrupt addiction's grip or process trauma's scars, a one-time intervention where traditional methods may fall short.

The Science Behind It
Ibogaine interacts with the brain's wiring—touching serotonin, dopamine, and opioid systems, potentially reshaping pathways tied to dependence and distress. It may dampen withdrawal, quiet cravings, or open a window to revisit pain with new clarity. For vets, it's not about the chemistry alone—it's the possibility of breaking cycles that years of service etched in deep. Research offers glimpses—small studies suggest real shifts—but the evidence is early, incomplete, and shadowed by serious risks, especially to the heart.

The Impact of Ibogaine on Veterans' Health
- Wellness Benefits: It's proposed to ease addiction's hold, soften trauma's edge, restore mental balance—gains vets seek when conventional roads run dry.

- Consequences of Ignoring It: Without it, substance use, haunting memories, or fog may persist—loads that test even the strongest.

Identifying and Analyzing Your Struggles
- Self-Assessment: Take stock—what's weighing you down? A reliance on pills

to numb pain? Relentless echoes of combat? A mind dulled by injury? Write it down—name your fight.

- Setting Priorities: Order the battles—addiction if it's consuming you, trauma if it's unrelenting, clarity if you're lost. Start with the heaviest; the rest will follow.

Fostering the Ibogaine Approach
- Set Goals: Define it clearly—e.g., "Pursue ibogaine to address my opioid use this year." Precise, like a mission objective—focus, act.

- Building a Support System: Bring in trusted allies—a fellow vet, a counselor, a medical team—to anchor you before and after the experience.

Implementation Strategies
- Single-Use Focus: This isn't a daily regimen—it's a rare, deliberate step, perhaps once or twice in a lifetime. Treat it like a critical operation, planned with intent.

- Habit Stacking: Align it with a transition—after a therapy milestone or a sober stretch—to integrate it into your broader recovery.

Targeted Protocols for Veterans' Wellness
Here's how to approach ibogaine for specific needs, with supplies for each—serious, vet-centered, and practical:

1. Addiction - Opioids
- What: Arrange a single clinic session, one dose (10–20 mg/kg) with magnesium support.

- Why: Opioids from pain or escape tightening their grip? Ibogaine may ease withdrawal and weaken that pull—a chance to reclaim control.

- How: Seek a reputable clinic—Mexico or Costa Rica—requiring a heart check (EKG) and liver test first. No drugs for 48 hours prior. Take the dose, endure 24 hours of intense effects under supervision, then rest. One session—assess if the need lessens soon after. If your pulse feels off, medics are there.

- Supplies Needed: Clinic access ($5,000–$10,000), EKG and lab tests, travel funds, a VA contact for follow-up.

2. PTSD
- What: Undergo one guided dose with post-session counseling.

- Why: Memories of service cutting deep? It might let you face them with distance—process without breaking.

- How: Choose a clinic with experience—screen heart and liver, take the dose, ride out the visions for a day, then talk it through with a pro. One treatment—

feel if the burden shifts in days. If it's too heavy, lean on support.

- Supplies Needed: Clinic cost, travel essentials, a counselor (VA or private), a journal.

3. Depression and Anxiety

- What: One ibogaine session, monitored for 24–48 hours, followed by weekly check-ins.

- Why: A persistent darkness or tension wearing you down? It could offer relief—lift the weight vets carry silently.

- How: Medical team in place—dose it, navigate the experience, reflect afterward with guidance. One attempt—sense a calm in weeks? If it stirs unease, reach out fast.

- Supplies Needed: Clinic fee, magnesium supplement, travel gear, a trusted vet ally.

4. Traumatic Brain Injury (TBI)

- What: One dose with professional oversight, tracking mental gains after.

- Why: Head injuries clouding your focus? It might sharpen what's dulled—restore a vet's edge.

- How: Clinic with cardiac monitoring—EKG cleared, dose taken, watched for a day. Note memory or focus shifts—improved in a month? If fog lingers, consult your doc.

- Supplies Needed: Clinic payment, a wearable tracker (e.g., Fitbit), a log, VA follow-up.

5. Resilience and Recovery

- What: One treatment, paired with rest and nutrition adjustments.

- Why: Worn thin from years of strain? It could renew your strength—keep you vet-ready.

- How: Screened clinic—dose it, recover with medics, then build back with sleep and solid chow. One go—energy return in days? If it's rough, ease into routine.

- Supplies Needed: Clinic, travel resources, protein-rich food, a quiet rack spot.

Eliminating Barriers to Consideration

- Identify Triggers: Pinpoint what holds you back—"Too dangerous," "Too costly," "Unproven." Acknowledge it—then weigh it soberly.

- Replace Hesitation: Shift "Not now" to "One careful step"—approach it like a recon mission. Trade uncertainty for "What might it heal?"—assess, decide.

- Veteran-Specific Substitutes:

  - Safety: Replace "I'll crash" with "I've got pros"—rely on medical oversight, like a squad's trust.

  - Doubt: Swap "No proof" for "My call"—judge it by your need, not just the labs.

Mindfulness and Self-Regulation
- Techniques: Prepare with purpose—breathe steady (5-5-5), set your aim: "Release the past." After, anchor with reflection or quiet. It keeps you centered, not adrift.

- Benefits: You'll recognize when you're breaking—signal the move. Awareness is your strength, honed by service.

Seeking Professional Help
- When Needed: Heart concerns or mental fragility surfacing? Consult your VA doctor first—ibogaine demands a clear baseline.

- Resources: VA cardiology, mental health teams, or vetted programs like VETS, Inc.—they're built for vets, ready to guide or caution.

Maintaining and Sustaining the Outcome
- Track Progress: Record the shifts—less reliance, calmer nights? Note it: "Took it, found ground."

- Overcome Plateaus: No change? Deepen counseling or adjust habits—push forward like a stalled advance.

- Build Resilience: Each gain reinforces you—layer it up, and you're stronger, beyond old wounds.

Bottom Line
Ibogaine offers a serious prospect—easing addiction's chains, softening trauma's scars, lifting mental burdens, sharpening cognition, bolstering resilience—through a single, intense dose in a supervised clinic ($5,000–$10,000). For vets bearing substance struggles, PTSD, or injury's toll, it's a potential turning point, drawing from ancient rites and modern desperation. Reports call it transformative—breaking cycles where others falter; science sees flickers of hope—small studies hint at relief—but solid evidence lags, and the heart risk is real, with over 30 deaths tied to its use in decades. It's not a standalone answer—experts demand oversight and screening—so consult your VA provider, pursue it only with pros (EKG, medical watch), and balance it against proven care. Powerful, perilous, it's a tool for the determined—approach it with respect and readiness.

Inflammation

Inflammation is a natural biological response to injury, illness or infection and is essential for the body's defense mechanism. It involves the release of various signaling molecules and the activation of immune cells, which work together to eliminate harmful pathogens and repair damaged tissue. However, when the inflammatory response persists for an extended period, it can have significant negative impacts on our health.

Chronic inflammation has been linked to several serious diseases and conditions, including cardiovascular disease, type 2 diabetes, cancer, Alzheimer's disease and rheumatoid arthritis. It also contributes to the aging process and can lead to an increased risk of disability and death.

The good news is that there are several ways to minimize the risks associated with inflammation and promote overall health. Here are some strategies that can help:

• *Eat an anti-inflammatory diet:* A diet rich in fruits, vegetables, whole grains, lean protein and healthy fats can help reduce chronic inflammation and promote overall health. Foods that are high in anti-inflammatory compounds include berries, leafy greens, fatty fish, nuts and seeds. On the other hand, foods that can contribute to inflammation include sugar, refined carbohydrates, trans fats and processed meats.

• *Exercise regularly:* Regular physical activity has been shown to reduce inflammation and promote overall health. Exercise can help regulate the immune system, improve cardiovascular health and reduce the risk of chronic diseases. Aim for at least 30 minutes of moderate physical activity every day, such as brisk walking, cycling or swimming.

• *Manage stress:* Chronic stress has been linked to increased inflammation and a range of health problems, including cardiovascular disease and depression. Effective stress management strategies include exercise, mindfulness meditation, deep breathing and spending time in nature.

• *Get enough sleep:* Sleep plays a critical role in regulating the immune system and reducing inflammation. Aim for 7-9 hours of quality sleep each night and establish a regular bedtime routine to help you fall asleep more easily.

• *Avoid smoking and excessive alcohol consumption:* Smoking and excessive alcohol consumption have both been linked to increased inflammation and a range of health problems. If you are a smoker, quitting can help reduce the risk of chronic diseases and improve your overall health. If you drink alcohol, limit your consumption to moderate levels.

• ***Supplement your diet with anti-inflammatory nutrients:*** Certain nutrients have been shown to have anti-inflammatory effects, including omega-3 fatty acids, Vitamin D, turmeric and ginger. Talk to your doctor about incorporating these nutrients into your diet through dietary changes or supplements.

• ***Maintain a healthy weight:*** Being overweight or obese can increase inflammation and the risk of chronic diseases. Aim for a healthy body weight by maintaining a balanced diet and engaging in regular physical activity.

Bottom Line

Chronic inflammation is a major contributor to several serious diseases and conditions. By following a healthy lifestyle and adopting anti-inflammatory strategies, it is possible to minimize the risks associated with inflammation and promote overall health. It is important to talk to your doctor if you are concerned about the risks associated with chronic inflammation and to discuss an appropriate plan of action to reduce your risk.

Infrared Sauna

An infrared sauna is a type of sauna that uses infrared heaters to emit infrared light waves, which penetrate the skin and heat the body directly, rather than heating the air around you. This type of sauna has several benefits, both for overall health and wellness and for specific medical conditions.

• ***Detoxification:*** One of the main benefits of using an infrared sauna is the ability to detoxify the body. When the body is exposed to infrared heat, it causes an increase in sweat production. Sweating is one of the body's natural ways of eliminating toxins and using an infrared sauna can help to flush out toxins and impurities from the body.

• ***Pain relief:*** Infrared saunas can also be used for pain relief. The deep penetrating heat of infrared light can help to increase blood flow and reduce inflammation, which can be beneficial for people with conditions such as arthritis, fibromyalgia and chronic pain.

• ***Weight loss:*** Regular use of an infrared sauna can also aid in weight loss. The high heat of the sauna can cause an increase in heart rate, which can lead to an increase in calorie burn. Additionally, sweating can help to eliminate water weight.

• ***Relaxation and Stress relief:*** Using an infrared sauna can also help to promote relaxation and reduce stress. The heat and the quiet, relaxing environment of the sauna can help to soothe the mind and promote a sense of calm and well-being.

• **Improving skin:** Infrared saunas can also improve the appearance of the skin. The heat and sweating can help to open up pores and remove impurities, leaving the skin looking and feeling smoother and clearer.

• **Cardiovascular health:** Regular use of an infrared sauna can also benefit cardiovascular health. The heat can cause an increase in heart rate, which can help to improve circulation and lower blood pressure.

• **Immune system support:** Infrared saunas can also help to boost the immune system. The heat can help to increase the production of white blood cells, which can help to fight off infection and illness.

• **Anti-aging:** Infrared saunas can also have anti-aging benefits. The heat can help to increase collagen production, which can help to firm and tighten the skin, giving it a more youthful appearance.

It's also important to note that before using an infrared sauna, it's best to consult with a doctor, especially if you have any medical conditions or are pregnant. And make sure the sauna is clean, safe and well-maintained before use. Additionally, it's important to stay hydrated by drinking plenty of water before and after using the sauna.

Bottom Line
The infrared sauna offers a wide range of health benefits, from helping to detoxify the body and providing pain relief, to promoting relaxation and reducing stress. Regular use of an infrared sauna can also improve cardiovascular health, boost the immune system and have anti-aging benefits for the skin.

Intentions and Intention Setting

Veterans know the weight of purpose—missions gave it, service demanded it, and leaving can strip it bare. Intentions and intention setting offer a way back: a quiet, deliberate choice to steer your mind and days toward something real—peace, strength, healing. It's not just wishing or chasing checklists—it's grounding yourself in what matters, moment by moment. For vets navigating the fog of post-service life—PTSD's grip, a lost compass, or battered health—it's a tool to reclaim control and clarity. This section lays out what intentions are, why they hit home for warriors, and how to make them stick, all with a vet's steel.

Understanding Intentions and Intention Setting
An intention's a commitment you set inside—a clear aim like "I'll stay steady to-

day" or "I'll mend what's broken." It's less about hitting a target—like dropping pounds—and more about how you move through the day, aligning your head and heart. Rooted in old practices and sharpened by modern mind work, it's a daily reset. For Veterans, it's a way to cut through the noise of transition, trauma, or drift, anchoring you when the ground feels shaky.

The Science Behind It
Your brain thrives on direction—without it, stress and clutter take over. Setting an intention lights a path: it steadies your focus, calms the chaos, nudges habits into line. It's not magic—think of it as tuning your internal comms, keeping the signal strong. For vets, it's less about lab proof and more about feel—does it quiet the storm, lift the haze? Research backs it some—small groups find sharper minds and lighter loads—but it's your resolve that turns it real.

The Impact of Intentions on Veterans' Health
- Wellness Benefits: It's pitched to clear your thoughts, toughen your spirit, ease the strain—stuff vets need when the past echoes or the future blurs.

- Consequences of Ignoring It: Skip it, and fog, fragility, or tension dig in—extra drag on a frame built to push.

Identifying and Analyzing Your Needs
- Self-Assessment: Take stock—what's off? Mind scattered from TBI? Soul raw from combat? Drive gone post-service? List it—know your fight.

- Setting Priorities: Rank the loads—clarity if you're lost, resilience if you're cracking, calm if stress rules. Start where it's heaviest; the rest follows.

Fostering the Intention Habit
- Set Goals: Keep it tight—e.g., "Set one intention each morning this week to stay grounded." Clear, like a patrol plan—lock, move.

- Building a Support System: Pull in a vet brother, kin, or counselor—they've got your flank, keeping you honest when the intent's set.

Implementation Strategies
- Daily Practice: Weave it in—morning words, evening pause. Start small; steady beats a rush, like pacing a ruck.

- Habit Stacking: Tie it to routine—set it with coffee, reflect post-PT. Anchors it to what's solid, keeps it real.

Targeted Protocols for Veterans' Wellness
Here's how to set intentions for specific needs, with supplies for each—vet-ready, no frills:

1. Mental Clarity and Focus

- What: Set a daily intent—"I'll keep my head clear"—5 minutes each morning.

- Why: Fog from blasts or stress clouding you? It cuts through—sharpens a vet's edge.

- How: Sit quiet, say it—"I intend to focus"—write it if it sticks better. Five minutes, eyes shut or on paper—feel the clutter fade in a day. If it drifts, repeat it firm.

- Supplies Needed: Nothing fancy—chair, pen and pad (optional), silence.

2. Emotional Resilience

- What: Morning intent—"I'll stand strong"—with 10-minute journaling, thrice weekly.

- Why: PTSD or loss rocking you? It steadies the core—builds vet grit inside out.

- How: Write it—"I intend to endure"—then spill what's up, 10 minutes. Three days a week—feel tougher in a week? If it's heavy, talk it out too.

- Supplies Needed: Notebook, pen, quiet corner.

3. Stress Reduction

- What: Evening intent—"I'll let it go"—with 10-minute breath work, daily.

- Why: Transition or ghosts stressing you? It dials it back—eases a vet's load.

- How: Set it—"I intend to release"—breathe slow (4-7-8), 10 minutes before rack time. Daily—calm hit in days? Too wired? Shift to morning.

- Supplies Needed: Spot to sit, timer (phone), dark room.

4. Behavioral Change

- What: Weekly intent—"I'll choose better"—with 15-minute visualization, twice weekly.

- Why: Booze or junk habits sticking? It guides the shift—steers vet will to new tracks.

- How: Picture it—"I intend to heal"—see yourself strong, 15 minutes, twice a week. Feel the pull ease in weeks—slipping? Tighten the image.

- Supplies Needed: Quiet space, chair, mind's eye.

5. Purpose and Motivation

- What: Daily intent—"I'll find my why"—with 20-minute meditation, thrice weekly.

- Why: Lost your north star post-service? It lights it up—fires a vet's drive.

- How: Set it—"I intend to connect"—sit, breathe, repeat it silent, 20 minutes, three days. Purpose spark in a month? If it's dim, lean on a vet pal.

- Supplies Needed: VA app (Mindfulness Coach, free), cushion, calm spot.

Eliminating Barriers to Setting

- Identify Triggers: Spot what blocks you—"Too soft," "No time," "Pointless." Name it—then face it square.

- Replace Hesitation: Swap "Later" for "Five minutes now"—quick hit, done. Trade doubt for "What's it build?"—test, own it.

- Veteran-Specific Substitutes:

  - Skepticism: Swap "Touchy-feely" for "Mission mind"—frame it as focus, vet-style.

  - Rush: Trade "Too busy" for "Short burst"—fit it tight, like a field fix.

Mindfulness and Self-Regulation

- Techniques: Lock on the intent—breathe it in (5-5-5), feel it settle. It's your anchor, cutting "it's bunk" chatter. Vets know discipline—use it here.

- Benefits: You'll spot when you're slipping—cue the set. Awareness keeps you in the driver's seat, steering your course.

Seeking Professional Help

- When Needed: PTSD or addiction overwhelming? Hit your VA shrink—intentions lift, but don't solo the big stuff.

- Resources: VA therapy, mindfulness programs, vet groups—free, ready, they'll back it or adjust it.

Maintaining and Sustaining the Practice

- Track Progress: Log the wins—clearer head, steadier heart? Mark it: "Set it, felt it."

- Overcome Plateaus: Flat? Shift words or add ritual—push like a stalled march.

- Build Resilience: Each intent's a brick—stack 'em, and you're tougher, past the drift.

Bottom Line

Intentions and setting them offer vets a steady hand—sharpening focus, building grit, easing stress, shifting habits, finding purpose—through simple acts like words, breath, or writing. For warriors hauling trauma, addiction, or a lost why, it's a mindful anchor, drawn from old ways and head science, giving direction when life's a haze. Some swear it—grounds you, lifts you; studies hint—focus and calm grow—but big proof's thin, and it's no cure if you just wish. It's not a lone fix—pros say pair it with real care—so hit your VA crew, start with five minutes daily (free), and weave it into your fight. Quiet, strong, it's a tool in your kit—use it steady and true.

Intimacy

Playing a crucial role in helping Veterans deal with common issues such as depression, PTSD and relationship problems, intimacy can foster a safe and supportive environment where Veterans feel understood, heard and accepted, intimacy can provide Veterans with a sense of comfort and security that is essential for their emotional and mental well-being.

Depression is a common issue among Veterans and it can be exacerbated by feelings of loneliness and isolation. Intimacy can help to mitigate these feelings by creating a sense of connection and belonging. For example, a trusted friend or romantic partner can provide Veterans with a listening ear and support, which can be essential for managing depression. Additionally, intimacy can also help Veterans feel more confident and secure in their own skin, leading to a more positive outlook on life.

PTSD (Post-Traumatic Stress Disorder) is another common issue among Veterans. This condition can make it difficult for Veterans to form close relationships, as they may be plagued by feelings of anxiety, fear and distrust. However, intimacy can help to counter these negative feelings by providing a sense of comfort and security. A trusted friend or partner can help Veterans to open up about their experiences and feelings, which can be an important step in the process of healing from PTSD.

Intimacy can also help Veterans deal with relationship problems, which are often a result of the challenges associated with re-adjusting to civilian life after serving in the military. For example, Veterans may struggle to communicate effectively with their spouse or partner or they may feel disconnected from their friends and family. However, intimacy can help to bridge these gaps by fostering a sense of connection and understanding. Through close and open communication, Veterans can feel heard and valued, which can be essential for maintaining healthy relationships.

Bottom Line
Intimacy plays a crucial role in helping Veterans deal with common issues such as depression, PTSD and relationship problems. By fostering a safe and supportive

environment where Veterans feel understood, heard and accepted, intimacy can provide Veterans with a sense of comfort and security that is essential for their emotional and mental well-being. If you are a Veteran who is struggling with these issues, it is important to seek out supportive relationships and intimate connections that can help you to heal and move forward in life.

Inversion Tables

An inversion table is a piece of equipment that allows individuals to hang upside down by their feet or ankles, providing a range of benefits for the body. Inversion therapy has been used for centuries, with early practitioners using ropes and pulleys to achieve the same effect. Today, inversion tables are a popular and convenient way to experience the benefits of inversion therapy.

Here are some of the benefits of using an inversion table:

• ***Improved spinal health:*** Inversion therapy has been shown to improve spinal health by reducing compression of the spinal discs and increasing the space between vertebrae. This can help reduce back pain and improve overall spinal function.

• ***Improved joint health:*** The use of an inversion table can help improve joint health by reducing inflammation and improving circulation. This can be particularly beneficial for individuals with arthritis or other joint problems.

• ***Reduced stress and anxiety:*** The practice of inversion therapy can help reduce stress and anxiety by promoting relaxation and improving overall mood.
• ***Improved circulation:*** Inversion therapy has been shown to improve circulation by increasing blood flow to the brain and other areas of the body.

• ***Improved posture:*** The use of an inversion table can help improve posture by decompressing the spine and reducing tension in the back and neck.

• ***Improved flexibility:*** Inversion therapy can help improve flexibility by increasing the range of motion in the joints and reducing muscle tension.

• ***Improved lymphatic function:*** The use of an inversion table can help improve lymphatic function by promoting lymphatic drainage and reducing inflammation.

When using an inversion table, it's important to start slowly and work your way up to longer sessions. Beginners should start with just a few minutes at a time and gradually increase the length of their sessions over time. It's also important to stay hydrated and avoid eating or drinking immediately before or after using the table.

There are a few different types of inversion tables on the market, each with its own unique features and benefits. Some of the most popular types include:

• **Standard inversion tables:** These are the most common type of inversion table and are designed to be used in a horizontal position. They typically feature a padded backrest and ankle holders to help keep you in place while inverting.

• **Gravity boots:** These are special boots that are designed to be worn while inverting. They attach to the ankles and allow you to hang upside down without the need for a table.

• **Inversion chairs:** These are designed to provide the benefits of inversion therapy while in a seated position. They are often recommended for individuals with mobility issues or those who find it difficult to use a standard inversion table.

When using an inversion table, it's important to follow the manufacturer's instructions carefully and to ensure that the table is set up correctly before using it. It's also important to consult with a healthcare professional before starting inversion therapy, particularly if you have a history of back or neck problems or any other health concerns.

Bottom Line
The use of an inversion table can offer a range of benefits for the body, including improved spinal and joint health, reduced stress and anxiety, improved circulation, improved posture, improved flexibility and improved lymphatic function. When using an inversion table, it's important to start slowly, follow the manufacturer's instructions carefully and consult with a healthcare professional to ensure that it's safe and appropriate for your individual health needs. With regular use, an inversion table can be a powerful tool for improving overall health and wellness.

Iodine

Iodine is an essential mineral that plays a crucial role in thyroid function, metabolism, cognitive health, and immune support. For Veterans, factors like stress, environmental toxin exposure, and dietary changes post-service can contribute to iodine imbalances, leading to fatigue, brain fog, weight fluctuations, or thyroid disorders. Unlike other micronutrients, iodine deficiency develops subtly, making it essential to recognize signs early and implement targeted corrections. This section explores iodine's role, symptoms of imbalance, and practical strategies for Veterans to optimize their iodine intake.

Understanding Iodine

Iodine is a trace element primarily stored in the thyroid gland, where it is required for the production of thyroid hormones (T3 and T4). These hormones regulate metabolism, energy levels, and neurological function. Key sources of iodine include:

- Seafood (fish, seaweed, shellfish): Richest natural sources.

- Dairy Products (milk, cheese, yogurt): Contains iodine due to animal feed fortification.

- Iodized Salt: A common dietary source but often avoided in processed foods.

- Eggs & Vegetables: Provide smaller but beneficial amounts, depending on soil content.

The Science of Iodine Deficiency

Iodine deficiency remains a global health issue, with research in Thyroid Health Journal (2021) indicating that mild deficiency affects cognitive function and metabolism. Studies have also linked iodine levels to stress resilience and immune function. Veterans may be at risk due to dietary shifts post-service, high-stress environments impacting thyroid function, or exposure to iodine-disrupting chemicals like fluoride and bromine.

Why Iodine Matters for Veterans

- Thyroid & Metabolism: Proper iodine levels ensure optimal thyroid function, preventing sluggish metabolism and weight gain.

- Cognitive Function: Iodine supports mental clarity, focus, and memory, reducing brain fog and fatigue.

- Energy & Fatigue Resistance: Thyroid hormones regulate stamina and endurance, aiding recovery from physical strain.

- Immune Health: Iodine has antimicrobial properties and supports immune function, helping Veterans combat illness.

- Detoxification: Iodine helps flush heavy metals and toxins, crucial for Veterans exposed to environmental hazards.

Identifying Iodine Deficiency

- Common Signs: Fatigue, difficulty concentrating, weight fluctuations, dry skin, cold intolerance.

- Veteran-Specific Triggers: Field rations (low iodine content), stress-related thyroid suppression, toxin exposure.

- Assessment Tools: Symptom tracking, checking dietary intake, observing energy levels.

- Medical Testing: Urinary iodine tests, thyroid function tests (TSH, T3, T4) via VA or private clinics ($50–$200).

Strategies for Optimal Iodine Intake

- Dietary Sources: Incorporate iodine-rich foods like seaweed (1–2 servings weekly), seafood, eggs, and iodized salt.

- Cooking Adjustments: Use unprocessed iodized salt in home meals; avoid excess processed foods that lack iodine.

- Hydration Balance: Filtered water (free from fluoride and chlorine) supports thyroid health and iodine absorption.

Targeted Corrections for Veterans

1. Thyroid Support (Metabolism, Fatigue)
- What: Add seaweed (e.g., nori, kelp) to meals 1–2 times weekly.

- Why: Provides natural iodine to sustain thyroid function.

- How: Use in soups, salads, or sushi.

- Supplies: Dried seaweed, grocery list.

2. Cognitive Boost (Brain Fog, Focus)
- What: Consume iodine-rich dairy or eggs at breakfast.

- Why: Supports neurotransmitter function and cognitive clarity.

- How: Include yogurt, cheese, or boiled eggs in morning meals.

- Supplies: Meal plan, grocery adjustments.

3. Immune & Detox Support (Environmental Toxins, Resilience)
- What: Increase water intake (8–12 cups daily) with iodine-rich foods.

- Why: Enhances detoxification and immune strength.

- How: Track daily hydration and include seafood weekly.

- Supplies: Reusable water bottle, meal tracker.

4. Weight & Energy Stability (Thyroid Regulation)
- What: Replace processed salt with iodized or sea salt in meals.

- Why: Ensures consistent iodine intake without excess additives.

- How: Use 1/4 tsp daily in home cooking.

- Supplies: Iodized or sea salt, seasoning guide.

Supplementation and Medical Support
- Iodine Supplements: Available as potassium iodide pills (150 mcg daily, $5–$15 per bottle), effective for consistent intake.

- Roll-On Iodine Liquid: Applied topically for absorption through the skin ($10–$20, check concentration and usage instructions).

- Multivitamins with Iodine: Provides balanced intake ($10–$25, check ingredient label).

- Professional Guidance: Over-supplementation can disrupt thyroid function; consult healthcare providers before taking high doses.

Integrating Iodine into Daily Life
- Set SMART Goals: Example: "Consume seafood twice weekly for the next 4 weeks to support thyroid health."

- Build a Routine: Pair iodine-rich meals with existing habits (e.g., eggs at breakfast, seaweed in soup).

- Leverage Veteran Support: VA nutrition programs, telehealth consultations, online Veteran wellness groups.

Bottom Line
Iodine plays a vital role in thyroid health, metabolism, cognitive function, and immunity. Veterans facing stress, dietary shifts, or toxin exposure can benefit from optimizing iodine intake through whole foods, supplementation (pills or roll-on iodine), hydration, and medical oversight. Research supports iodine's role in energy balance, brain function, and immune resilience, though excessive intake should be avoided. Start with simple, cost-effective dietary adjustments—monitor symptoms, improve food choices, and consult healthcare providers for personalized guidance. Maintaining iodine balance is a long-term investment in overall wellness and vitality.

Ionized Water Protocols

Water is a cornerstone of life, but for Veterans, it can be more than just hydration—it can be a tool for reclaiming health and well-being. Ionized water, created through a process that adjusts its pH to suit specific needs, offers a practical way to support physical recovery, mental clarity, and daily resilience. This section explores how Veterans can use ionized water protocols to enhance their wellness. By understanding the science behind ionization, mastering a basic daily routine, and applying targeted strategies, Veterans can integrate this approach into their lives for better health outcomes.

Understanding Ionized Water
Ionized water isn't your average tap or bottled stuff—it's water transformed by electrolysis, a process that splits it into alkaline (pH 8.5–11.5) and acidic (pH 2.5–6.0) streams using an ionizer machine. Each type has a purpose: alkaline water hydrates and balances, while acidic water cleans and soothes. For Veterans, this versatility can address both the wear-and-tear of service and the stresses of civilian life.

The Science of Ionization
Electrolysis happens in an ionizer's chambers, where electrodes charge water, shifting its pH. Alkaline water gains electrons, acting as a mild antioxidant—potentially reducing oxidative stress from years of physical strain or trauma. Acidic water, with a positive charge, becomes a disinfectant, tackling bacteria or inflammation. Research, like a 2018 study in *Medical Gas Research*, suggests alkaline water may ease oxidative stress, while acidic water's antimicrobial power is well-documented. For Veterans, this means a dual-purpose tool: internal support and external care.

Why Pre-Filtering Matters
Before ionization, water must be clean. Tap water often carries chlorine, fluoride, or metals—remnants Veterans might recognize from field conditions. Pre-filtering with a carbon filter or reverse osmosis (RO) system removes these, ensuring ionized water's purity. Without it, contaminants could weaken results or harm your ionizer. Think of it like prepping gear: start with a solid base, and the mission succeeds.

The Impact of Ionized Water on Veterans' Health
- Wellness Benefits: Regular use of alkaline water can hydrate deeply, support digestion, and reduce fatigue—key for Veterans managing chronic pain or stress. Acidic water aids skin healing and hygiene, vital for those with service-related injuries.

- Health Risks of Ignoring It: Skipping pre-filtering or overusing strong pH levels (like pH 11.5 internally) can irritate tissues or waste potential. Balance is critical—Veterans know overdoing it rarely works.

Basic Ionized Water Protocol
- What: Drink 16–20 oz of pH 9.0–9.5 alkaline water daily, split into two sessions.

- Why: This hydrates, mimics blood's pH (7.4), and counters acidity from stress or poor diet—common post-service struggles.

- How: Pre-filter water, ionize it fresh, sip slowly (10–15 minutes per glass), room temp. Morning (pre-coffee) and mid-afternoon (3 p.m.) are ideal—away from meals (30 minutes before, 2 hours after).

- Supplies Needed: Ionizer (pH 9.0–9.5), pre-filter (carbon or RO), glass or stainless steel tumbler.

Identifying and Analyzing Your Water Needs

- Self-Assessment: Track hydration, energy, or skin issues in a journal or app. Note triggers—stress, diet, or old injuries—that signal where ionized water might help.

- Setting Priorities: Focus on high-impact areas first: digestion for PTSD-related gut issues, skin for scars, or fatigue for transition burnout.

Fostering Ionized Water Habits

- Set Goals: Use SMART goals—e.g., "Drink 8 oz of pH 9.5 alkaline water every morning for 30 days to boost energy." Start small, scale up.

- Building a Support System: Share your plan with family or a battle buddy—accountability keeps you on track, just like in uniform.

Implementation Strategies

- Daily Integration: Add the basic protocol to your routine—like PT or chow time. Start with one glass, then two. Gradual beats abrupt—Veterans know pacing wins battles.

- Habit Stacking: Pair ionized water with existing habits—sip pH 9.5 while reading the news or stretching post-workout.

Targeted Protocols for Veterans' Wellness
Here's how to tailor ionized water to specific needs, with supplies for each:

1. Skin Conditions (Scars, Rashes)

- What: Rinse with pH 5.5 acidic water twice daily; spot-treat scars or rashes with pH 2.5 acidic water.

- Why: pH 5.5 matches skin's natural barrier, soothing irritation from old wounds. pH 2.5 kills bacteria, aiding healing—think field cuts turned scars.

- How: Splash 4–6 oz of pH 5.5 over affected areas, air dry. For spots, dab pH 2.5 with a cotton pad for 30 seconds, rinse with pH 5.5. Twice daily—consistency heals.

- Supplies Needed: Ionizer (pH 5.5 and 2.5), pre-filtered water, cotton pads, small glass dish.

2. Mental Clarity (Stress, Fatigue)

- What: Sip 8 oz of pH 9.5 alkaline water mid-morning and mid-afternoon.

- Why: Stress spikes acidity—pH 9.5 counters it, hydrating brain cells taxed by hypervigilance or sleep loss.

- How: Pour fresh, sip over 10 minutes, pair with deep breathing (5-5-5 method). Daily—watch clarity creep back.

- Supplies Needed: Ionizer (pH 9.5), pre-filtered water, glass tumbler.

3. Digestive Health (PTSD Gut Issues)
- What: Drink 8 oz of pH 9.5 alkaline water 30 minutes before meals.

- Why: Stress and meds can wreck digestion—pH 9.5 buffers acid, easing reflux or bloating from irregular chow.

- How: Sip slowly, room temp, three times daily. If bloating hits, cut to 4 oz—adjust to your gut.

- Supplies Needed: Ionizer (pH 9.5), pre-filtered water, glass.

4. Joint and Muscle Recovery
- What: Soak sore spots in pH 5.5 acidic water, 10 minutes daily; drink pH 9.0 alkaline water post-exercise.

- Why: pH 5.5 reduces inflammation from old injuries; pH 9.0 hydrates and flushes lactic acid.

- How: Fill a basin with 8 oz of pH 5.5, soak, pat dry. Sip 8 oz of pH 9.0 after PT—daily for stiffness.

- Supplies Needed: Ionizer (pH 5.5 and 9.0), pre-filtered water, basin, glass.

5. Oral Health (Tobacco Use)
- What: Gargle pH 2.5 acidic water, rinse with pH 9.0 alkaline water, twice daily.

- Why: pH 2.5 kills bacteria from smoking; pH 9.0 freshens and balances.

- How: Swish 1 oz of pH 2.5 for 30 seconds, spit, then 1 oz of pH 9.0 for 30 seconds. Post-brushing works best.

- Supplies Needed: Ionizer (pH 2.5 and 9.0), pre-filtered water, two shot glasses.

Eliminating Barriers to Use
- Identify Triggers: Spot excuses—cost, time, doubt. Counter with facts: ionizers last years, protocols take minutes, results build trust.

- Replace Habits: Swap soda or coffee with pH 9.5 water—same ritual, better outcome. For skin, ditch harsh soaps for pH 5.5 rinses.

- Veteran-Specific Substitutes:

  - Smoking: Sip pH 9.5 during cravings—hydrates and calms. Pair with gum or a quick walk.

  - Overeating: Pre-meal pH 9.5 cuts appetite; swap chips for nuts with pH 5.5-soaked hands to slow snacking.

Mindfulness and Self-Regulation
- Techniques: Use mindfulness—focus on water's taste or the rinse's coolness—to curb impulses like skipping protocols. Breathe through cravings (4-7-8 method) while sipping.

- Benefits: Awareness builds control—Veterans thrive on discipline, and this channels it.

Seeking Professional Help
- When Needed: If ionized water doesn't dent chronic pain, fatigue, or dental woes, tap VA resources or a doc. It's a tool, not a fix-all.

- Resources: VA clinics, telehealth, or vet support groups can guide integration with meds or therapy.

Maintaining and Sustaining Protocols
- Track Progress: Log energy, pain, or skin changes in a notebook or app. Celebrate a week of clear skin or steady guts—small wins fuel momentum.

- Overcome Plateaus: Hit a stall? Switch protocols (e.g., digestion to joints) or up volume slightly—patience beats frustration.

- Build Resilience: Consistent use mirrors military grit—each glass or rinse strengthens adaptability and hope.

Bottom Line
Ionized water protocols are a transformative option for Veterans seeking wellness. By mastering the science of ionization, starting with a basic routine, and targeting specific health needs, Veterans can harness water's potential to rebuild physically and mentally. This isn't about quick fixes—it's about steady, practical steps toward a healthier, more resilient life. Grab your ionizer, pre-filter your water, and take charge—one sip at a time.

JB Maintenance Workout

Designed to be the bare minimum to maintain strength, the JB Maintenance Workout works best if you ensure the weights are not too heavy for the exercises. If you are unfamiliar with the moves, consult a workout manual or YouTube for clarification. Of course, consult a doctor prior to engaging in a new exercise workout.

Back and Biceps

Wide lat pulldown	3x12
Pushups	3x10
Reverse grip pulldown	3x12
Diamond pushups	3x10
Bent over rows	3x12
Superman	3x20
Cardio - elliptical 20 seconds high intensity and 40 seconds low intensity for 20 minutes	

Chest/Triceps/Shoulders

Dumbbell incline bench press	3x12
Dumbbell lateral raises	3x12
Dumbbell decline bench press	3x12
Dumbbell front raises	3x12
Triceps kickbacks	3x12
Dumbbell overhead press	3x15
Plank	3x45 seconds
Cardio – treadmill 15% for 30 minutes	

Legs

Walking lunges	3x8 each leg
3way calf raises (in, neutral, out)	3x20 each
Straight leg dumbbell	3x12
Step ups	3x12
Glute bridge Raises	3x15
Reverse lunges	3x8 each leg
Plank	30 sec, 45 sec and 60 seconds
Cardio – bike hill 8 for 30 minutes	

Journaling

Journaling is a simple and effective tool that can help Veterans to manage their mental health and well-being. By providing a space for self-expression, reflection and problem-solving, journaling can offer a range of benefits for Veterans, especially those who have experienced trauma and are struggling with mental health conditions such as post-traumatic stress disorder (PTSD).

One of the key benefits of journaling for Veterans is that it can help to reduce symptoms of anxiety and depression. Writing about traumatic experiences can provide a sense of release and catharsis, allowing Veterans to process their emotions and gain a greater understanding of their experiences. This can help to reduce symptoms of anxiety and depression, as Veterans are better able to manage their emotions and feelings.

In addition, journaling can help Veterans to identify and understand patterns of thought and behavior. By reflecting on their experiences and emotions, Veterans can gain a deeper understanding of the underlying causes of their symptoms, such as negative beliefs and thought patterns. This can help them to develop more effective coping strategies and improve their overall mental health and well-being.

Journaling also can be a powerful tool for self-discovery and personal growth. By reflecting on their experiences, Veterans can gain a greater sense of self-awareness, which can lead to increased self-confidence and a more positive self-image. This can be especially important for Veterans who have experienced trauma, as it can help them to overcome feelings of shame and self-blame and to view themselves in a more positive light.

Another benefit of journaling for Veterans is that it can help to improve their sleep. Writing about traumatic experiences before bed can help to process and release negative emotions, making it easier for Veterans to fall asleep and stay asleep. This can be especially important for Veterans with PTSD, as sleep disturbances are a common symptom of the condition.

Journaling can help Veterans who are struggling with substance abuse or addiction. Writing about their experiences and emotions can help Veterans to gain a deeper understanding of their triggers and to develop more effective coping strategies. This can be especially important for Veterans who have experienced trauma, as substance abuse is often used as a way to cope with the effects of trauma.

Journaling also can help Veterans who are in therapy. By writing about their experiences and emotions, Veterans can prepare for therapy sessions and make the most of their time with their therapist. In addition, journaling can provide a space for Veterans to reflect on their progress and to track their symptoms, allowing them to see the positive changes in their mental health over time.

And journaling can help Veterans who are seeking to build resilience and improve their overall well-being. By writing about their experiences and emotions, Veterans can develop a greater sense of self-awareness, which can help them to identify and overcome negative thought patterns and behaviors. This can lead to improved mental health and well-being, as well as increased resilience in the face of future challenges.

There is no right or wrong way to journal. The goal is to create a space for self-expression and reflection, so find what works best for you and stick with it. The benefits of journaling will come with time and consistency. Here are some steps to get started with journaling:

• *Choose a journal and writing implement:* Choose a journal that feels comfortable to write in and a writing implement that you enjoy using. Some people prefer a physical journal and pen, while others prefer to journal on a computer or tablet.

• *Set aside time:* Choose a time each day or week to journal. Make it a regular part of your routine to help you develop the habit.

• *Write freely:* Start by writing freely about whatever comes to mind. Don't worry about grammar or punctuation, just write whatever you are feeling or thinking.

• *Reflect on your experiences:* After writing freely, take some time to reflect on your experiences and emotions. Write about your thoughts and feelings, what you learned about yourself and what you would like to work on in the future.

• *Focus on gratitude:* Take some time to write about the things you are grateful for. This can help to shift your focus away from negative experiences and improve your overall mood and well-being.

• *Use prompts:* If you are struggling to know what to write about, try using prompts. You can find lists of journaling prompts online or you can create your own.

• *Be honest and authentic:* Write from the heart and be honest with yourself. Journaling is a safe space where you can express your true thoughts and feelings.

• *Make it a habit:* Journaling is most effective when it becomes a regular habit. Set aside time each day or week to journal and stick to it as much as possible.

Bottom Line

Journaling is a powerful tool that can offer a range of benefits for Veterans, especially those who have experienced trauma and are struggling with mental health conditions such as PTSD. By providing a space for self-expression, reflection and problem-solving, journaling can help Veterans to manage their emotions and improve their overall mental health and well-being. Whether used on its own or in combination with other forms of therapy, journaling is a valuable tool for Veterans seeking to overcome the impact of their traumatic experiences and build a brighter future.

Juicing

Fruit juicing is a popular method for detoxification and promoting overall health. By juicing fresh fruits, you can extract the vitamins, minerals and other nutrients that are beneficial for your health and consume them in a more concentrated form. In this article, we will explore the benefits of fruit juicing for detoxification and health and offer some tips for incorporating it into your diet.

Detoxification is the process of removing toxins from the body. Toxins can come from a variety of sources, including food, the environment and even our own bodies. Over time, these toxins can accumulate in the body, causing health problems such as fatigue, headaches and digestive issues. By drinking fresh fruit juices, you can help to remove these toxins from your body, giving your liver and other organs a break from the work of filtering out harmful substances.

In addition to detoxifying the body, fruit juicing can also have a positive impact on overall health. For starters, fresh fruit juices are rich in vitamins and minerals that are essential for good health. For example, vitamin C, which is found in many fruits, is important for boosting the immune system and fighting off infections. It also acts as an antioxidant, helping to protect the body from harmful free radicals that can cause damage to cells and contribute to the development of chronic diseases.

Another benefit of fruit juicing is that it can help to improve digestion. By breaking down the fiber in fruits, the juice can make it easier for your body to absorb the nutrients contained within. This can help to relieve digestive issues such as bloating, constipation and heartburn. Additionally, some fruit juices, such as apple juice, contain pectin, a type of fiber that can help to regulate digestion and improve gut health.

Fruit juicing can also be beneficial for weight management. By incorporating fresh fruit juices into your diet, you can help to reduce your calorie intake, while still getting the vitamins and minerals that your body needs. Additionally, many fruit juices are low in calories, which can help you to feel full and satisfied, reducing the urge to snack on unhealthy foods.

Finally, fruit juicing can have a positive impact on mental health. Many fruits, such as berries, are rich in antioxidants that can help to reduce inflammation in the brain, which has been linked to depression and anxiety. Additionally, some fruits, such as citrus fruits, are rich in vitamin C, which has been shown to boost mood and energy levels.

When incorporating fruit juicing into your diet, it is important to choose fresh organic fruits whenever possible. This will help to ensure that you are getting the maximum benefits from the juice, while avoiding the harmful pesticides and chemicals that are often found on non-organic produce. Additionally, be sure to use a variety of different fruits in your juices, as this will help to ensure that you are getting a wide range of vitamins and minerals.

It is also important to remember that fruit juicing should not be used as a substitute for a balanced diet. While fresh fruit juices can be a great way to supplement your diet, they should not replace whole fruits and vegetables, which are also important for overall health. Additionally, fruit juices are often high in sugar, so it is important to be mindful of your consumption of them, especially if you have a sweet tooth.

Remember to always use fresh organic fruits and vegetables whenever possible and to consult with a healthcare professional before starting any new diet or health program. By incorporating these fruit juicing recipes into your diet, you can help to promote overall health and wellness and reap the many benefits that fresh fruits have to offer. Check that you are not including any items to which you are allergic or are inflammatory to your system.

Bottom Line
Fruit juicing can be a great way to detoxify your body and promote overall health. By incorporating fresh organic fruits into your diet, you can help to remove toxins from your body, improve digestion, boost weight management and improve mental health. However, it is important to remember that fruit juicing should be used in conjunction with a balanced diet and that it should not replace whole fruits and vegetables. Additionally, it is recommended to limit your consumption of fruit juices, as they can be high in sugar. It's always best to consult with a healthcare professional before starting any new diet or health program. By making informed choices and incorporating fruit juicing into your diet in moderation, you can reap the many benefits it has to offer for detoxification and overall health.

- K -

Ketosis

Ketosis is a metabolic state in which the body burns fat for energy instead of carbohydrates. This state is achieved by following a low-carbohydrate, high-fat diet, also known as a ketogenic diet. In a ketogenic diet, the body is forced to burn fat for energy because it lacks the glucose from carbohydrates that it normally uses for energy.

The human body is designed to use either carbohydrates or fat for energy, depending on the availability of these nutrients. Normally, the body burns glucose from carbohydrates for energy, but when glucose is not available, the body will switch to burning fat for energy. In a state of ketosis, the body is able to efficiently burn fat for energy, leading to rapid weight loss and improved health.

One of the main health benefits of ketosis is weight loss. In a state of ketosis, the body burns fat for energy instead of carbohydrates, leading to a rapid reduction in body fat. The ketogenic diet has been shown to be effective for weight loss in numerous studies and has been shown to be more effective than traditional low-fat diets.

In addition to weight loss, ketosis has also been shown to have numerous other health benefits. For example, it has been shown to improve blood sugar control in people with type 2 diabetes, reduce inflammation and oxidative stress and improve brain function. The ketogenic diet has also been shown to be beneficial for people with neurological disorders such as epilepsy, as it can help to reduce seizures.

Another benefit of ketosis is improved heart health. The ketogenic diet has been shown to lower total cholesterol levels, triglycerides and low-density lipoprotein (LDL) cholesterol, which is often referred to as the "bad" cholesterol. Additionally, the ketogenic diet has been shown to increase high-density lipoprotein (HDL) cholesterol, which is often referred to as the "good" cholesterol.

The ketogenic diet has also been shown to have anti-inflammatory effects in the body, which can help to reduce the risk of chronic diseases such as heart disease, cancer and Alzheimer's disease. Inflammation is a major contributor to many chronic diseases and the anti-inflammatory effects of the ketogenic diet can help to reduce the risk of these diseases.

One of the key benefits of the ketogenic diet is improved brain function. The ketones produced during ketosis are a source of energy for the brain and the diet has been shown to improve cognitive function, memory and mood. Additionally, the ketogenic diet has been shown to reduce the risk of neurological disorders such as Alzheimer's disease, Parkinson's disease and multiple sclerosis.

The ketogenic diet has also been shown to have positive effects on athletic performance as it can help to improve energy levels, endurance and strength. The diet can also help to reduce recovery time after exercise, as it can help to reduce inflammation and oxidative stress in the body.

In order to achieve and maintain ketosis, it is important to limit carbohydrate intake and increase fat intake. This can be achieved by consuming foods such as meats, fish, eggs, dairy products, oils and non-starchy vegetables. It is also important to limit the intake of processed and high-carbohydrate foods, such as bread, pasta and sweets.

There are several ways to track the level of ketosis, including measuring blood ketone levels, using breath ketone analyzers and monitoring physical symptoms such as increased energy levels and reduced hunger. These tools can help to ensure that individuals are following the diet correctly and achieving the desired level of ketosis.

Despite the numerous health benefits of ketosis, it is important to remember that the ketogenic diet is not for everyone. People with certain medical conditions such as liver or kidney disease, pancreatic disease and type 1 diabetes should not follow a ketogenic diet, as it can be harmful to their health. Additionally, pregnant women and children should not follow a ketogenic diet, as it can be harmful to their growth and development.

Bottom Line
Ketosis is a metabolic state in which the body burns fat for energy instead of carbohydrates. The ketogenic diet can help to achieve this state, leading to numerous health benefits. However, it is important to remember that the ketogenic diet should only be followed under the supervision of a healthcare professional and should be used in conjunction with a balanced diet. By tracking the level of ketosis, individuals can ensure that they are following the diet correctly and achieving the desired level of ketosis.

Key Health Numbers Every Veteran Should Know

As veterans, maintaining optimal health is critical to living a fulfilling and active life after service. Understanding the standard health metrics for a healthy adult can empower you to take charge of your wellness, monitor your body's signals, and work with your healthcare provider to address any concerns. Below is a list of key health numbers to know, based on widely accepted medical guidelines. Always consult your doctor or VA healthcare provider for personalized guidance.

Essential Health Metrics for Veterans

These ranges are for the average healthy adult and may vary depending on factors like age, sex, and individual health conditions.

1. Blood Pressure: Less than 120/80 mmHg
- Normal blood pressure is under 120/80 mmHg. A range of 120-129/<80 mmHg is considered elevated, and 130/80 mmHg or higher may indicate hypertension. Regular monitoring can help prevent heart disease, a common concern for veterans.

2. Resting Heart Rate (Pulse): 60-100 beats per minute (bpm)
- A healthy resting heart rate is typically 60-100 bpm. Fit individuals, including many veterans who maintain an active lifestyle, may have a lower rate of 50-70 bpm. Check your pulse in the morning for the most accurate reading.

3. Body Temperature: 97°F to 99°F (36.1°C to 37.2°C)
- Normal body temperature averages around 98.6°F (37°C) but can range from 97°F to 99°F. Variations may occur based on the time of day or measurement method (oral, forehead, etc.).

4. Respiratory Rate: 12-20 breaths per minute
- At rest, a healthy adult typically breathes 12-20 times per minute, with 12-16 being common. If you notice changes in your breathing, especially with a history of service-related respiratory exposure, consult your doctor.

5. Hemoglobin:
  - Men: 13.5-17.5 g/dL
  - Women: 12.0-15.5 g/dL
- Hemoglobin levels indicate your blood's oxygen-carrying capacity. Low levels may signal anemia, which can affect energy and recovery.

6. Cholesterol:
  - Total Cholesterol: Less than 200 mg/dL
  - LDL ("bad" cholesterol): Less than 100 mg/dL (optimal)
  - HDL ("good" cholesterol): Greater than 60 mg/dL (optimal)

- Veterans may be at higher risk for heart disease due to stress or lifestyle factors, so keeping cholesterol in check is key.

7. Potassium: 3.5-5.0 mEq/L
- Potassium supports muscle and nerve function. Abnormal levels can affect heart rhythm, so regular blood tests are important.

8. Sodium: 135-145 mEq/L
- Sodium balance is crucial for hydration and nerve function. Dehydration, common during physical activity, can affect sodium levels.

9. Triglycerides: Less than 150 mg/dL
- High triglycerides (150 mg/dL or more) can increase the risk of heart disease. A healthy diet and exercise can help keep levels in check.

10. Blood Volume: 4.5-6 liters
- The average adult has 4.5-6 liters of blood, depending on body size. Staying hydrated supports healthy blood volume and circulation.

11. Fasting Blood Glucose: 70-99 mg/dL
- Normal fasting blood sugar is 70-99 mg/dL. Levels of 100-125 mg/dL indicate prediabetes, and 126 mg/dL or higher may suggest diabetes. Regular screening is vital, especially if you have a family history or service-related risk factors.

12. Serum Iron: 60-170 mcg/dL
- Iron levels reflect your body's ability to produce red blood cells. For dietary intake, men need about 8 mg/day, while women of reproductive age need 18 mg/day. Low iron can lead to fatigue, a common complaint among veterans.

13. White Blood Cells (WBC): 4,000-11,000 per microliter
- A normal WBC count helps your body fight infections. Abnormal levels may indicate an underlying issue, such as an infection or immune system concern.

14. Platelets: 150,000-450,000 per microliter
- Platelets are essential for blood clotting. If you're on blood thinners or have a history of injury, monitoring platelet levels is important.

15. Red Blood Cells (RBC):
  - Men: 4.5-5.9 million per microliter
  - Women: 4.1-5.1 million per microliter
- RBCs carry oxygen throughout your body. Low counts can lead to fatigue or shortness of breath.

16. Calcium: 8.6-10.3 mg/dL
- Calcium supports bone health, which is critical for veterans who may have experienced physical strain during service. Low levels can also affect muscle function.

17. Vitamin D (25-hydroxyvitamin D): 20-50 ng/mL (30-50 ng/mL optimal)

- Vitamin D is essential for bone health, mood, and immune function. Many veterans, especially those with limited sun exposure, may need supplements to maintain optimal levels.

18. Vitamin B12: 200-900 pg/mL

- Vitamin B12 supports nerve health and energy production. Deficiency can cause fatigue or neurological symptoms, which may be mistaken for other conditions like PTSD.

Bottom Line

These numbers provide a general benchmark for health, but your personal "normal" may differ based on your age, medical history, or service-related conditions. For example, veterans exposed to burn pits or other environmental hazards may need more frequent monitoring of respiratory or blood metrics. Work closely with your VA healthcare provider to establish a baseline for your health and address any concerns. Regular checkups, a balanced diet, physical activity, and mental health support are all part of a holistic approach to wellness after service.

Liver and Gallbladder Cleanse

A detoxification program designed to cleanse the liver and gallbladder of accumulated toxins and waste products, liver and gallbladder cleansing was popularized by Andreas Moritz in his book, <u>The Liver and Gallbladder Miracle Cleanse: An All-Natural, At-Home Flush to Purify and Rejuvenate Your Body</u>.

The liver and gallbladder cleanse involves drinking a mixture of olive oil and lemon juice on an empty stomach, followed by a series of flushes and dietary changes. The main idea behind this cleanse is that the olive oil and lemon juice will help to loosen and flush out accumulated waste products, including gallstones, from the liver and gallbladder. (Note: A detailed account of the 2-day cleanse may be found in **Annex E—Alternate Approaches**)

While the Liver and Gallbladder Miracle Cleanse has been promoted as a safe and effective way to detoxify the liver and gallbladder, it should be noted that there is limited scientific evidence to support these claims. Additionally, the cleanse involves drinking large amounts of oil and salt, which can be dangerous and have potential side effects such as nausea, diarrhea and dehydration.

Furthermore, the cleanse can also cause the release of gallstones, which can lead to blockages in the bile ducts or other complications. It is important to consult a healthcare professional before attempting this cleanse, especially if you have any underlying health conditions or are taking any medications.

Bottom Line
The Liver and Gallbladder Miracle Cleanse is a popular detoxification program that claims to cleanse the liver and gallbladder of accumulated toxins and waste products. While it may offer some benefits, it is important to understand the potential risks and side effects of this cleanse and to consult a healthcare professional before attempting it.

Loneliness

Loneliness is a feeling of isolation and disconnection from others and it is a growing concern in modern society. With technology and social media being prevalent in people's lives, many people are feeling increasingly lonely despite being more connected than ever. Loneliness can have a profound impact on mental and physical health, leading to depression, anxiety and even chronic health problems such as heart disease and stroke.

Fortunately, there are several strategies that people can use to mitigate loneliness and improve their overall well-being. Here are some of the most effective ways to combat loneliness:

- **_Connect with others:_** One of the best ways to combat loneliness is to connect with others. This can be done through social activities, volunteer work, joining clubs or groups with shared interests or simply reaching out to friends and family members. The key is to make an effort to connect with people on a regular basis, even if it feels uncomfortable at first.

- **_Get physical:_** Exercise is a powerful way to reduce loneliness. It increases endorphins, the feel-good chemicals in the brain and it also provides opportunities to connect with others. Whether it's joining a gym, participating in a sport or simply going for a walk, physical activity can help people feel more connected and less isolated.

- **_Volunteer:_** Volunteering is a great way to meet new people and connect with others who share similar values and interests. Whether it's helping at a local food bank, volunteering at a pet shelter or participating in a community cleanup effort, volunteering can provide a sense of purpose and fulfillment that can help combat loneliness.

- **_Take up a new hobby:_** Trying new things and exploring new interests can help people feel more connected to others and less isolated. Whether it's learning a new language, taking up photography or joining a local book club, taking up a new hobby can provide a sense of accomplishment and help people form new relationships.

- **_Use technology wisely:_** While technology and social media can contribute to feelings of loneliness, they can also be a valuable tool for connecting with others. Joining online forums, participating in social media groups and using video conferencing to connect with friends and family members can help people feel more connected and less isolated.

- **_Seek professional help:_** If loneliness is affecting mental health, it may be necessary to seek professional help. A therapist or counselor can help people identify the root causes of their loneliness and develop strategies to manage it. In some cases, medication may also be recommended to help manage depression and anxiety.

• **Practice self-care:** Taking care of oneself is important for overall well-being and it can also help reduce feelings of loneliness. Engaging in activities such as reading, journaling, meditating or simply taking a relaxing bath can help people feel more connected to themselves and less isolated.

Bottom Line

Loneliness is a common feeling that can have a profound impact on mental and physical health. By connecting with others, engaging in physical activity, volunteering, taking up new hobbies, using technology wisely, seeking professional help and practicing self-care, people can reduce feelings of loneliness and improve overall well-being. Loneliness is a growing concern in modern society, but it is a problem that can be effectively addressed.

Lyme Disease

Lyme disease is a bacterial infection caused by the bacterium *Borrelia burgdorferi* in North America and parts of Europe and is transmitted to humans through the bite of infected black-legged ticks. The disease is prevalent in certain regions of the United States, Europe and Asia and is a growing concern for people who enjoy outdoor activities. Other subspecies of *Borrelia* bacteria cause the disease as well in Europe and Asia.[10]

• **Diagnosis:** The early stages of Lyme disease can present as a flu-like illness with symptoms like fever, headache, fatigue, muscle and joint aches and swollen lymph nodes. The hallmark of the disease is a bull's eye rash that appears at the site of the tick bite, which is called *erythema migrans* (EM) rash. However, not everyone with Lyme disease develops a rash and many of the symptoms can be vague and non-specific, making it difficult to diagnose the disease. In such cases, a doctor may rely on a patient's history of exposure to infected ticks, presence of EM rash or other physical symptoms and laboratory testing.

• **Laboratory Testing:** The diagnosis of Lyme disease typically starts with a blood test, which can detect antibodies to the *Borrelia* bacteria. There are two types of blood tests used to diagnose Lyme disease:

   • **Enzyme-linked immunosorbent assay (ELISA):** This is a screening test that is used to detect the presence of antibodies to the Lyme disease bacteria in a patient's blood.

   • **Western blot test:** This test is used to confirm the results of an ELISA test. It is more specific and can distinguish between different strains of the Lyme disease bacterium.

These tests are not perfect and can sometimes produce false negative results, especially in the early stages of the disease. A negative test result does not rule out Lyme disease and a doctor may need to consider other factors when making a diagnosis.

• **Treatment:** Lyme disease is treatable with antibiotics and early treatment is essential to prevent the progression of the disease and reduce the risk of long-term complications.

> • The most commonly used antibiotics for Lyme disease include doxycycline, amoxicillin, ceftriaxone and cefuroxime. The choice of antibiotics and the duration of treatment will depend on the stage and severity of the disease, the location of the infection and the patient's age and overall health.[11]

> • Early localized Lyme disease: This stage of the disease is characterized by the presence of a bull's eye rash and symptoms like fever, headache, fatigue, muscle and joint aches and swollen lymph nodes. The disease can be treated with a 2-4 week course of antibiotics, which can be taken orally.

> • Early disseminated Lyme disease: This stage of the disease is characterized by the spread of the bacterium to other parts of the body, such as the heart, nervous system and joints. The disease can be treated with a 2-4 week course of antibiotics, which can be taken orally or intravenously.

> • Late Lyme disease: This stage of the disease is characterized by persistent symptoms like fatigue, muscle and joint aches and neurological problems. The disease can be treated with a longer course of antibiotics, which can be taken orally or intravenously.

In some cases, the symptoms of Lyme disease may persist even after treatment with antibiotics. This is referred to as post-treatment Lyme disease syndrome (PTLDS) and the cause is not well understood. Treatment options for PTLDS may include pain relievers, physical therapy and cognitive behavioral therapy.

It is important for individuals who live in or visit areas where Lyme disease is common to take precautions to reduce the risk of tick bites such as wearing protective clothing, using insect repellent and conducting regular tick checks. If you develop symptoms of Lyme disease, see a doctor immediately for a thorough evaluation and appropriate treatment.

In addition, it is important for individuals to educate themselves about Lyme disease and its symptoms, as well as to communicate any concerns or questions with their healthcare provider. With proper awareness and treatment, Lyme disease can be effectively managed and the risk of long-term complications can be reduced.

Bottom Line
Lyme disease is a growing concern for people who enjoy outdoor activities and is a potentially serious condition that can cause long-term health problems if left untreated. The key to successful treatment is early diagnosis and prompt initiation of appropriate antibiotics. However, the symptoms of Lyme disease can be non-specific and may not develop immediately after the tick bite, making it difficult to diagnose the disease.

Lymph Detox

Veterans carry the load of service—toxins from burn pits, fatigue from long hauls, inflammation from old wounds. Lymph detox steps in as a quiet ally, tuning up the body's waste-clearing system—vessels and nodes that sweep out junk and bolster your fight. It's not a doc's fix for swollen limbs—it's a hands-on wellness play, using moves, chow, or rubs to keep things flowing. For vets wrestling post-service wear—pain that lingers, energy that's gone, or a system bogged down—it's a way to feel lighter and tougher. This section breaks down why lymph detox matters, what it offers, and how to work it, all with a vet's resolve.

Understanding Lymph Detox
Lymph detox means nudging your lymphatic system—think pipes and filters under your skin—to clear waste, fluids, and muck that pile up. It's not a pill or a cure—just daily or weekly habits like brushing, walking, or eating right to keep it moving. For Veterans, it's a low-key shot at shaking off the sludge of deployment stress, inactivity, or field grit, a wellness boost rooted in old healing ways and new health hacks.

The Science Behind It
Your lymph's a cleanup crew—hauling out trash and guarding against bugs, but it needs a push; it doesn't pump on its own. Stress, scars, or toxins can clog it, leaving you puffy or worn. Detox tricks—motion, pressure, water—kick it into gear, easing the load. For vets, it's less about lab charts and more about feel—does it cut the drag, lift the haze? Science nods at the basics—movement and rubs help flow—but the big detox talk's more hope than hard fact.

The Impact of Lymph Detox on Veterans' Health
- Wellness Benefits: It's pitched to shrink swelling, sharpen immunity, boost juice—stuff vets need when the body's beat and the fight's still on.

- Consequences of Skipping It: Ignore it, and bloat, weakness, or fog settle in—extra weight on a frame built to roll.

Identifying and Analyzing Your Load
- Self-Assessment: Scope your sitrep—what's heavy? Legs puffed from old injuries? Tired from who-knows-what? Sick too often? List it—know your red zone.

- Setting Priorities: Rank the hits—swelling if you're stiff, energy if you're flat, immunity if you're down. Start where it's loudest; the rest lines up.

Fostering the Lymph Detox Habit
- Set Goals: Keep it tight—e.g., "Brush or walk 10 minutes daily this week to feel lighter." Clear, like a range call—aim, fire.

- Building a Support System: Tell a vet pal or VA doc you're on it—they've got your six, keeping you steady when you start.

Implementation Strategies
- Daily Integration: Slot it in—morning rub, evening stroll. Start easy; steady beats a sprint, like pacing a hump.

- Habit Stacking: Pair it with routine—brush with coffee, walk post-chow. Ties it to what's locked in, keeps it real.

Targeted Protocols for Veterans' Wellness
Here's how to run lymph detox for specific needs, with supplies for each—vet-ready, no fluff:

1. Reduced Swelling
- What: Dry brush 5–10 minutes daily or massage 15 minutes thrice weekly.

- Why: Puffy hands or feet from scars or stress? It nudges fluid out—eases a vet's frame.

- How: Grab a brush ($10–$30), sweep up from toes to chest, light and firm, 5 minutes daily. Or hands-on—stroke toward your heart, 15 minutes, three days. Feel looser in a week—too rough? Soften it.

- Supplies Needed: Brush or hands, quiet spot, shower after.

2. Improved Immunity
- What: Rebound or walk 20–30 minutes, 3–5 times weekly.

- Why: Colds hitting hard post-service? Pumping lymph might toughen your guard—keeps a vet in the fight.

- How: Bounce on a trampoline ($50–$100) or stride out—30 minutes, three days. Sweat it up—sick less in weeks? If it's flat, up the pace.

- Supplies Needed: Shoes or mini-trampoline, open space, water.

3. Increased Energy
- What: Hydrate with 8–12 cups water daily, brush 5 minutes, 3 times weekly.

- Why: Dragging from field wear? Clearing muck could lift you—puts gas back in a vet's tank.

- How: Sip water all day—greens or citrus if you can—brush light, 5 minutes, three days. Perk up in a week—still beat? Add a walk.

- Supplies Needed: Water bottle, brush, fruit stash.

4. Detoxification Support
- What: Walk 30 minutes daily, breathe deep 10 minutes, 3 times weekly.

- Why: Burn pit crud sticking around? Moving lymph might flush it—lightens a vet's load.

- How: Step out—30 minutes steady—then sit, breathe slow (5-5-5), 10 minutes, three days. Cleaner feel in weeks—too much? Ease off breath.

- Supplies Needed: Shoes, quiet nook, timer (optional).

5. Stress Relief
- What: Massage self 15–30 minutes or pro ($50–$100), weekly.

- Why: Transition buzz frying you? Lymph flow might calm it—steadies a vet's nerves.

- How: Rub up from feet to neck, light, 15 minutes weekly—or book a pro. Tension drop in days—too sore? Go gentler.

- Supplies Needed: Hands or clinic cash, calm space.

Eliminating Barriers to Detox
- Identify Triggers: Spot what stalls you—"Too weird," "No juice," "No proof." Name it—then square it up.

- Replace Hesitation: Swap "Later" for "Ten minutes now"—quick hit, done. Trade doubt for "What's it shift?"—try, judge.

- Veteran-Specific Substitutes:

  - Skepticism: Swap "Hocus-pocus" for "Field tune"—frame it as upkeep, vet-style.

  - Fatigue: Trade "Too tired" for "Light lift"—start small, build it.

Mindfulness and Self-Regulation
- Techniques: Focus on the move—feel the brush, count the breaths. It's your anchor, cutting "it's bunk" noise. Vets know focus—lock it here.

- Benefits: You'll spot when you're bogged—cue the flow. Awareness keeps you in command, steering your frame.

Seeking Professional Help
- When Needed: Swelling's bad or heart's off? Hit your VA doc—detox's gentle, but not for every scar.

- Resources: VA physio, primary care, telehealth—free, vet-ready, they'll clear or tweak it.

Maintaining and Sustaining the Practice
- Track Progress: Log the wins—less puff, more pep? Mark it: "Brushed, felt light."

- Overcome Plateaus: No shift? Up the minutes or mix moves—push like a stalled op.

- Build Resilience: Each flow's a brick—stack 'em, and you're tougher, shedding what slows you.

Bottom Line
Lymph detox offers vets a quiet boost—easing swelling, sharpening immunity, lifting energy, flushing junk, calming stress—through rubs, brushes, walks, water, or breath. For warriors hauling pain, fatigue, or field grit, it's a hands-on play to feel steadier, rooted in old cures and wellness smarts. Some swear it—lightens the load, perks you up; science sees bits—flow and swelling shift—but big detox claims lean on feel over facts. Risks? Overdo it, and you're sore—watch it if you're beat up. It's no cure—pros say back it with care—so check your VA doc if you're dicey, start free with walks or breath, add a brush ($10–$30) if it fits. Simple, steady, it's a tool in your kit—use it smart and calm.

- M -

Macronutrients and Micronutrients

Both are essential for maintaining good health, but they serve different purposes.

Macronutrients are the nutrients that the body needs in large amounts to function properly. They include carbohydrates, proteins and fats. Carbohydrates are the body's main source of energy and they are found in foods such as grains, fruits and vegetables. Proteins are essential for the growth and repair of tissues and they are found in foods such as meat, fish, eggs and dairy products. Fats are also important for energy and for the absorption of certain vitamins and minerals. They are found in foods such as oils, nuts and avocados.

Micronutrients are the nutrients that the body needs in smaller amounts. These include vitamins and minerals. Vitamins are essential for the proper functioning of the body's metabolism and for maintaining good health. They include Vitamin A, Vitamin C, Vitamin D, Vitamin E and Vitamin K. Minerals are also essential for maintaining good health and are important for the proper functioning of the body's metabolism. They include calcium, iron, zinc and iodine.

A balanced diet should include a combination of macronutrients and micronutrients. The specific macronutrient ratios that are right for you will depend on your age, sex, body composition and physical activity level. In general, a balanced diet should include:

45-65% of your calories from carbohydrates

10-35% of your calories from proteins

20-35% of your calories from fats

It is also important to consume a variety of micronutrients to ensure that you are getting all the vitamins and minerals your body needs. This can be done by eating a variety of fruits, vegetables, whole grains, lean proteins and healthy fats.

Consuming too much or too little of certain macronutrients can have negative effects on health. For example, consuming too many carbohydrates can lead to weight gain, while consuming too little protein can lead to muscle loss. Similarly, consuming too much or too little of certain micronutrients can also have negative effects on health. For example, consuming too little iron can lead to anemia, while consuming too much Vitamin A can lead to liver damage.

Here are some strategies for ensuring that you are getting the proper balance of macronutrients and micronutrients in your diet:

• ***Consult with a registered dietitian or a nutritionist:*** They can help you determine the specific macronutrients and micronutrients for your individual needs and goals and create a personalized meal plan.

• ***Focus on whole, unprocessed foods:*** Whole, unprocessed foods are typically more nutrient-dense than processed foods. Examples include fruits, vegetables, whole grains, lean proteins and healthy fats. Often times, supermarkets are laid out with the whole, unprocessed foods located around the edges of the store and the processed foods—typically prepackaged meals and foods with preservatives and additives—located towards the center of the store.[12]

• ***Incorporate a variety of protein sources:*** Consuming a variety of protein sources can help ensure that you are getting all the essential amino acids your body needs. Examples include meat, fish, poultry, eggs, beans and lentils.

• ***Include healthy fats in your diet:*** Healthy fats such as those found in nuts, seeds, avocados and olive oil, are important for absorption of certain vitamins and minerals, as well as for heart health.

• ***Eat a variety of fruits and vegetables:*** Fruits and vegetables are excellent sources of vitamins and minerals and eating a variety can help ensure that you are getting a wide range of micronutrients.

• ***Choose whole grains over refined grains:*** Whole grains are a good source of fiber and other important nutrients, while refined grains are often stripped of many important nutrients.

• ***Limit processed and sugary foods:*** Processed and sugary foods are often high in added sugars and lack important nutrients. It is best to limit these foods in your diet.

• ***Take a multivitamin:*** Taking a multivitamin can help fill any nutrient gaps in your diet. However, it's always best to consult with a healthcare professional before starting any supplement.

• ***Cook and prepare your own meals as much as possible:*** By cooking your own meals, you have more control over the ingredients and can make sure that you are getting the proper balance of macronutrients and micronutrients.

Bottom Line:
There are many strategies for ensuring that you are getting the proper balance of

macronutrients and micronutrients in your diet. It's important to consult with a registered dietitian or nutritionist, focus on whole, unprocessed foods, incorporate a variety of protein sources, include healthy fats, eat a variety of fruits and vegetables, choose whole grains over refined grains, limit processed and sugary foods, take a multivitamin and cook and prepare your own meals as much as possible. These strategies will help you to achieve a healthy and balanced diet. Macronutrients and micronutrients are both essential for maintaining good health. Macronutrients provide the body with the energy it needs to function properly, while micronutrients are important for the proper functioning of the body's metabolism and maintaining good health. A balanced diet should include a combination of macronutrients and micronutrients and it is important to consume a variety of foods to ensure that you are getting all the nutrients your body needs. It's also important to avoid consuming too much or too little of certain macronutrients and micronutrients to prevent negative effects on health.

Magnetic e-Resonance Therapy

Otherwise known as MeRT, it is a cutting-edge therapy that uses magnetic fields to target specific areas of the brain. The therapy has been found to be highly effective in treating a wide range of conditions, including post-traumatic stress disorder (PTSD), traumatic brain injuries (TBIs) and depression.

Traditional therapies, such as medication and talk therapy, can be effective in treating certain conditions but they often have a broad effect on the brain and can have unintended side effects. MeRT, on the other hand, uses magnetic fields to specifically target areas of the brain that are associated with specific conditions, such as the hippocampus for memory and the amygdala for fear and anxiety. This allows for highly targeted treatment that is less likely to have unintended side effects.

MeRT is also non-invasive and does not require the use of drugs. This makes it a safe and effective alternative to traditional therapies. MeRT is also a relatively quick treatment, taking only 30-40 minutes per session. This makes it an ideal treatment option for Veterans who may have limited time and resources.

MeRT has been found to be particularly effective in treating PTSD, a condition that affects many Veterans. PTSD is characterized by a wide range of symptoms, including flashbacks, nightmares and avoidance behaviors. Traditional therapies for PTSD, such as talk therapy and medication, can be effective but they can also take a long time to work. MeRT, on the other hand, has been found to have a rapid effect on PTSD symptoms, often providing significant improvement after just a few sessions.

MeRT has also been found to be effective in treating TBIs, which are common among Veterans. TBIs can cause a wide range of symptoms, including memory loss, difficulty concentrating and mood swings. MeRT has been found to be particularly effective in improving memory and concentration, which can greatly improve quality of life for Veterans with TBIs.

MeRT has also been found to be effective in treating depression, which is a common condition among Veterans. Depression can be caused by a wide range of factors, including PTSD, TBIs and the stress of combat. MeRT has been found to be particularly effective in treating depression that is associated with PTSD and TBIs, providing Veterans with a much-needed alternative to traditional antidepressants.

Application of the Magnetic e-Resonance Therapy to Veterans

This typically involves a series of treatment sessions that are tailored to the individual's specific needs.

The first step in the process is a thorough evaluation by a qualified healthcare professional, such as a neurologist or psychiatrist. This evaluation will typically include a review of the Veteran's medical history, as well as a physical and cognitive examination. The healthcare professional will also assess the Veteran's symptoms and determine which areas of the brain are most likely to be affected by the condition being treated.

Based on the results of the evaluation, a treatment plan will be developed. This will typically include a series of MeRT sessions, which will be administered by a trained technician. The sessions will typically last between 30-40 minutes and will be administered on a regular basis, usually several times a week. The number of sessions required will depend on the individual's condition and response to treatment.

During the MeRT session, the Veteran will be seated in a chair and will be fitted with a helmet that contains the magnetic coils. The magnetic field will then be directed at the specific areas of the brain that have been identified as being involved in the Veteran's condition. The Veteran will not feel any pain or discomfort during the session and will typically be able to return to their normal activities immediately afterwards.

MeRT is generally considered to be a safe and well-tolerated treatment, with few side effects. Some Veterans may experience a mild headache or dizziness following a session, but these symptoms are typically short-lived and can be easily managed with over-the-counter pain medication.

It is important to note that MeRT should be used in conjunction with other therapies, such as talk therapy, medication and rehabilitation. The MeRT treatment is not a replacement for other treatments that might be required for the Veterans condition.

Bottom Line
MeRT is a cutting-edge therapy that offers a wide range of benefits for Veterans, particularly those suffering from PTSD, TBIs and depression. It is non-invasive, does not require the use of drugs and is highly effective in targeting specific areas of the brain. With MeRT, Veterans can see rapid improvement in their symptoms, which can greatly improve their quality of life. It is a promising therapy that should be considered as a treatment option for Veterans.

MDMA

Veterans know the unseen wounds—PTSD that grips like a vice, depression that dims the light, a rift from the world that grows wider with time. MDMA, born in a lab over a century ago, isn't the rave pill of old tales—it's a deliberate tool, paired with therapy, to crack open what's sealed shut. It stirs empathy, softens fear, and pulls you into the moment, offering a way to face what's buried without breaking. For vets carrying trauma's weight, a shadowed mood, or the ache of isolation post-service, it's a guided path to mend, not a reckless high. This section lays out what MDMA brings, why it resonates with warriors, and how to approach it, all with a vet's steady gaze.

Understanding MDMA
MDMA—3,4-methylenedioxymethamphetamine—started as a chemist's experiment in 1912, later finding its place in therapy before the law locked it down. It's a synthetic compound that floods your system with serotonin, dopamine, and oxytocin, sparking connection and clarity for 3–6 hours per dose. In a clinic, it's a capsule swallowed under watchful eyes, not a street snort or party mix. For Veterans, it's less about the buzz and more about the breakthrough—a chance to process combat's toll or life's drift with a pro steering the wheel, distinct from the wild trips of psychedelics like LSD.

The Science Behind It
Your mind's a locked bunker—MDMA hands you the key. It quiets the fear center, lifts the chemical tide, and lets you sit with pain or loss without the flinch. It's not just feeling good—it's seeing clear, talking straight, rewiring what service or its aftermath bent out of shape. For vets, it's a shot at cutting through trauma's static or

isolation's chill, a tool science is proving out—trials show it shifts the headspace, steadies the heart—but only when guided right, with risks you can't ignore.

The Impact of MDMA on Veterans' Health
- Wellness Benefits: It's pitched to unravel trauma, brighten mood, weave bonds—gains vets chase when the past haunts or the present fades.

- Consequences of Missing It: Skip it, and the echoes, gloom, or distance hold fast—burdens a warrior doesn't need to shoulder alone.

Identifying and Analyzing Your Struggles
- Self-Assessment: Take a hard look—what's weighing you? Night terrors from the field? A heavy gray that won't shift? A wall between you and yours? Write it down—name your enemy.

- Setting Priorities: Sort the load—trauma if it's screaming, mood if it's crushing, connection if you're cut off. Hit the deepest first; the rest falls in line.

Fostering the MDMA Approach
- Set Goals: Make it real—e.g., "Pursue MDMA therapy this year to quiet the noise." Sharp, like a mission brief—lock, load.

- Building a Support System: Bring in your VA doc, a vet brother, or a clinic crew—they've got your back, keeping you grounded through the ride.

Implementation Strategies
- Therapy Focus: This isn't a weekend fling—plan 2–3 sessions over months, guided by pros, not a solo run. Space it like a long patrol, deliberate and paced.

- Habit Stacking: Link it to your recovery—after a therapy stretch, before a deep talk. Fits it into your fight, keeps it steady.

Targeted Protocols for Veterans' Wellness
For trauma, MDMA's your sit-down with the past—80–125 mg swallowed in a quiet room, two therapists at your side, talking you through 6–8 hours of raw truth. You'll face the sandbox ghosts or convoy blasts, fear dialed down, trust dialed up, repeating twice over a few months. It's not about forgetting—it's about filing it right, letting the weight ease off your chest. If it stirs too much, the follow-ups catch you.

When the gray's got you—depression or anxiety choking the days—MDMA lifts it slow. Start with 80 mg, a booster of 40 mg a couple hours in, guided over two sessions weeks apart. You'll feel the haze thin, the buzz soften, talking it out with pros who know the terrain. It's a reset, not a cure—check in after if the dark creeps back.

If you're cut off—family, squad, or just the world feeling miles away—MDMA rebuilds the bridge. One 100 mg dose, 6 hours with a team, opens the gates; you'll feel the walls drop, words flow, trust grow. One session might shift it—closer ties in days—but lean on a vet pal after to hold it.

For resilience, when the cracks show, it's two 120 mg hits, 3–5 weeks apart. You'll sift the hurt with pros, reframing it into something you can carry, tougher each time. It's building armor, not dodging blows—talk it solid after, scale back if it's too loud.

Addiction's pull—booze or pills—gets a crack with one 100 mg session. You'll feel the crave fade under guidance, clarity cutting through, weekly talks to lock it in. It's a hand up, not a free pass—hit support hard if the itch returns.

Eliminating Barriers to Use
- Identify Triggers: Pin what stops you—"Too dangerous," "Can't get it," "Not my way." Call it out—then weigh it straight.

- Replace Hesitation: Shift "Not yet" to "One move now"—scout it like a new LZ. Trade doubt for "What's it fix?"—judge, act.

- Veteran-Specific Substitutes:

  - Risk: Swap "I'll crash" for "Guides hold it"—trust the pros, like a squad's got you.

  - Access: Trade "It's locked" for "Trials open"—find the lane, vet-style.

Mindfulness and Self-Regulation
- Techniques: Prep with purpose—breathe deep (5-5-5), set your aim: "See it clear." After, ground with talk or silence. Keeps you steady, not spinning.

- Benefits: You'll spot when you're sinking—signal the shift. Awareness is your steel, vet-forged.

Seeking Professional Help
- When Needed: Ticker's off or mind's frayed? Hit your VA doc—MDMA's no game for the shaky.

- Resources: VA mental health, MAPS trials, legal retreats—vet-ready, they'll green-light or wave off.

Maintaining and Sustaining the Gains
- Track Progress: Note the lift—trauma softer, ties tighter? Log it: "Faced it, felt it."

- Overcome Plateaus: Stall out? Deepen the talks or lean on routine—push like a bogged-down march.

- Build Resilience: Each step's a brick—stack 'em, and you're tougher, past the old breaks.

Bottom Line
MDMA hands vets a real shot—unpacking trauma, chasing gloom, mending bonds, forging grit, loosening cravings—through a few guided doses (80–125 mg) with therapy, not street chaos. For warriors hauling PTSD, depression, or drift, it's a deep play to heal, born from lab roots and clinic care, opening what's clamped shut. Some call it a game-changer—shifts the fight; science proves it—trials show relief—but it's the pro hands that make it hold, with risks like heart strain or burn-out you can't shrug off. It's no solo fix—docs say tie it tight to oversight—so hit your VA crew, chase trials (free–$500) or retreats ($2,000–$5,000), and root it in your fight. Strong, guided, it's a tool in your kit—use it steady and sure.

Meditation

Meditation is a practice that involves sitting quietly and focusing the mind on a particular object, thought or activity to increase awareness and achieve a mentally clear and emotionally calm state. Meditation has been practiced for thousands of years in different cultures and traditions and has been found to have a wide range of benefits for both the mind and body.

- **Stress reduction:** One of the most well-known benefits of meditation is its ability to reduce stress and anxiety. Regular meditation can help to decrease the activity of the body's stress response, which can lead to a reduction in symptoms of anxiety and stress.

- **Improved focus and concentration:** By training the mind to focus on one thing at a time, meditation can help to improve attention span and concentration, which can be beneficial for both personal and professional life.

- **Increased emotional regulation:** By training the mind to be more aware of emotions and how to manage them, meditation can help to reduce emotional reactivity and increase emotional resilience.

- **Improved sleep:** By reducing stress and anxiety and promoting relaxation, meditation can help to improve the quality of sleep and reduce symptoms of insomnia.

- **Improved immune function:** Meditation may also have a positive impact on the immune system. Studies have found that regular meditation can increase the activity of natural killer cells, which are important for fighting off infections and cancer cells.

- **Decreased blood pressure:** Regular meditation practice may also lead to a decrease in blood pressure, which can reduce the risk of heart disease and stroke.

- **Improved overall well-being:** By reducing stress, improving focus and increasing emotional regulation, meditation can help to improve overall happiness and satisfaction with life.

It's important to note that meditation is not a one-size-fits-all practice and different techniques may be more effective for different people. Additionally, it's best to start with short sessions, gradually increasing the duration of the practice as you become more comfortable with it. Furthermore, it's important to find a quiet and comfortable place to meditate and to not be discouraged if your mind wanders, it's a normal part of the process.

Bottom Line

Meditation is an ancient practice that can have a wide range of benefits for both the mind and body. It can help to reduce stress and anxiety, improve focus and concentration, increase emotional regulation, improve sleep and improve overall well-being. It's important to find a technique that works best for you and to start with short sessions and gradually increase the duration. Find a quiet and comfortable place to meditate and do not be discouraged if your mind wanders, it's a normal part of the process.

Mental Health

Maintaining good mental health is essential for overall well-being. Here are some benefits of mental health maintenance:

- **Improved mood:** Regularly maintaining good mental health can help to improve mood, reduce feelings of depression and anxiety and increase overall well-being.

- **Increased resilience:** Taking care of mental health can help to increase resilience in the face of stress and adversity.

- **Increased productivity:** Maintaining good mental health can help to improve focus, concentration and productivity in work and other areas of life.

• **Stronger relationships:** Good mental health can help to improve communication, empathy and emotional intelligence, resulting in stronger relationships with others.

• **Improved physical health:** Maintaining good mental health can help to improve physical health by reducing the risk of chronic diseases such as obesity, diabetes and heart disease.

• **Increased creativity and problem-solving:** Maintaining good mental health can help to boost creativity, improve problem-solving skills and enhance decision-making abilities.

• **Better sleep:** Good mental health can help to promote better sleep by reducing stress and anxiety.

Regularly maintaining good mental health can help to increase self-awareness and self-esteem, which can lead to more fulfilling and satisfying relationships and experiences. Maintaining good mental health is a continuous process that involves self-care and self-awareness and it's different for everyone. Some ways to maintain good mental health include getting enough sleep, eating a healthy diet, exercise, developing healthy relationships, setting boundaries and seeking professional help if necessary.

Jordan Peterson, a clinical psychologist and bestselling author, has written extensively about the importance of addressing mental health needs. According to Peterson, mental health is not just about the absence of mental illness, but about achieving a state of well-being and fulfillment.

Peterson argues that addressing mental health needs is crucial for individuals to be able to take control of their lives and achieve their goals. He emphasizes the importance of taking responsibility for one's own mental health and taking action to improve it.

One key aspect of addressing mental health needs, according to Peterson, is addressing negative thoughts and emotions. He suggests using techniques such as cognitive-behavioral therapy to challenge and change negative thought patterns. Peterson also emphasizes the importance of setting and working towards goals, as well as developing a sense of purpose and meaning in life. He suggests that by setting goals and working towards them, individuals are able to take control of their lives and improve their mental well-being.

Another important aspect of addressing mental health needs is developing healthy habits and routines. Peterson suggests taking care of one's physical health through regular exercise, eating a healthy diet and getting enough sleep. He also suggests developing a regular meditation practice to help reduce stress and anxiety.

Peterson also emphasizes the importance of connecting with others and building a support system. He suggests seeking out friends and family, as well as professional help if necessary.

Here is a suggested routine for maintaining good mental health:

- Wake up at the same time every day and establish a regular sleep schedule.

- Start the day with a healthy breakfast and make sure to eat regularly throughout the day.

- Engage in regular physical activity, such as going for a walk or run or doing a workout at home or gym.

- Practice mindfulness and meditation techniques, such as deep breathing or yoga, to reduce stress and anxiety.

- Make time for hobbies or activities that you enjoy, such as reading, writing or playing an instrument.

- Connect with friends and family, whether through phone calls, text messages or social media, to build a support system.

- Try to avoid excessive use of electronic devices before bedtime, establish a bedtime routine and create a comfortable sleeping environment.

- Seek professional help if necessary, such as counseling or therapy, if you are experiencing symptoms of mental illness or distress.

Review your progress regularly and adapt the routine as needed. It's important to keep in mind that maintaining good mental health is a continuous process and it's different for everyone. It's important to find what works best for you and to be patient and kind to yourself. It's also important to remember that seeking professional help is a sign of strength.

Properly dealing with life's challenges

Life is full of challenges and it's important to have strategies in place for dealing with them effectively. Here are some suggestions for properly dealing with life's challenges:

- ***Identify and acknowledge the problem:*** The first step in dealing with a challenge is to identify and acknowledge it. Take the time to understand the problem and what is causing it.

- **Develop a plan of action:** Once you have identified the problem, develop a plan of action to address it. Break the problem down into smaller, manageable steps and set specific, achievable goals.
- **Take action:** It's important to take action, rather than just thinking about the problem. Take the steps necessary to address the problem and work towards your goals.

- **Practice self-care:** Taking care of yourself is important during times of stress. Make sure to get enough sleep, eat a healthy diet and engage in regular physical activity.

- **Seek support:** Don't be afraid to reach out for help if you need it. Talk to friends and family or seek professional help if necessary.

- **Learn from the experience:** Life's challenges can provide valuable learning opportunities. Reflect on the experience and try to identify any lessons that can be learned from it.

- **Be flexible:** Be open to different solutions and be willing to adapt your plan if it's not working.

- **Find a positive perspective:** Try to find a positive perspective on the situation, it can help you to feel more resilient and optimistic.

- **Have a sense of humor:** Laughing at yourself, life challenges and its craziness, can help you to feel less stressed and more in control. Remember that challenges are a normal part of life and it's important to be kind and patient with yourself. It's also important to keep in mind that you are not alone and that help is available.

Exercise and nutrition have a significant impact on mental health.

- **Exercise and physical activity:** Regular exercise has been shown to reduce symptoms of depression and anxiety, improve mood and overall well-being and help to increase self-esteem and self-confidence. Exercise also releases endorphins, which are chemicals in the brain that act as natural painkillers and mood elevators.

- **Nutrition:** Eating a balanced diet that is rich in fruits, vegetables and whole grains can help to support mental health by providing the body with the necessary nutrients to function properly. Studies have shown that a diet that is high in sugar, processed foods and saturated fats can increase the risk of depression and anxiety.
- **Combination of exercise and nutrition:** When exercise and nutrition are combined together, the results are even more powerful. Nutrition provides the fuel for the body to exercise, while exercise helps to improve the body's ability

262

to use that fuel effectively. This combination can help to improve mood, reduce symptoms of anxiety and depression and promote overall well-being.

• **Weight management:** Maintaining a healthy weight through regular exercise and a balanced diet can help to reduce the risk of developing weight-related conditions such as diabetes and heart disease, which in turn can improve mental health by reducing stress and anxiety.

Bottom Line

It is important to note that every individual is different and there is no one-size-fits-all solution for exercise and nutrition. It's important to consult with a professional nutritionist or a trainer to find the best approach that suits you and your goals. Additionally, it's important to remember that exercise and nutrition should be part of a holistic approach to mental health which includes therapy and medication if necessary.

Methylene Blue

A synthetic dye, Methylene Blue, that has gained attention for its potential therapeutic benefits in various fields including medicine and neuroscience. Recent research suggests that combining the activation of methylene blue with red light can enhance its effects and unlock additional benefits. This combination therapy holds promise in areas such as neuroprotection, cognitive enhancement and overall brain health.

• **Neuroprotection:** Methylene blue, when activated with red light, has shown promising neuroprotective effects. It has been found to help protect brain cells from damage, reduce oxidative stress and promote cellular energy production. These effects can potentially slow down the progression of neurodegenerative diseases such as Alzheimer's and Parkinson's.

• **Cognitive Enhancement:** Combining methylene blue with red light has been studied for its potential in enhancing cognitive function. Methylene blue has been shown to improve memory, attention and overall cognitive performance. When activated with red light, it may further enhance these effects by promoting neuroplasticity and synaptic activity in the brain.

• **Mitochondrial Function:** Mitochondria are responsible for producing cellular energy and their dysfunction is implicated in various diseases and aging. Activation of methylene blue with red light has been found to enhance mitochondrial activity and increase the production of adenosine triphosphate (ATP), the energy currency of cells.

• **Anti-inflammatory Effects:** Activation of methylene blue with red light has shown anti-inflammatory effects. It can help reduce inflammation in the body and alleviate symptoms associated with inflammatory conditions. By modulating the immune response, this combination therapy has the potential to improve overall health and reduce the risk of chronic diseases linked to inflammation.

• *Antioxidant Activity:* Methylene blue when activated with red light exhibits potent antioxidant activity. It helps neutralize harmful free radicals and reduce oxidative stress, which can damage cells and contribute to various diseases. This antioxidant effect is crucial for maintaining cellular health and protecting against age-related conditions.

• *Pain Relief:* Combining methylene blue with red light has shown potential in reducing pain and inflammation. This therapy can modulate pain pathways, decrease inflammatory markers and promote tissue healing. It has been explored for managing chronic pain conditions, musculoskeletal disorders and post-operative pain.

• *Skin Health:* Red light stimulates collagen production, improves skin elasticity and promotes wound healing. When combined with methylene blue, these effects can be enhanced, leading to improved skin appearance, reduced wrinkles and faster healing of wounds or skin conditions.

It's important to note that the combination therapy of methylene blue with red light is an emerging area of research and more studies are needed to fully understand its mechanisms and optimize its applications. The specific parameters, such as light intensity, duration and wavelength, need to be carefully calibrated to ensure safety and effectiveness.

In addition, it's recommended to consult with healthcare professionals or experts in the field before considering the use of methylene blue and red light activation for specific purposes. They can provide guidance on appropriate dosages, treatment protocols and potential interactions with other medications.

Bottom Line
The combination of methylene blue with red light activation holds great potential for a range of benefits, including neuroprotection, cognitive enhancement, mitochondrial function improvement, anti-inflammatory effects, antioxidant activity, pain relief and skin health. As research in this area continues to evolve, we can expect to uncover more about the mechanisms and applications of this promising therapy, ultimately leading to improved health outcomes in various domains.

Mindfulness

Mindfulness is the practice of being present and fully engaged in the current moment, without judgment. It is a simple yet powerful technique that can help to improve mental and physical well-being. Mindfulness can be practiced in many different ways, including through meditation, yoga and other mindful movement practices. It can also be practiced by focusing on the task at hand or on the conversation you may be having at the moment. Setting aside mobile devices, turning off the TV or radio, muting your phone and staying off the internet while working may all help when initially learning to be mindful in your actions and thoughts.

Self-care is the practice of taking care of one's own physical, emotional and mental well-being. It is important to prioritize self-care in order to maintain good health and overall well-being. Self-care practices can include things like getting enough sleep, eating a healthy diet, exercising regularly and taking time for relaxation and stress management. This may also include removing oneself from a toxic or unhealthy environment or relationship.

One of the most effective ways to practice mindfulness and self-care is through meditation. Meditation is a simple practice that can be done anywhere and at any time and it can help to reduce stress, improve focus and promote a sense of calm and inner peace. There are many different types of meditation, including mindfulness meditation, loving-kindness meditation and movement meditation.

Another effective way to practice mindfulness and self-care is through yoga. Yoga is a form of mindful movement that combines physical postures, breathing exercises and meditation. The practice of yoga can help to improve flexibility, strength and balance, as well as promoting relaxation and reducing stress.

Mindful movement practices such as tai chi and qigong are also effective ways to practice mindfulness and self-care. These practices focus on slow, flowing movements and deep breathing and they can help to improve balance and coordination, as well as promoting relaxation and reducing stress.

Self-care also includes taking care of your physical health. Eating a healthy diet, getting enough sleep and regular physical activity are all important aspects of self-care. Drinking enough water, avoid smoking, limit alcohol and caffeine intake and getting regular checkups and screenings can help you maintain a good physical health.

In addition to physical self-care, it is also important to take care of your emotional and mental well-being. This can include setting boundaries, developing healthy relationships and practicing self-compassion.

It is also important to make time for relaxation and stress management. This can include reading, listening to music, spending time in nature or engaging in a hobby.

Bottom Line
Mindfulness and self-care practices are essential for maintaining good health and overall well-being. Mindfulness can be practiced through meditation, yoga and other mindful movement practices and self-care can include things like getting enough sleep, eating a healthy diet, exercising regularly and taking time for relaxation and stress management. It is important to prioritize self-care in order to maintain good health and overall well-being.

Mold in the Body

Mold exposure affects Veterans through time spent in damp barracks, humid deployment zones, or near burn pits, where spores and mycotoxins—toxic byproducts of fungi—can enter the body via inhalation or ingestion. This isn't about cleaning a building; it's about addressing internal health effects, such as chronic fatigue, respiratory issues, or inflammation, that may persist after exposure. Veterans with unexplained symptoms post-service can use detection and removal methods to improve vitality. Detection involves recognizing symptoms and confirming with tests; removal includes detox, dietary changes, or medical treatment. Benefits claimed include symptom relief, increased energy, and reduced inflammation, supported by clinical observations and limited studies, though evidence for systemic mold illness remains debated, and risks like over-diagnosis are real.

Mold in the body refers to health problems from spores or mycotoxins, detected through persistent symptoms like fatigue, sinus congestion, or joint pain—common among Veterans—or via tests such as urine mycotoxin screens or blood antibody checks. Removal targets these effects with binders, antifungals, or lifestyle adjustments. Awareness of mold-related illness grew in the 1990s with "sick building syndrome," linked to damp environments, and expanded in the 2000s as mycotoxin research tied exposure to chronic conditions, though medical consensus is divided. Veterans face higher exposure risks from substandard housing or field conditions; a VA report noted many lived in water-damaged spaces, and burn pit exposure adds to the load.

Symptoms driving the need to remove mold include ongoing tiredness, brain fog, breathing difficulties, or aches—issues Veterans often report. These can signal mold effects, especially after time in mold-prone settings. Detection starts with tracking these signs, then moves to lab work. Urine mycotoxin tests from labs like

RealTime or Great Plains ($200–$400) measure toxins like ochratoxin; blood tests ($100–$300) check for immune responses to mold. Environmental sampling of home air or dust ($50–$200) confirms exposure sources, critical for Veterans in damp quarters. Doctors diagnose mold illness by combining history, symptoms, and test results, prescribing antifungals if confirmed.

Removal aims to clear these effects and improve health. Benefits include better respiratory function—easing asthma or allergies—increased energy by reducing toxic burden, lower inflammation tied to mycotoxins, improved mental clarity from less brain fog, and balanced immunity to fight infections. Risks involve over-diagnosis from vague tests leading to unneeded treatment, or side effects like constipation from binders; Veterans with kidney or heart issues need caution with antifungals. Evidence supports treatment for confirmed mold exposure—small studies show relief—but the broader "mold illness" concept lacks large-scale validation. Veterans with chronic symptoms or past exposure can explore this, starting with VA resources or private labs, and escalate based on findings.

Targeted Protocols for Veterans' Wellness

Veterans noticing persistent fatigue, sinus trouble, or joint pain after living in moldy barracks or deployment zones should consider mold's role. Begin by logging symptoms—when they hit, how long they last—especially if tied to damp billets or burn pit stints. Move to testing: urine mycotoxin screens from labs like RealTime or Great Plains ($200–$400) detect toxins in your system; blood tests ($100–$300) reveal immune reactions to mold. VA labs can run basic checks, or functional doctor offices—sometimes backed by foundations like the Gary Sinise Foundation or Wounded Warrior Project—offer funding support for Veterans, covering costs if you qualify. Home air or dust tests ($50–$200) pinpoint exposure sources, a must if quarters feel off.

If tests confirm mold, start removal with detox binders—charcoal or bentonite clay, a daily dose ($20–$50)—to trap mycotoxins and flush them out through digestion. A VA doctor or functional practitioner might prescribe antifungals like itraconazole, one pill daily for 4–12 weeks, to kill lingering spores; this needs medical oversight. Shift your diet to cut mold's fuel—drop grains and aged cheese, stick to meat and greens—to starve it out. Progress shows in weeks—breathing eases, energy ticks up—if not, retest or adjust with a pro.

For respiratory issues, common after field exposure, sweat it out. Infrared saunas or steady walks, 30–60 minutes three to five times a week, push toxins through your skin; deep breathing, 5–15 minutes daily, boosts lymph flow to clear the lungs. Energy improves as the load lightens—check it over a month; if it drags, tweak the routine.

Inflammation—aching joints or gut unrest—drops with binders and antifungals, but add natural fighters like garlic or oregano oil to your meals. Symptoms should soften in weeks; if they hold, consult a doctor for stronger options. Mental clarity lifts as fog fades—vital for Veterans with TBI—track it close and adjust if needed. Immunity strengthens with mold gone—fewer sick days—keeping you steady over time.

Consult a healthcare provider before starting, especially with kidney, heart, or chronic conditions, to confirm mold's role and avoid risks. VA resources or functional doctors with foundation backing (like Gary Sinise or Wounded Warrior) can guide testing and treatment, keeping it safe and affordable—free through VA or $20–$400 private. Start with symptom logs and diet shifts, escalate to tests and detox if signs point to mold, and remediate home exposure sources to seal the effort. Track changes—better breath, less pain—over 4–12 weeks, adjusting with professional input if progress stalls.

Bottom Line
Mold in the body detection and removal target health effects from spores or mycotoxins, offering respiratory relief, energy boosts, inflammation reduction, mental clarity, and immune balance through symptom checks, tests like urine mycotoxins, and methods such as binders, antifungals, or dietary changes. Veterans with exposure from barracks, burn pits, or chronic symptoms like fatigue can use this to address persistent issues, with small studies showing relief in confirmed cases over weeks. It focuses on internal impact, not just environmental fixes. Evidence supports treatment for verified exposure, but systemic "mold illness" lacks broad consensus, relying on clinical reports; testing accuracy varies. Risks include over-diagnosis or treatment side effects, notable for Veterans with health complexities. It's not a routine fix without confirmed mold—professionals advise evidence first—so consult a VA or functional doctor (some foundation-supported, like Gary Sinise), test via VA or labs ($100–$400), and remove with care (free–$50), integrating with VA oversight. It's effective when mold's proven, not a blanket detox, requiring precision and follow-through.

Movement

Movement is an effective tool that can help to improve physical and mental well-being. For Veterans, who might experience a range of physical and mental health concerns related to their service, movement can provide a range of benefits including reduced stress and anxiety, improved sleep, pain management, improved mental health and improved overall well-being. Some of the benefits of movement are:

• **Reduced stress and anxiety:** Movement can help to reduce stress and anxiety by promoting the release of endorphins, which are natural chemicals in the body that promote feelings of well-being and happiness. Walking, dancing and active meditation can all be effective in reducing stress and anxiety.

• **Improved sleep:** Sleep disturbances are common among Veterans with PTSD and other mental health conditions. Movement can help to promote better sleep by reducing stress and tension in the body and calming the mind. Walking, dancing and active meditation can all be effective in promoting better sleep.

• **Pain management:** Chronic pain is a common issue for many Veterans, particularly those who have experienced physical injuries or trauma during their service. Movement can help to reduce pain and improve physical function in those with chronic pain conditions such as back pain, neck pain and joint pain. Walking and active meditation can be particularly effective in reducing pain.

• **Improved mental health:** Movement can help to improve overall mental health and well-being. It can reduce symptoms of anxiety and depression, improve mood and promote a greater sense of calm and balance. Dancing and active meditation can be particularly effective in improving mental health.

• **Improved overall well-being:** Movement can help to improve overall health and well-being by promoting physical fitness, flexibility and strength. Walking, dancing and active meditation can all be effective in improving overall well-being.

Examples of movement practices that Veterans can use to promote physical and mental well-being:

• **Walking:** Walking is a simple and effective way to get moving and promote overall well-being. It can be done anywhere, at any time and can be easily incorporated into daily routines.

• **Dance:** Dancing is a fun and energizing way to get moving and promote overall well-being. It can be done alone or with others and can be tailored to different levels of fitness and ability.

• **Active meditation:** Active meditation involves combining physical movement with mindfulness techniques to promote relaxation and reduce stress. It can be done through practices like yoga, tai chi or qigong.

To enhance the benefits of movement, Veterans can employ several strategies:

• **Start slowly:** It is important to start slowly and gradually increase the intensity and duration of movement practices. This can help to avoid injury and prevent burnout.

• *Find activities that are enjoyable:* It is important to find movement practices that are enjoyable and sustainable. This can help to maintain motivation and promote long-term adherence to the practice.

• *Work with a professional:* Working with a trained and experienced fitness professional or movement therapist can help to ensure that movement practices are safe and effective.

• *Practice regularly:* To achieve the maximum benefits of movement, it is important to practice regularly. This can help to promote overall well-being and improve physical and mental health.

Bottom Line

Movement practices such as walking, dancing and active meditation can provide a range of benefits for Veterans, including reduced stress and anxiety, improved sleep, pain management, improved mental health and improved overall well-being. By incorporating movement practices into their daily routines, Veterans can improve their physical and mental health and promote overall well-being. Movement practices are a powerful tool for managing the physical and mental health concerns related to service and can complement traditional medical therapies. Veterans should always consult with their healthcare provider before starting any new movement practices and should work with trained professionals to ensure that the practices are safe and effective. By incorporating movement practices into their daily routines, Veterans can improve their physical and mental health, reduce stress and promote overall well-being.

Mycotoxins

Mycotoxins are toxic compounds produced by molds like Aspergillus or Fusarium, found in damp buildings, contaminated food, or airborne particles, entering the body through inhalation, ingestion, or skin contact. Unlike allergens, these are chemical toxins that can cause inflammation, immune disruption, and chronic symptoms, requiring testing to detect and treatments to remove. Veterans, exposed to mold in aging barracks, burn pit fumes, or humid deployment zones, may face persistent issues like fatigue or respiratory distress that mycotoxins could explain. Testing identifies exposure; treatments aim to eliminate the toxins from the body and environment. Benefits claimed include reduced inflammation, increased energy, and improved immunity, backed by clinical observations and small studies, though comprehensive evidence is limited, and risks like overtreatment are noted.

Mycotoxins, such as aflatoxins, ochratoxin A, and trichothecenes, are secondary mold metabolites detectable in urine, blood, or tissues. Their health impact emerged in the 1960s with food contamination findings and grew in the 1990s with "sick building syndrome," linking them to chronic conditions by the 2000s, though medical agreement varies. Veterans encounter them in mold-prone settings—poorly ventilated housing or tropical posts—where symptoms like fatigue, brain fog, or breathing problems often linger unexplained. Testing uses urine mycotoxin panels, blood antibody checks, or environmental sampling to confirm presence; treatments range from detox binders to home remediation.

The need for testing stems from mycotoxins' hidden effects—fatigue, cognitive issues, or lung irritation—that standard care might miss, especially in Veterans with service-related exposures. Urine tests from labs like RealTime or Great Plains ($200–$400) measure recent exposure through metabolites like ochratoxin A; blood IgG/IgE tests ($100–$300) detect immune responses, available via VA or private labs. Environmental sampling of home air, dust, or surfaces ($50–$200) traces the source, vital for Veterans in damp spaces. A doctor assesses symptoms alongside results to guide treatment.

Elimination targets these toxins to improve health. Reduced inflammation can ease joint pain or soreness; restored energy counters chronic tiredness; better immunity strengthens defenses against infections; mental clarity lifts brain fog; improved breathing relieves lung strain. Risks include digestive upset from binders or misdiagnosis from unclear tests; Veterans with kidney or liver conditions need caution during detox. Small studies suggest symptom relief with testing and treatment, but large-scale evidence is lacking, and benefits lean on clinical practice over definitive proof. Veterans with ongoing symptoms can start with affordable tests and treatments, escalating with professional input if mycotoxins are confirmed.

Targeted Protocols for Veterans' Wellness
Veterans experiencing persistent fatigue, brain fog, sinus problems, or joint pain after time in moldy barracks, burn pit zones, or humid deployments should consider mycotoxins as a factor. Begin by noting symptoms—when they occur, how long they last—especially if linked to past damp conditions. Urine mycotoxin tests from labs like RealTime or Great Plains ($200–$400) check for toxins like ochratoxin A in your system; blood tests ($100–$300) look for immune reactions to mycotoxins. VA labs offer basic options, or functional doctor offices—sometimes supported by foundations like the Gary Sinise Foundation or Wounded Warrior Project—can cover costs for qualifying Veterans. Home air or dust tests ($50–$200) confirm environmental exposure, essential if housing feels off.

If mycotoxins show up, start elimination with detox binders—activated charcoal or bentonite clay, 500–1000 mg daily ($20–$50)—to bind toxins in the gut and remove them through digestion. Doctors might prescribe liver support like glutathione or milk thistle, 200–500 mg daily for a month, to help process and clear the load; this needs medical clearance. Shift your diet to limit mycotoxin intake—cut nuts, coffee, and processed foods, focus on fresh meat and vegetables—while drinking 8–12 cups of water daily to flush the system. Symptoms may ease—energy rises, inflammation drops—within weeks; if not, retest or consult a pro.

Breathing issues, frequent after mold exposure, improve with sweating. Saunas or exercise, 30–60 minutes three to five times weekly, push toxins out through sweat; steady hydration supports the effort. Energy increases as the burden lightens—track it over a month; adjust if progress slows. Inflammation affecting joints or overall soreness reduces with binders and liver aids; dietary changes reinforce the effect. Check relief over weeks—persistent issues mean a doctor's input.

Mental clarity improves as toxins clear—less fog, sharper focus—crucial for Veterans with cognitive struggles. Sweating and diet changes drive this; monitor progress and tweak if needed. Immunity benefits follow—fewer infections, stronger resistance—as the toxic stress lifts, keeping you steadier long-term. Home remediation seals the plan—professional mold removal ($500–$5,000) or DIY fixes like dehumidifiers ($50–$200) stop the source, a one-time or ongoing task for Veterans in affected spaces.

Consult a healthcare provider before starting, especially with kidney, liver, or chronic conditions, to verify mycotoxins and avoid complications. VA resources or functional doctors with foundation support—like Gary Sinise or Wounded Warrior—guide testing and treatment, keeping costs manageable—free through VA or $20–$400 private. Begin with symptom tracking and diet adjustments, move to tests and binders if signs point to mycotoxins, and remediate home exposure to lock it down. Assess changes—better breathing, less fatigue—over 1–3 months, refining with professional oversight if results falter.

Bottom Line
Mycotoxins, toxic mold byproducts, require testing and treatments to eliminate their effects, offering reduced inflammation, restored energy, better immunity, mental clarity, and improved breathing through urine/blood tests, binders, liver support, sweating, diet shifts, and home fixes. Veterans with fatigue, pain, or exposure risks from service can address unexplained symptoms this way, with small studies and clinical reports suggesting relief over weeks to months. Unlike allergens, mycotoxins are chemical threats needing specific removal. Evidence supports benefits in confirmed cases—small trials show promise—but lacks large-scale backing; detox relies heavily on practice, not definitive proof, with gaps in long-term data. Risks include digestive upset or misdiagnosis, plus costs ($50–$5,000), a concern for Veterans with health or financial limits. It's not a primary solution without clear exposure—professionals recommend evidence first—so consult a VA or functional

doctor (some foundation-supported, like Gary Sinise), test via labs ($200–$400), and treat with affordable steps (e.g., binders, $20–$50), integrating with VA care. It's effective when mycotoxins are verified, not a broad fix, requiring careful execution.

NAC

N-Acetyl Cysteine (NAC) is a derivative of the amino acid cysteine and is used as a supplement for its various health benefits. NAC is known to have antioxidant, anti-inflammatory and mucolytic properties, making it a popular supplement for a wide range of health conditions.

One of the most well-known benefits of NAC is its ability to support respiratory health. NAC helps break down mucus in the lungs, making it easier to cough up and remove from the airways. This makes it a popular supplement for individuals with conditions such as chronic bronchitis, cystic fibrosis and other respiratory conditions. NAC improves lung function and reduces the frequency of respiratory infections.[13]

NAC is beneficial to mental health. It reduces symptoms of anxiety and depression and improves symptoms of obsessive-compulsive disorder (OCD). NAC works by increasing levels of glutamate, which is a neurotransmitter that is important for mood regulation and cognitive function.[14]

NAC has benefits for cardiovascular health. It reduces oxidative stress and inflammation, both of which are important factors in the development of cardiovascular disease. NAC also reduces cholesterol and triglyceride levels, making it a popular supplement for individuals at risk for heart disease.[15]

NAC also benefits liver health. It protects the liver from damage caused by drugs and other toxic substances and improves liver function in individuals with liver disease. NAC also benefits individuals with non-alcoholic fatty liver disease (NAFLD), a condition characterized by an accumulation of fat in the liver.[16]
NAC benefits skin health as well. It improves symptoms of skin conditions such as acne and psoriasis, as well as skin hydration and elasticity. NAC works by reducing oxidative stress and inflammation, which are important factors in the development of skin aging and skin conditions.

NAC has a positive effect in the treatment of COVID-19 although further studies are needed.[17]

NAC is generally considered safe when taken in recommended doses, although it can cause side effects such as nausea, vomiting and diarrhea in some individuals. NAC can also interact with certain medications, therefore it is important to consult with a healthcare professional before taking NAC if you are taking any medications.

Bottom Line
N-Acetyl Cysteine (NAC) is a versatile supplement that has a wide range of health benefits. From supporting respiratory health to improving mental health, liver health and skin health, NAC is a popular supplement for individuals looking to support their overall health and wellness. As with any supplement, it is important to consult with a healthcare professional before taking NAC to ensure that it is safe and appropriate for you.

Neural Pathway Integration

Neural Pathway Integration (NPI) focuses on optimizing the brain's neural connections—networks of about 86 billion neurons linked by synapses—to improve physical, mental, and emotional health. It uses the brain's ability to adapt and rewire, known as neuroplasticity, a concept from Donald Hebb's 1949 theory that neurons firing together strengthen their links. Veterans, dealing with chronic pain, stress, or trauma from service, can use NPI to restore function and resilience by repairing or enhancing pathways disrupted by injury or habits. Benefits claimed include pain relief, better physical function, mental clarity, emotional resilience, faster recovery, holistic healing, and improved adaptability, supported by neuroscience principles and integrative methods like chiropractic care or cognitive exercises, though evidence for specific NPI techniques varies, and risks like time demands or individual differences apply.

NPI involves deliberately reconnecting or strengthening neural pathways to address dysfunction, distinct from standard therapy by its holistic approach. It stems from Hebb's neuroplasticity work, with modern use growing in integrative fields like chiropractic and psychotherapy since the 2000s. Chronic pain, stress, and trauma, common among Veterans, drive interest in NPI to rewire pathways beyond symptom relief. Combat injuries, stress, and toxin exposure can disrupt neural signals; NPI targets these to restore brain-body communication. Symptoms like pain, fatigue, mental fog, or emotional distress indicate pathway issues, which NPI aims to repair or reroute.

Techniques include chiropractic adjustments, cognitive exercises, and physical therapy to leverage plasticity. Practitioners assess dysfunction through exams or history, taking 1–2 hours, to identify pathways needing work. Adjustments or acupressure (20–60 minutes weekly) realign nerves; visualization or reframing (15–30 minutes daily) reshape thought patterns; guided movements (30–60 minutes, 3–5 times weekly) reinforce motor pathways. Daily or weekly practice over

4–12 weeks solidifies changes, with symptom tracking adjusting the approach. Risks involve the time and consistency required, which may not suit all, and some proprietary methods lack proven efficacy; Veterans with complex conditions need tailored plans. Neuroscience supports plasticity benefits, with small studies on related therapies showing promise, but branded NPI lacks large trials. Pain, PTSD, and adjustment struggles make it relevant for Veterans, who often explore integrative healing.

Targeted Protocols for Veterans' Wellness

Veterans with chronic pain, fatigue, or emotional strain from service can explore NPI to address disrupted neural pathways. Start with a practitioner—chiropractor or therapist ($50–$150)—who evaluates your history and symptoms over 1–2 hours to pinpoint issues like pain from old injuries or stress from combat. VA referrals can connect you to care, or functional providers with foundation support, like the Gary Sinise Foundation or Wounded Warrior Project, may offset costs for qualifying Veterans. Track symptoms—pain levels, focus, mood—in a log to guide the process.

For pain relief, chiropractic adjustments, 20–60 minutes weekly, target spinal alignment to ease hypersensitive pathways; Veterans with lingering discomfort from service can expect reduced soreness over weeks. Add daily visualization, 15–30 minutes, imagining pain fading to reinforce relief signals—consistency over 4–12 weeks shows if it's working; adjust with the provider if progress lags. Physical function improves with guided movements—30–60 minutes, three to five times weekly—like stretches or strength drills to boost brain-muscle coordination; Veterans rebuilding mobility after injuries see steadier steps in a month, refining with feedback.

Mental clarity comes from cognitive exercises—15–30 minutes daily—focusing on clear thoughts or reframing negative loops, strengthening prefrontal pathways. Veterans with post-service fog can sharpen focus over weeks; if it's slow, pair with therapy. Emotional resilience builds through similar reframing, targeting amygdala-driven stress—daily practice over a month eases anxiety or lifts mood for Veterans carrying trauma's weight; check in with a pro if it stalls.

Recovery speeds up with a mix of adjustments and movements—weekly sessions and three daily drills—to restore connections disrupted by injury; Veterans healing from service wounds prevent bad habits in weeks, adjusting intensity if needed. Holistic healing ties it together—chiropractic, exercises, and mindfulness (10–20 minutes daily)—to boost vitality across systems; Veterans seeking overall wellness feel steadier over a month, tweaking based on logs. Adaptability grows with consistent practice—daily or weekly efforts over 4–12 weeks—enhancing plasticity for future stress; Veterans facing new challenges gain flexibility, refining with provider input.

Consult a healthcare provider before starting, especially with chronic pain, PTSD, or injuries, to ensure safety and alignment with VA care. VA therapy or integrative providers with foundation backing (like Gary Sinise or Wounded Warrior) guide the process, keeping costs manageable—free through VA or $50–$150 private. Begin with an assessment, add adjustments or exercises (15–60 minutes daily), and monitor progress—less pain, clearer head—over 4–12 weeks, adjusting with professional oversight if results falter.

Bottom Line

Neural Pathway Integration (NPI) aims to enhance neural connections for pain relief, improved physical function, mental clarity, emotional resilience, faster recovery, holistic healing, and adaptability by using neuroplasticity through chiropractic adjustments, cognitive exercises, or physical therapy. Veterans with pain, PTSD, or stress from service can target disrupted pathways non-invasively, with neuroscience and small studies suggesting relief over weeks to months. It's a holistic approach, distinct from standard treatments, relying on plasticity principles. Evidence supports the concept—synaptic strengthening and neurogenesis are established—but specific NPI techniques lack large-scale trials, drawing from related research like CBT. Risks include time demands or unproven methods, a factor for Veterans needing fast outcomes or with complex needs. It's not a standalone treatment—professionals suggest pairing with VA care due to limited data and variability—so consult a healthcare provider, start with accessible steps (e.g., $50–$150 sessions), and integrate with therapy or exercise, approaching with patience and realistic expectations. It's a potential aid for some, not a complete solution, needing steady effort and oversight.

Neurogenesis

The process of creating new neurons or brain cells, neurogenesis is an important process for maintaining brain health and cognitive function and has been shown to be particularly important for people who have experienced trauma, including Veterans.

There are several ways to enhance neurogenesis, which can help to improve cognitive function and overall brain health for Veterans. These include:

• *Exercise:* Exercise has been shown to be one of the most effective ways to enhance neurogenesis. Studies have shown that regular exercise can increase the number of new neurons in the hippocampus, a part of the brain that is important for memory and learning. Exercise can also help to reduce inflammation in the brain, which can contribute to cognitive decline.

- **Diet:** A healthy diet can also help to enhance neurogenesis. Diets that are high in fruits, vegetables and whole grains have been shown to be beneficial for brain health, while diets that are high in processed foods and saturated fats can have a negative impact on neurogenesis. Specific nutrients that have been shown to enhance neurogenesis include omega-3 fatty acids, which are found in fatty fish and some plant-based foods, and flavonoids, which are found in colorful fruits and vegetables.

- **Stress reduction:** Chronic stress can have a negative impact on neurogenesis, so finding ways to reduce stress can be beneficial for brain health. Techniques like meditation, yoga and deep breathing exercises can help to reduce stress and improve overall well-being.

- **Socialization:** Socialization has been shown to be an important factor in enhancing neurogenesis. Spending time with friends and family, joining clubs or organizations and volunteering can all help to improve social connections and enhance brain health.

- **Mental stimulation:** Keeping the brain active through mental stimulation can also enhance neurogenesis. Activities like reading, doing crossword puzzles or Sudoku and learning new skills or languages can help to keep the brain active and promote the growth of new neurons.

For Veterans, who might have experienced trauma or other challenges that can impact brain health, enhancing neurogenesis can be particularly important. Studies have shown that Veterans with post-traumatic stress disorder (PTSD) may have reduced neurogenesis, which can contribute to symptoms like memory loss and cognitive decline. Enhancing neurogenesis can be a key part of a comprehensive approach to treating PTSD and other conditions that impact brain health.

In addition to the strategies listed above, there are several other approaches that may be particularly helpful for Veterans looking to enhance neurogenesis:

- **Cognitive behavioral therapy (CBT):** CBT is a type of talk therapy that has been shown to be effective for treating PTSD and other mental health conditions. CBT can help Veterans to reframe negative thoughts and emotions, which can reduce stress and improve overall brain health.

- **Exposure therapy:** Exposure therapy is a type of therapy that is used to help people with PTSD overcome their fear and anxiety by gradually exposing them to the source of their trauma. This type of therapy has been shown to be effective for enhancing neurogenesis in Veterans with PTSD.

- **Mindfulness-based interventions:** Mindfulness-based interventions, like mindfulness meditation, have been shown to be effective for reducing stress and enhancing brain health. Mindfulness meditation can help to reduce anxiety, improve mood and enhance neurogenesis.

- **Complementary and alternative therapies:** Complementary and alternative therapies, like acupuncture and massage, may also be helpful for enhancing neurogenesis and reducing stress. These therapies can help to improve circulation, reduce inflammation and promote relaxation, which can all contribute to better brain health.

Bottom Line

Enhancing neurogenesis is an important aspect of maintaining brain health and cognitive function, particularly for Veterans who may have experienced trauma or other challenges that can impact brain health. Strategies like exercise, diet, stress reduction, socialization and mental stimulation can all be helpful in enhancing neurogenesis and improving brain health for Veterans.

Niacin[18]

Also known as Vitamin B3, niacin is a water-soluble vitamin that is essential for human health. It plays a crucial role in energy production, maintaining healthy skin and improving cognitive function. One of the most well-known benefits of niacin is its ability to cause a niacin flush, which is a temporary skin redness and warmth that is caused by the dilation of blood vessels.

Some of the benefits of niacin:

- **Lowers cholesterol:** Niacin has been shown to lower total cholesterol levels and low-density lipoprotein (LDL) cholesterol, also known as "bad" cholesterol. This helps reduce the risk of heart disease and stroke.

- **Improves cardiovascular health:** Niacin has been shown to improve overall cardiovascular health by reducing inflammation, improving blood flow and preventing the buildup of plaque in the arteries.

- **Boosts energy levels:** Niacin is involved in energy production and a deficiency can lead to fatigue and decreased energy levels. Taking a niacin supplement can help improve energy levels and combat fatigue.

- **Helps with depression and anxiety:** Niacin has been shown to have a positive effect on mood and some studies have suggested that it may help with depression and anxiety.

• *Supports skin health:* Niacin is essential for maintaining healthy skin and a deficiency can lead to skin problems such as pellagra. Taking a niacin supplement can help improve skin health and prevent skin problems.

• *Improves cognitive function:* Niacin has been shown to improve cognitive function, including memory and attention and may help prevent age-related cognitive decline.

• *Supports digestive health:* Niacin is involved in the production of digestive juices and a deficiency can lead to digestive problems such as peptic ulcers. Taking a niacin supplement can help improve digestive health and prevent digestive problems.

The niacin flush is a well-known side effect of niacin supplementation and occurs when blood vessels dilate, causing increased blood flow and resulting in a temporary skin redness and warmth. Although the niacin flush can be uncomfortable, it is generally harmless and typically subsides within 30 minutes to an hour.

Some of the benefits of the niacin flush:

• *Helps improve blood flow:* The niacin flush is caused by increased blood flow and regular use of niacin has been shown to improve overall blood flow and circulation.

• *Supports healthy skin:* The niacin flush can help improve skin health by increasing blood flow and oxygenation to the skin. This can help promote a healthy, radiant complexion.

• *Supports healthy joints:* The niacin flush can help improve joint health by increasing blood flow and reducing inflammation.

• *Supports healthy eyes:* The niacin flush can help improve eye health by increasing blood flow and oxygenation to the eyes. This can help prevent age-related vision problems.

• *Supports healthy brain function:* The niacin flush can help improve brain function by increasing blood flow and oxygenation to the brain. This can help improve cognitive function and prevent age-related cognitive decline.

It's important to note that not everyone experiences the niacin flush and the severity and frequency of the flush can vary depending on the individual and the dose of niacin taken. In some cases, taking a lower dose of niacin or gradually increasing the dose over time can help minimize the severity of the niacin flush.

Bottom Line

Niacin is an essential nutrient that offers a range of health benefits, including improving energy levels, reducing cholesterol and supporting skin and cognitive health. The niacin flush, while uncomfortable, can also offer additional benefits such as improved blood flow, skin health, joint health, eye health and brain function. It's important to consult a healthcare professional before starting a niacin supplement to ensure it's safe and appropriate for you and to determine the appropriate dosage.

NMN

Also known as nicotinamide mononucleotide, NMN is a naturally occurring molecule that is a form of vitamin B3. It is found in a variety of foods, including mushrooms, avocados and tomatoes and it is also available as a dietary supplement.

One of the primary health benefits of NMN is its ability to support healthy aging. NMN has been found to increase levels of NAD (nicotinamide adenine dinucleotide), which is a molecule that declines with age and is essential for energy production and cell repair. By increasing NAD levels, NMN has been shown to improve energy production and support cellular repair, which may help to slow the aging process.[19]

NMN benefits cardiovascular health. It improves the function of blood vessels, reduces oxidative stress and lowers blood pressure. These effects may help to reduce the risk of cardiovascular disease, which is a leading cause of death and disability.

NMN also benefits brain health. It improves cognitive function and reduces the risk of neurodegenerative diseases such as Alzheimer's and Parkinson's. NMN helps protect the brain from damage caused by oxidative stress, which is a key factor in the development of neurodegenerative diseases.

NMN is also good for skin health. It improves skin hydration, elasticity and overall appearance. NMN may also help to reduce the appearance of fine lines and wrinkles, making it a popular supplement for individuals looking to maintain healthy, youthful-looking skin.

NMN is generally considered safe when taken in recommended doses, although it can cause side effects such as nausea, headache and skin irritation in some individuals. NMN can also interact with certain medications, so it is important to consult with a healthcare professional before taking NMN if you are taking any medications.

Bottom Line

NMN is a naturally occurring molecule with a variety of potential health benefits. From supporting healthy aging to improving cardiovascular and brain health and skin health, NMN is a popular supplement for individuals looking to support their overall health and wellness. As with any supplement, it is important to consult with a healthcare professional before taking NMN to ensure that it is safe and appropriate for you. Further research is needed to fully understand the potential health benefits of NMN and to determine its long-term safety and efficacy.

Obesity

Obesity is a serious health concern for Veterans, as it can increase the risk of a range of health problems including heart disease diabetes and stroke. In addition to these health risks, obesity can also have a negative impact on mental health and overall quality of life.

Dangers of obesity for Veterans

- *Increased risk of chronic health problems:* Obesity can increase the risk of a range of chronic health problems, including heart disease, diabetes, stroke and certain types of cancer. These health problems can have a significant impact on quality of life and may require ongoing medical treatment.

- *Mental health problems:* Obesity can increase the risk of mental health problems, such as depression, anxiety, and low self-esteem. These mental health problems can have a significant impact on overall quality of life and may require treatment.

- *Reduced mobility:* Obesity can make it difficult to move around, which can impact daily activities and reduce overall mobility. This can have a negative impact on independence and overall quality of life.

- *Reduced life expectancy:* Obesity has been linked to reduced life expectancy, meaning that Veterans who are obese may have a shorter life expectancy than those who maintain a healthy weight.

Strategies for reducing obesity

- *Healthy eating:* A healthy diet is essential for maintaining a healthy weight. Veterans should aim to eat a balanced diet that includes plenty of fruits, vegetables, whole grains, lean protein and healthy fats. They should also avoid foods that are high in saturated and trans fats, added sugars and salt.

- *Regular exercise:* Regular exercise is essential for maintaining a healthy weight and reducing the risk of chronic health problems. Veterans should aim to get at least 30 minutes of moderate-intensity exercise most days of the week. This can include activities such as walking, cycling, swimming, or strength training.

• **Support groups:** Joining a support group can provide Veterans with the motivation and accountability they need to maintain a healthy weight. Support groups can also provide emotional support and a sense of community.

• **Behavioral therapy:** Behavioral therapy can be effective for helping Veterans to develop healthy habits and stick to a healthy eating and exercise plan. This may involve working with a therapist or counselor to identify triggers and develop strategies for managing cravings and emotional eating.

• **Medications:** In some cases, medications may be prescribed to help Veterans lose weight. These medications work by suppressing appetite or reducing the absorption of fat.

• **Weight loss surgery:** Weight loss surgery may be an option for Veterans who are severely obese and have not been successful with other weight loss methods. This may include procedures such as gastric bypass or sleeve gastrectomy.

Bottom Line
Obesity is a serious health concern for Veterans that can increase the risk of chronic health problems, mental health problems, reduced mobility and reduced life expectancy. Strategies for reducing obesity include healthy eating, regular exercise, support groups, behavioral therapy, medications and weight loss surgery. Veterans should work with their healthcare provider to develop a personalized weight loss plan that is safe and effective for their individual needs. By maintaining a healthy weight, Veterans can reduce their risk of health problems, improve overall quality of life, and enjoy greater physical and mental well-being.

Oil-Pulling[21]

An ancient practice that involves swishing edible oil in the mouth for several minutes, this simple but effective technique has been used for centuries in traditional Indian medicine to improve oral health and overall well-being. Today, oil-pulling is gaining popularity as a natural and holistic approach to oral care.

Benefits

• **Improves Oral Health:** Oil-pulling is believed to help remove harmful bacteria from the mouth, which can lead to improved oral health. By removing harmful bacteria, oil pulling can help prevent tooth decay, gum disease, and bad breath.

• **_Boosts Immune System:_** Oil-pulling is also believed to help boost the immune system by removing toxins from the body. When you swish oil in your mouth, it binds to harmful bacteria, viruses and toxins, which are then removed from the body when you spit the oil out.

• **_Promotes Healthy Skin:_** Oil-pulling is believed to have a positive impact on the skin. The practice of oil pulling is said to help remove toxins from the body that can cause skin problems such as acne and eczema.

• **_Reduces Inflammation:_** Oil-pulling is also believed to help reduce inflammation in the body. Inflammation is a key factor in many health problems including heart disease, arthritis and cancer. By removing harmful bacteria and toxins from the mouth, oil pulling can help reduce inflammation and improve overall health.

• **_Enhances Energy Levels:_** Oil-pulling is believed to help enhance energy levels by removing toxins from the body. When toxins are removed, the body is able to function more efficiently, leading to increased energy levels.

Oil-pulling how-to

Oil-pulling is a simple and easy practice that can be done in the comfort of your own home.

• **_Choose the Right Oil:_** The most commonly used oil for oil-pulling is coconut oil. However, you can also use sesame oil, olive oil or sunflower oil. Choose an oil that is high-quality and organic, if possible.

• **_Put Oil in Your Mouth:_** Take a tablespoon of oil and place it in your mouth. Do not swallow the oil.

• **_Swish Oil Around Mouth:_** Swish the oil around your mouth for 15-20 minutes. Be sure to move the oil through all parts of your mouth, including your teeth and gums.

• **_Spit Out Oil:_** After 15-20 minutes, spit the oil into a trash can (or plastic bag). Do not spit the oil down the sink as it can clog pipes.

• **_Rinse Mouth with Water:_** Rinse your mouth with water to remove any remaining oil.

• **_Brush Teeth:_** Brush your teeth as you normally would.

It is recommended to oil-pull first thing in the morning, before eating or drinking anything. It is also important to remember that oil-pulling is not a substitute for brushing and flossing your teeth. It is best used as an additional step in your oral care routine.

Bottom Line
Oil-pulling is an ancient practice that has been used for centuries to improve oral health and overall well-being. The benefits of oil-pulling include improved oral health, a boost to the immune system, healthy skin, reduced inflammation and enhanced energy levels

<u>Omega 3[22]</u>

A type of essential fatty acid that are critical for human health, Omega-3 fatty acids are found in a variety of foods including fatty fish such as salmon, mackerel and sardines, as well as in plant-based sources such as flaxseed and chia seeds. Omega-3 fatty acids are also available as dietary supplements.

One of the primary health benefits of Omega-3 fatty acids is their ability to support heart health. Omega-3 fatty acids have been shown to reduce the risk of heart disease by lowering levels of triglycerides and blood pressure and by decreasing the formation of blood clots. They also help to reduce inflammation in the body, which is a key factor in the development of heart disease.

Omega-3 fatty acids have also been found to have benefits for brain health. They have been shown to improve cognitive function, reduce the risk of neurodegenerative diseases such as Alzheimer's and Parkinson's and to improve mood and reduce symptoms of depression and anxiety. Omega-3 fatty acids help to protect the brain from damage caused by oxidative stress and they are important for the growth and development of brain cells.

Omega-3 fatty acids have also been found to have benefits for joint health. They have been shown to reduce joint pain and stiffness and to improve mobility in individuals with osteoarthritis. Omega-3 fatty acids help to reduce inflammation in the joints, which can play a role in the development of osteoarthritis.

Omega-3 fatty acids have also been found to have benefits for eye health. They have been shown to reduce the risk of age-related macular degeneration, a leading cause of blindness in the elderly and to improve visual acuity and visual function in individuals with dry eye syndrome.

Omega-3 fatty acids are generally considered safe when taken in recommended doses although they can cause side effects such as gastrointestinal upset, heartburn, and diarrhea in some individuals. Omega-3 fatty acids can also interact with certain medications, therefore it is important to consult with a healthcare professional before taking Omega-3 fatty acids if you are taking any medications.

Bottom Line
Omega-3 fatty acids are an essential type of fatty acid that are critical for human health. From heart health to improving brain health, joint health and eye health, Omega-3 fatty acids are a popular supplement for individuals looking to support their overall health and wellness. As with any supplement, it is important to consult with a healthcare professional before taking Omega-3 fatty acids to ensure that they are safe and appropriate for you. Further research is needed to fully understand the potential health benefits of Omega-3 fatty acids and to determine their long-term safety and efficacy.

Operator Syndrome

Special operations Veterans were often exposed to traumatic events and prolonged stress, which can take a toll on their mental health. The nature of their work, which often included covert operations and intense combat, can make it difficult for them to process and cope with the traumatic experiences they have been through. Additionally, the physical and emotional demands of special operations training can contribute to the development of mental health issues. This feeling stems from the individual no longer being part of a high functioning and challenging team conducting a very specialized, dangerous and important mission supporting the higher goal of an overall operation.

Symptoms of operator syndrome can include flashbacks, nightmares, difficulty sleeping, irritability and feelings of guilt or shame. These symptoms can make it difficult for special operations Veterans to readjust to civilian life and can have a negative impact on their relationships and overall well-being.

PTSD is one of the most common mental health issues associated with operator syndrome. This condition can be caused by exposure to traumatic events, such as combat or the loss of a fellow service member. Symptoms of PTSD can include flashbacks, nightmares and avoidance of certain places or people that remind the individual of the traumatic event.

Depression and anxiety are also common among special operations Veterans. These conditions can be caused by the prolonged stress of combat and the emotional demands of special operations training. Symptoms of depression can include feelings of hopelessness, fatigue and loss of interest in activities, while symptoms of anxiety can include panic attacks, excessive worry and difficulty sleeping.

Treatment for operator syndrome typically includes therapy, medication and support from peers and family members. Therapy can help special operations Veterans process and cope with the traumatic experiences they have been through, while medication can help alleviate symptoms of depression and anxiety. Support from peers and family members can also be beneficial, as they can provide a sense of understanding and validation for the individual.

It is important to note that not all Veterans will experience operator syndrome and not everyone who experiences it will have the same symptoms. Additionally, not all Veterans seek help for these conditions, for a variety of reasons, including stigmas associated with mental health issues and a lack of access to appropriate care.

Bottom Line

Operator syndrome is a term that describes a range of mental health issues that can affect special operations Veterans. These conditions can include PTSD, depression and anxiety and can be caused by the intense and prolonged stress of combat, as well as the physical and emotional demands of special operations training. Special operations Veterans need to be provided with appropriate mental health care, counseling and support to help them cope with their experiences and overcome the challenges they face. It is important that society, Veterans organizations and the government work together to ensure that special operations Veterans have access to the care they need.

Other Types of Treatment

There are several alternative or complementary methods that may help Veterans suffering from post-traumatic stress disorder (PTSD) and other mental health conditions. Some of these methods include:

• *Yoga and mindfulness-based practices:* These practices can help reduce stress, improve mood and increase physical and mental resilience.

• *Art therapy:* Art therapy uses creative expression to help individuals process and cope with traumatic experiences.

• *Equine therapy:* Equine therapy involves working with horses to promote physical, emotional and mental well-being.

• *Outdoor activities:* Outdoor activities such as hiking, camping and fishing can help Veterans connect with nature and reduce stress.

• *Acupuncture:* Acupuncture is a traditional Chinese medicine technique that involves inserting needles into specific points on the body to promote healing and relaxation.

• *Aromatherapy:* Aromatherapy involves using essential oils to promote physical and emotional well-being.

• *Music therapy:* Music therapy involves using music to help individuals cope with emotional and psychological difficulties.

It's important to note that these alternative methods should not be seen as a substitute for evidence-based treatments for PTSD, such as therapy and medication. Individuals with PTSD should seek the guidance of mental health professionals to determine the best course of treatment for their needs.

Ozone Therapy[23]

Ozone therapy is a complementary and alternative medical treatment that uses ozone, a naturally occurring gas, to improve health and wellness. Ozone therapy has been used for over 100 years and is becoming increasingly popular as a natural and effective way to treat a variety of conditions.

Here are some of the benefits of ozone therapy:

• *Improved immune system:* Ozone therapy has been shown to boost the immune system by increasing the production of white blood cells, which are the body's first line of defense against illness and disease. The therapy also helps to activate and regulate the immune system, making it more effective in fighting off infection and disease.

• *Reduced inflammation:* Ozone therapy has anti-inflammatory properties that can help reduce inflammation and swelling, making it an effective treatment for conditions such as arthritis, rheumatism and other inflammatory disorders.

• *Improved circulation:* Ozone therapy can help improve circulation by increasing the production of red blood cells and oxygenation. This can help reduce symptoms of conditions such as diabetes, peripheral artery disease and other circulatory disorders.

• *Improved oxygenation:* Ozone therapy can help improve oxygenation and increase the delivery of oxygen to cells, tissues and organs. This can help improve energy levels and overall health.

• **Reduced pain:** Ozone therapy has been shown to reduce pain in a variety of conditions, including back pain, neuropathic pain and other chronic pain conditions. The therapy works by reducing inflammation and improving circulation, which can help reduce pain and discomfort.

• **Improved wound healing:** Ozone therapy has been shown to improve wound healing and reduce the appearance of scars. The therapy increases blood flow and oxygenation to the wound site, which helps promote healing and reduces inflammation.

• **Improved dental health:** Ozone therapy has been shown to improve dental health by reducing plaque and gum inflammation and improving overall oral hygiene. The therapy can also help treat periodontitis and other gum diseases.

When performed properly, ozone therapy is a safe and non-invasive treatment that can be performed in a doctor's office or at home using an ozone generator. The treatment typically involves administering ozone gas into the body through a variety of methods, including intravenous injection, ozone sauna and rectal or vaginal insufflation.

Bottom Line
Ozone therapy has numerous health benefits and can be used as a complementary or alternative treatment for a variety of conditions. Whether you are looking to improve your immune system, reduce pain, improve wound healing or simply improve your overall health, ozone therapy is worth considering. However, it is important to consult with a healthcare provider before starting any new treatment, especially if you have any pre-existing health conditions.

Parasite Elimination

Parasite elimination involves identifying and treating infections from organisms like worms, protozoa, or flukes that live in or on the body, as well as the alternative health practice of periodic "cleansing" to address perceived parasitic burdens. These parasites can enter through contaminated food, water, or soil, often tied to travel, diet, or environmental exposure, and differ from routine hygiene by requiring specific interventions. Veterans, who may have faced parasites during deployments in regions with poor sanitation or experienced chronic symptoms post-service, can use this approach to tackle health issues. Benefits claimed include improved digestion, increased energy, and enhanced immunity, supported by medical evidence for confirmed infections and anecdotal reports for cleanses, though scientific support for routine elimination in healthy individuals is limited, and risks like over-treatment apply.

Parasites include giardia, tapeworms, and hookworms, detectable through stool tests or bloodwork, with treatments using drugs like ivermectin or fenbendazole, herbs, diets, or supplements. Treatment dates back to ancient herbal purges, with modern antiparasitics like ivermectin (1980s) and fenbendazole (1970s, originally for animals) emerging later; alternative cleanses grew from 20th-century naturopathy. Veterans are at risk from deployments—poor water quality in places like Iraq or Afghanistan increases exposure, and burn pit fumes may worsen gut issues, though not directly parasitic. Symptoms like diarrhea, fatigue, or malnutrition signal infection, often misdiagnosed, driving the need for elimination.

Testing confirms parasites via VA-ordered stool or blood tests; treatments aim to clear them with medical drugs or alternative methods. Improved digestion comes from removing parasites causing bloating or IBS-like issues; energy increases as nutrient drains lift; immunity strengthens with less parasitic stress; mental clarity improves by reducing gut-related fog; weight stabilizes with better absorption. Risks include nausea or diarrhea from drugs or herbs, and misdiagnosis delaying care; Veterans with heart or kidney issues need caution. Evidence confirms benefits for diagnosed infections, but routine cleanses lack large trials, relying on anecdotal claims. Deployment exposure, gut troubles, and fatigue make this relevant for Veterans, who can start with VA testing and escalate as needed.

Targeted Protocols for Veterans' Wellness
Veterans with ongoing diarrhea, fatigue, or bloating after deployments in tropics or war zones with poor sanitation should consider parasites as a cause. Start with a symptom log—note when issues flare, especially if tied to past field conditions.

VA labs offer stool tests or bloodwork ($0–$50 copay) to confirm infections like giardia or roundworm; results take days and guide treatment. Functional doctor offices, sometimes backed by foundations like the Gary Sinise Foundation or Wounded Warrior Project, can provide testing or funding support for qualifying Veterans if VA access lags.

For confirmed infections, ivermectin (3–12 mg, 1–2 days, $10–$50) clears worms like strongyloides or protozoa, prescribed by a doctor; it's effective in most cases within days. Fenbendazole (222 mg daily, 3–7 days, $20–$100), originally for animals, is used off-label for worms like pinworms—Veterans source it through alternative channels, with relief possible in a week, though human data is thin. Digestive health improves fast—less bloating, steadier gut—check progress in weeks; if symptoms hold, retest or adjust with a provider.

Energy lifts with a low-sugar, high-fiber diet—vegetables, pumpkin seeds, no processed carbs—to starve parasites while flushing the gut; add this daily for 4–6 weeks alongside treatment. Immunity benefits follow—fewer infections as the load drops—track sick days over a month; if no change, consult a doctor. Mental clarity gains come from clearing gut inflammation—daily diet shifts and treatment reduce fog in weeks, key for Veterans with cognitive struggles; monitor and tweak if needed.

Weight regulation stabilizes with parasite removal—nutrient absorption evens out—pair treatment with diet and check shifts over a month; persistent issues mean further testing. Herbs like wormwood, black walnut, or cloves (500 mg daily, 2–4 weeks, $20–$50) offer an alternative cleanse—Veterans buy kits online, with relief possible in weeks, though effects may vary. Coffee or saline enemas (1–2 cups, weekly) aim to expel lower colon parasites—some report ease in days, but evidence is weak; use sparingly to avoid gut strain.

Medical treatment is short—1–14 days—for infections; alternative cleanses run monthly or quarterly but risk imbalance if overdone. Consult a healthcare provider before starting, especially with chronic symptoms or medications, to confirm parasites and avoid side effects like nausea or liver strain from drugs or herbs; ivermectin or fenbendazole overdoses can cause neurotoxicity, rare but serious. VA care or functional doctors with foundation support (like Gary Sinise or Wounded Warrior) keep costs low—free through VA or $10–$100 private. Begin with symptom tracking and diet, test via VA if issues persist, treat with prescribed drugs or herbs, and monitor—less fatigue, better gut—over 1–3 months, adjusting with professional input if results stall.

Bottom Line
Parasite elimination targets infections or perceived burdens, offering improved di-

gestion, energy, immunity, mental clarity, and weight regulation through drugs like ivermectin (highly effective), fenbendazole (anecdotal relief), herbs, diet, or enemas. Veterans with deployment exposure risks, gut issues, or fatigue can address chronic symptoms, with studies showing relief in confirmed cases over weeks. It's a targeted approach, distinct from general detox, using medical or alternative methods. Evidence supports treatment for diagnosed infections—drugs clear most cases—but routine cleanses lack large-scale proof, relying on anecdotal reports; fenbendazole's human efficacy is untested in trials. Risks include side effects like nausea or neurotoxicity from over-treatment, and misdiagnosis, a concern for Veterans with complex health needs. It's not recommended as a preventive or standalone treatment without confirmed infection—professionals require evidence—so consult a healthcare provider, confirm parasites via VA testing before using ivermectin or fenbendazole, and pair with VA care, approaching with caution and oversight. It's effective when parasites are present, but routine cleansing lacks justification.

PEMF (Pulsed Electromagnetic Field) Therapy

Pulsed Electromagnetic Field (PEMF) therapy uses low-frequency electromagnetic waves, delivered through devices like mats, coils, or handheld units, to stimulate cellular repair, improve circulation, and support wellness. These devices pulse energy in controlled bursts, typically 1–100 Hz at low intensity, differing from static magnets by mimicking the Earth's natural magnetic fields to affect cell function. Veterans, dealing with chronic pain, inflammation, or mental health issues from service, can use PEMF as a non-invasive, drug-free method to aid recovery and resilience. It addresses cellular dysfunction, with benefits claimed including pain relief, reduced inflammation, better sleep, stress reduction, and enhanced recovery, supported by clinical studies and growing use in integrative medicine, though evidence varies by condition, and risks like overstimulation apply.

PEMF began in the 1950s with research on bone healing, receiving FDA approval in 1979 for fractures; its use expanded to broader wellness in the 2000s, with Veteran applications for pain and stress emerging by the 2010s. Chronic pain, fatigue, and stress, common among Veterans, drive interest in PEMF to manage symptoms not fully addressed by standard treatments. Combat injuries, toxin exposure, and prolonged stress disrupt cellular health; PEMF targets these by boosting energy at the cell level. Pain, inflammation, and sleep issues indicate wear that PEMF aims to repair, focusing on root causes rather than just symptoms.

Devices include full-body mats ($500–$5,000), localized coils ($200–$1,000), or wearable bands ($100–$500), used for 10–60 minutes daily. Sessions run pre-set programs or custom settings, applied 1–2 times daily over weeks to months. Benefits include less pain through better blood flow, lower inflammation via cellular repair, improved sleep by regulating patterns, reduced stress by calming nerves, and faster healing with enhanced energy. Risks involve mild dizziness or fatigue from overuse; Veterans with pacemakers or severe heart conditions need caution due to electromagnetic interference. Studies confirm pain and bone healing benefits, with smaller trials and user reports supporting sleep and stress relief, though large-scale evidence is limited. Pain, fatigue, and stress make PEMF relevant for Veterans, who can integrate it with VA care for practical results.

Targeted Protocols for Veterans' Wellness

Veterans with chronic pain, poor sleep, or ongoing stress from service can use PEMF to support cellular health. Start with a device—full-body mats ($500–$5,000) cover overall wellness, lying flat for 10–60 minutes daily; localized coils ($200–$1,000) target areas like knees or back, 15–30 minutes daily; wearable bands ($100–$500) offer low-intensity pulses during activities, worn for hours. VA clinics may offer rentals ($50–$150 per session), or functional doctor offices with foundation support—like the Gary Sinise Foundation or Wounded Warrior Project—can offset costs for qualifying Veterans. Track symptoms—pain levels, sleep hours, tension—in a log to measure progress.

For pain relief, use a coil on sore spots like joints or old injuries, 15–30 minutes daily; mats work for widespread aches, 30–60 minutes once or twice daily. Sessions at 5–10 Hz calm nerve signals and boost blood flow—Veterans with lingering discomfort notice less ache in weeks; adjust time or frequency with a provider if it's slow. Inflammation drops with mat use, 30–60 minutes daily at 1–5 Hz, aiding cellular repair—Veterans with swelling from service demands see reduced soreness over a month; tweak settings if needed.

Sleep improves with evening mat sessions, 20–30 minutes at 8 Hz, regulating rest patterns—Veterans with insomnia or restless nights get deeper sleep in weeks; shift to morning if it drags. Stress eases with daily use—mats or wearables, 15–60 minutes at 5–10 Hz—calming the nervous system; Veterans carrying tension feel steadier over a month, pairing with relaxation if progress stalls. Recovery speeds up with coils on injury sites, 15–30 minutes daily, or mats for full-body support, 30–60 minutes—Veterans healing from service wounds gain strength faster in weeks; monitor and adjust with a pro.

Integrate PEMF with VA physical therapy or exercise—use after workouts or sessions—for better results, building a routine over 4–8 weeks. Consult a healthcare provider before starting, especially with pacemakers, heart conditions, or chronic issues, to ensure safety and compatibility with VA care. VA resources or foundation-backed providers (like Gary Sinise or Wounded Warrior) keep costs manageable—free rentals through clinics or $100–$5,000 for devices. Begin with a portable unit ($200–$1,000), apply 15–30 minutes daily, and assess—less pain, better rest—over 4–8 weeks, refining with professional input if outcomes falter.

Bottom Line

PEMF therapy uses pulsed electromagnetic fields through mats, coils, or wearables (10–60 minutes daily) to stimulate cellular health, offering pain relief, reduced inflammation, better sleep, stress reduction, and enhanced recovery. Veterans with pain, fatigue, or stress from service can benefit from this non-invasive approach, with studies showing pain and healing improvements over weeks, supported by user experiences for sleep and stress. It's a pulsed, low-frequency method, unlike static magnets. Evidence is solid for pain and bone repair—clinical trials confirm it—but sleep and stress benefits rely on smaller studies, lacking broad consensus. Risks include mild overstimulation or device interference, a concern for Veterans with implants, plus costs ($100–$5,000) that may strain budgets. It's not a stand-alone treatment for serious conditions—professionals recommend pairing with VA care due to mixed data and mild effects—so consult a healthcare provider, start with affordable devices ($200–$1,000), and integrate with existing routines, approaching with realistic goals and oversight. It's a practical tool for some, not a full fix, requiring consistent use.

Peptides

Peptides are short chains of amino acids, typically 2–50 units, that function as signaling molecules in the body to regulate hormone production, tissue repair, and immune response. They differ from proteins, which are longer, and are used therapeutically through injections, oral supplements, nasal sprays, or topicals to address health issues. Veterans, facing chronic pain, slow recovery, or mental health challenges from service, can use peptides to support healing and resilience. Benefits claimed include improved recovery, reduced inflammation, and enhanced cognitive function, supported by clinical research and growing use in regenerative medicine, though evidence varies by peptide, and risks like side effects or regulatory gaps apply.

Peptides emerged in medicine with insulin in the 1920s; synthetic versions like BPC-157 developed in the 1990s, with research expanding in the 2000s and Veteran-focused studies by the 2020s for recovery and stress. Chronic conditions—pain, disability, and fatigue—affect many Veterans, driving interest in peptides as a regenerative option. Combat injuries, stress, and toxin exposure accelerate tissue damage; peptides target these repair needs. Symptoms like PTSD, tiredness, and slow healing indicate areas peptides may address, acting in doses from micrograms to milligrams over days to months.

Delivery includes subcutaneous injections (200–500 mcg daily), oral capsules (5–10 g daily), nasal sprays (100–300 mcg daily), or topical creams (1–2 mg daily), used for 4–12 weeks. Benefits include tissue repair with peptides like BPC-157, reduced inflammation with TB-500, cognitive enhancement with Semax, mood improvement with Selank, and muscle growth with CJC-1295. Risks involve nausea or water retention; unregulated sources risk contamination, and Veterans with heart issues need caution. Studies show benefits in small trials, but human data for some peptides is limited, and few are FDA-approved beyond specific uses like insulin. Pain, brain injury, and stress make peptides relevant for Veterans, who can access them through VA or private providers.

Targeted Protocols for Veterans' Wellness

Veterans with chronic pain, slow healing, or mental strain from service can explore peptides to target specific needs. Begin with a functional medicine doctor or VA consultation ($0–$500) to assess symptoms—joint pain, fatigue, memory issues—and match peptides to goals; VA may cover diagnostics, or functional offices with foundation support, like the Gary Sinise Foundation or Wounded Warrior Project, can offset costs for qualifying Veterans. Track progress with logs—pain levels, energy, focus—to adjust over 4–12 weeks.

For tissue repair, BPC-157 injections (200–500 mcg daily, $50–$100/vial) target injuries—subcutaneous shots near the site, self-administered or by a clinician for 4–8 weeks; Veterans with lingering wounds see faster healing in weeks, tweaking dose with a doctor if needed. Inflammation reduces with TB-500 (500 mcg injections, 2–3 times weekly), calming swelling—Veterans with joint soreness notice less stiffness over a month; monitor and adjust if progress slows.

Cognitive enhancement uses Semax nasal spray (100–300 mcg daily, $30–$70/bottle), 1–2 doses for 1–4 weeks—Veterans with brain fog or TBI gain focus in days; extend or pair with therapy if effects fade. Mood improvement comes from Selank nasal spray (200 mcg daily), reducing anxiety over 3–4 weeks—Veterans with depression or stress feel calmer, checking logs to refine use. Muscle growth relies on CJC-1295 injections (2 mg weekly, $50–$100/vial), boosting strength—Veterans rebuilding physically see gains in 8 weeks; blood tests (IGF-1, $50–$100) track response.

Oral collagen peptides (5–10 g daily, $20–$50/month) support joints and gut, taken daily for months—Veterans with pain feel relief over 12 weeks; consistency matters. Topical GHK-Cu cream (1–2 mg daily, $30–$60/tube) aids scars or skin repair, applied daily for weeks—Veterans with visible service marks see improvement in a month. Blood tests or symptom logs monitor effects—adjust doses weekly or monthly with a provider; VA protocols suggest 4–12 week cycles.

Consult a healthcare provider before starting, especially with heart conditions,

PTSD, or medications, to ensure safety and VA alignment. VA care or foundation-backed providers (like Gary Sinise or Wounded Warrior) keep costs manageable—free through VA or $20–$500 private. Start with oral collagen or prescribed injections, dose daily or weekly, and assess—less pain, sharper mind—over 4–12 weeks, refining with professional input if results stall.

Bottom Line

Peptides, short amino acid chains, offer tissue repair, reduced inflammation, cognitive enhancement, mood improvement, and muscle growth through injections (e.g., BPC-157, 200–500 mcg), oral doses (e.g., collagen, 5–10 g), nasal sprays (e.g., Semax), or topicals, targeting health needs. Veterans with pain, TBI, or PTSD can use them for recovery, with studies showing 15–30% improvements in healing, cognition, and mood over 4–12 weeks. They're precise bioactive agents, unlike proteins. Evidence supports specific benefits—small trials (20–60 participants) and clinical use show promise—but many (e.g., BPC-157) lack large human RCTs; FDA approval is limited to a few like insulin. Risks include side effects (e.g., nausea) and unregulated sourcing, a concern for Veterans with complex needs. They're not a standalone treatment—professionals require oversight due to variable data and safety issues—so consult a healthcare provider, source via VA or trusted clinicians ($20–$500), and monitor with logs, integrating with VA care. They're a targeted tool for some, not a broad fix, needing informed application.

Personal Exercise Plan
(also, see Fitness)

Creating a personalized exercise plan can help you achieve your fitness goals and make exercise a sustainable part of your lifestyle. Here are some steps to consider when creating your own personalized exercise plan:

• *Assess your current fitness level:* Take into consideration your current physical activity level, any medical conditions or injuries and your overall health. This will help you set realistic and achievable goals for your exercise plan.

• *Set specific and measurable goals:* Your goals should be specific, measurable and time-bound. For example, instead of setting a goal to "lose weight," set a goal to "lose 10 pounds in 8 weeks."

• *Identify the types of exercise that you enjoy:* This is important because you are more likely to stick to an exercise plan if you enjoy the activities you are doing. Consider your personal interests and preferences when selecting activities.

- **Create a schedule:** It's important to include exercise in your daily routine. You can schedule your workouts for the same time each day or week to help make it a habit.

- **Gradually increase the intensity and duration of your workouts:** It's important to start with a workout that is appropriate for your current fitness level and gradually increase the intensity and duration as your fitness improves.

- **Monitor your progress:** Keep track of your progress by measuring your weight, body fat percentage and other relevant metrics. This will help you stay motivated and make any necessary adjustments to your exercise plan.

- **Get professional guidance:** It's always a good idea to consult a professional, such as a personal trainer, to help you create a personalized exercise plan that is safe and effective.

- **Be consistent:** Consistency is key when it comes to achieving your fitness goals. It's important to stick to your exercise plan, even on days when you may not feel like working out.

- **Have fun:** Remember that exercise should be enjoyable, not a chore. So, try to find activities that you enjoy and make sure to keep a positive attitude.

Bottom Line

Creating a personalized exercise plan can help you achieve your fitness goals and make exercise a sustainable part of your lifestyle. By assessing your current fitness level, setting specific and measurable goals, identifying the types of exercise that you enjoy, creating a schedule, gradually increasing the intensity and duration of your workouts, monitoring your progress, getting professional guidance, being consistent and having fun, you can create a plan that works for you.

Photon Sound Beam Therapy

Photon Sound Beam Therapy is a type of alternative therapy that uses light and sound frequencies to improve overall health and wellbeing. This therapy is based on the concept that the body is composed of energy and that the application of specific frequencies can help to balance and harmonize this energy, leading to improved health and wellness.

The Photon Sound Beam Therapy device generates light and sound frequencies, which are then applied to the body through various methods, such as through the skin or earlobes. The frequencies are said to penetrate the body and interact with the body's energy, helping to improve circulation, reduce inflammation, boost the immune system and promote overall health.

Benefits of Photon Sound Beam Therapy

• *Reduces inflammation:* Photon Sound Beam Therapy is said to reduce inflammation, which is a key factor in many chronic health conditions, including cancer, arthritis and heart disease.

• *Boosts the immune system:* The therapy is said to boost the immune system, helping to improve the body's ability to fight off infections and diseases. Improves circulation: Photon Sound Beam Therapy is said to improve circulation, which can help to deliver nutrients and oxygen to the cells and tissues and improve overall health.

• *Promotes relaxation:* The therapy is said to promote relaxation and reduce stress, which can help to improve overall health and wellbeing.

• *Supports the digestive system:* Photon Sound Beam Therapy is said to support the digestive system, helping to improve digestion, reduce bloating and support overall gut health.

• *Supports the nervous system:* The therapy is said to support the nervous system, helping to improve brain function, reduce anxiety and depression and improve overall mental health.

It is important to note that the benefits of Photon Sound Beam Therapy are largely anecdotal and there is limited scientific evidence to support the effectiveness of this therapy for treating cancer or any other condition.

Bottom Line
Photon Sound Beam Therapy is a type of alternative therapy that uses light and sound frequencies to improve overall health and wellbeing. While the therapy is said to provide a range of benefits, including reducing inflammation, boosting the immune system and improving circulation, the evidence supporting these claims is limited. It is important to discuss the use of Photon Sound Beam Therapy with a healthcare provider to determine if it is safe and appropriate for your individual needs.

Physical Health = Mental Health

The connection between physical health and mental health is a complex and intricate one, with each aspect of a person's well-being having a significant impact on the other. Physical health and mental health are intimately connected, with each aspect of a person's well-being influencing the other in various ways. This is why it is essential to take care of both physical and mental health in order to achieve optimal overall well-being.

One of the most significant ways in which physical health and mental health are connected is through the impact of chronic illnesses on mental well-being. Chronic illnesses such as diabetes, heart disease, cancer, COPD, TBI, and autoimmune disorders like fibromyalgia and rheumatoid arthritis can cause emotional distress and can lead to the development of mental health conditions such as depression and anxiety. The stress and uncertainty that come with having a chronic illness can also cause emotional distress. Additionally, physical symptoms associated with chronic illnesses, such as pain and fatigue, can also contribute to feelings of depression and anxiety.

The reverse is also true, with mental health conditions having a significant impact on physical health. Depression and anxiety, for example, can cause fatigue, headaches and changes in appetite, which can lead to weight gain or weight loss. These conditions can also lead to the development of chronic illnesses over time. Stress, which is a common symptom of mental health conditions, is also known to have a negative impact on physical health, as it can increase the risk of developing heart disease and other chronic illnesses.

The way a person takes care of their physical health can also have an impact on their mental well-being. Exercise, for example, is known to be an effective treatment for depression and anxiety as it releases serotonin and endorphins, two of the body's natural mood-boosters.[20] Eating a healthy diet, getting enough sleep and maintaining a healthy body weight are also important for maintaining good mental health. On the other hand, neglecting physical health can lead to the development of mental health conditions, as well as physical health problems.

Another way in which physical health and mental health are connected is through the impact of medication on both aspects of well-being. Medications used to treat physical health conditions, such as blood pressure medication, can also have an impact on mental health, as they can cause side effects such as drowsiness, fatigue and changes in mood. Medications used to treat mental health conditions, such as antidepressants, can also have an impact on physical health, as they can cause side effects such as changes in appetite and weight gain.

It is important to note that the connection between physical health and mental health is not a one-way street. There are numerous ways in which physical and mental well-being are interconnected and impact each other. In order to achieve optimal overall well-being, it is essential to take care of both physical and mental health. This can be achieved through a combination of healthy lifestyle choices, such as exercise, diet, and sleep, as well as through seeking professional help when needed.

Bottom Line

The connection between physical health and mental health is a complex and intricate one, with each aspect of a person's well-being having a significant impact on the other. Chronic illnesses can cause emotional distress and mental health conditions can affect physical health. The way a person takes care of their physical health can also have an impact on their mental well-being. Medications can also have an impact on both physical and mental health. It is essential to take care of both physical and mental health in order to achieve optimal overall well-being. This can be achieved through a combination of healthy lifestyle choices, such as exercise, diet, and sleep, as well as through seeking professional help when needed.

Preparedness

Preparedness is a state of readiness for any situation that may arise, whether it be a natural disaster, financial crisis or a personal emergency. For Veterans, preparedness can provide numerous benefits in their personal lives, helping them to better manage their daily activities and regain a sense of control and stability.

• *Provides structure and a sense of purpose:* Preparedness requires Veterans to develop a plan, set goals and take concrete steps to achieve them. This structured approach helps to give Veterans a sense of purpose and direction in their lives, as they work towards a goal that is meaningful to them.

• *Improves mental and physical well-being:* Preparedness activities such as outdoor recreation, exercise and skill-building can be therapeutic and help to improve Veterans' mental and physical well-being. Through these activities, Veterans can build resilience and develop positive coping skills that they can draw on in times of stress.

• *Develops coping skills for stress and trauma:* Preparedness activities can also provide a therapeutic outlet for Veterans struggling with the effects of trauma and stress. For example, outdoor recreation can help Veterans to decompress and refocus their thoughts, while skill-building can give them a sense of accomplishment and pride.

• *Builds self-sufficiency and independence:* Preparedness is about being self-sufficient and able to take care of oneself in any situation. By developing the skills and resources needed to meet their own needs, Veterans can become more independent and better able to manage their own lives.

• *Facilitates a successful transition back to civilian life:* The skills and experience that Veterans develop through preparedness can also be useful in their transition back to civilian life. By learning new skills, building a network of resources and gaining a sense of purpose and direction, Veterans can be better prepared to navigate the challenges of civilian life.

Building a preparedness plan

• *Assess your current needs:* Start by evaluating your current situation, including your personal needs, family responsibilities and financial status. This will help you determine what you need to prepare for and what resources you have available.

• *Set realistic goals:* Based on your assessment, set achievable goals that you want to work towards in your preparedness plan. This could be as simple as having a supply of non-perishable food and water or as complex as building a self-sufficient homestead.

• *Make a list of necessary supplies:* Make a list of the supplies and equipment that you will need to reach your preparedness goals. This may include food, water, medical supplies, tools, clothing and shelter.

• *Build a network of resources:* Connect with other Veterans, local organizations and community groups to build a network of resources that you can rely on in times of need.

• *Learn new skills:* Consider taking classes or attending workshops on skills that will be useful in a preparedness scenario. This could include first aid, outdoor survival skills or gardening.

• *Get involved in the community:* Join local preparedness groups and participate in community events and activities. This will help you to build relationships and connections with others in your community.

• *Plan and practice:* Once you have a solid plan in place, you should regularly practice your preparedness skills and strategies. This will help you to be better prepared and confident in your ability to respond in a real-life situation.

• *Review and update your plan:* Review and update your preparedness plan on a regular basis to ensure that it remains relevant and effective.

By following these steps, Veterans can build a comprehensive preparedness plan that will help them to be better prepared for any situation that may arise.

Bottom Line

Preparedness can be a valuable tool for Veterans as they work to regain control and stability in their lives. By providing structure, promoting mental and physical well-being, developing coping skills for stress and trauma, building self-sufficiency and independence and facilitating a successful transition back to civilian life, preparedness can help Veterans better organize their lives and move forward with confidence.

Probiotics

Live microorganisms beneficial to health when consumed in adequate amounts, probiotics are found in foods such as yogurt, kefir, sauerkraut and kimchi, as well as in supplement form. Probiotics can provide a range of health benefits, particularly for Veterans who may have unique health concerns related to their service.

One benefit of probiotics is their role in promoting gut health. The gut is home to trillions of bacteria, both beneficial and harmful. Consuming probiotics can help to increase the number of beneficial bacteria in the gut, which can improve digestive function and overall gut health. This can be particularly important for Veterans, who may experience gastrointestinal issues related to their service.

Probiotics also can help boost the immune system. The gut is home to a large portion of the body's immune system and consuming probiotics can help to support this system. Studies have shown that probiotics can help to reduce the risk of upper respiratory tract infections, as well as reduce the severity and duration of these infections when they do occur.

For Veterans, who could be at higher risk of infections and other health concerns due to their service, consuming probiotics can be an important part of maintaining overall health and well-being.

Another benefit of probiotics is their role in reducing inflammation in the body. Chronic inflammation is a contributing factor to many chronic diseases, including heart disease, arthritis and even cancer. Probiotics have been shown to help reduce inflammation in the body, which may help to prevent or manage these conditions.

Probiotics can have positive impacts on mental health. Studies have shown that probiotics can help to reduce symptoms of depression and anxiety, as well as improve overall mood and well-being. This may be due to the fact that the gut and brain are connected through the gut-brain axis and consuming probiotics can help to support this connection.

Another high risk to Veterans is a group of mental health conditions such as PTSD, depression and anxiety. Consuming probiotics can be an important part of maintaining overall mental health and well-being.

And probiotics can have positive impacts on skin health. The gut and skin are also connected through the gut-skin axis and consuming probiotics can help to support this connection. Studies have shown that probiotics can help to reduce symptoms of eczema and other skin conditions, as well as improve overall skin health and appearance.

For Veterans at higher risk of skin conditions related to their service, consuming probiotics can be an important part of maintaining overall skin health and well-being.

To enhance the benefits of probiotics, there are several strategies that Veterans can employ:

 • *Consume probiotic-rich foods:* Foods like yogurt, kefir, sauerkraut and kimchi are all good sources of probiotics. Including these foods in the diet on a regular basis can help to increase the number of beneficial bacteria in the gut.

 • *Take a probiotic supplement:* Probiotic supplements are available in a range of strains and dosages. Taking a probiotic supplement can help to ensure adequate intake of beneficial bacteria.

 • *Consume prebiotic-rich foods:* Prebiotics are a type of fiber that feeds beneficial bacteria in the gut. Foods like garlic, onions, bananas and asparagus are all good sources of prebiotics.

 • *Avoid excessive alcohol consumption:* Excessive alcohol consumption can have negative impacts on gut health and can disrupt the balance of beneficial bacteria in the gut.

 • *Reduce stress:* Chronic stress can have negative impacts on gut health and can disrupt the balance of beneficial bacteria in the gut. Finding ways to reduce stress, like meditation, yoga and deep breathing exercises, can be beneficial for gut health and overall well-being.

Consuming probiotics and enhancing their benefits can be an important part of a comprehensive approach to maintaining overall health and well-being for Veterans. By supporting gut health and the immune system, reducing inflammation and improving mental and skin health, probiotics can play a valuable role in promoting health and wellness for Veterans.

By consuming probiotic-rich foods, taking a probiotic supplement, consuming prebiotic-rich foods, avoiding excessive alcohol consumption and reducing stress, Veterans can enhance the benefits of probiotics and improve overall health and well-being.

It is important to note that not all probiotic supplements are created equal and it is important to choose a high-quality supplement that contains a variety of strains of beneficial bacteria. It is also important to consult with a healthcare provider before starting any new supplement, particularly if there are underlying health conditions or concerns.

Bottom Line

Probiotics are an important aspect of maintaining overall health and well-being, particularly for Veterans who may have unique health concerns related to their service. Probiotics can provide a range of benefits, including promoting gut health, boosting the immune system, reducing inflammation, improving mental health and enhancing skin health.

Processed Foods

A common staple in the modern American diet because they are convenient and often affordable, processed foods can have negative impacts on health, particularly for Veterans with unique health concerns related to their service.

Processed foods are defined as foods that have been altered from their natural state through techniques like canning, freezing, drying or baking. These foods often contain added preservatives, chemicals and sugars, which can have negative impacts on health. For Veterans, who may be more susceptible to certain health conditions due to their service, avoiding processed foods can be an important part of maintaining overall health and well-being.

One hazard of processed foods for Veterans is the potential for weight gain and obesity. Processed foods are often high in calories and low in nutrients like fiber, vitamins and minerals. This can lead to overconsumption, as the body craves more nutrients that are lacking in processed foods. In addition, processed foods often contain added sugars and unhealthy fats, which can contribute to weight gain and obesity.

Weight gain and obesity can be particularly problematic for Veterans, who may be more susceptible to certain health conditions like type 2 diabetes and cardiovascular disease. These conditions can be further exacerbated by excess weight and can have negative impacts on overall health and well-being.

Another hazard of processed foods for Veterans is the potential for inflammation. Many processed foods contain high levels of refined carbohydrates and omega-6 fatty acids, which can contribute to inflammation in the body. Inflammation is a contributing factor to many chronic diseases, including heart disease, arthritis and even cancer.

Inflammation can be a particular concern for Veterans who have experienced trauma or injury. Inflammatory conditions like arthritis and chronic pain are common among Veterans and consuming a diet high in processed foods can exacerbate these conditions.
Processed foods can have negative impacts on gut health, which is an important aspect of overall health and well-being. Many processed foods contain added preservatives and chemicals, which can disrupt the balance of healthy bacteria in the gut. This can lead to digestive issues like bloating, gas and constipation and can contribute to overall inflammation in the body.

For Veterans with unique health concerns related to their service, maintaining a healthy gut is particularly important. Many Veterans experience gastrointestinal issues related to their service and consuming a diet high in processed foods can exacerbate these conditions.

Processed foods can have negative impacts on mental health. Studies have shown that diets high in processed foods are associated with an increased risk of depression and anxiety. This may be due to the fact that processed foods are often low in nutrients like omega-3 fatty acids, which are important for brain health.

For Veterans, who could be at higher risk of mental health conditions such as PTSD, depression and anxiety, consuming a diet high in processed foods can have negative impacts on overall mental health and well-being.

Bottom Line
Processed foods can have significant hazards for Veterans, who may be more susceptible to certain health conditions due to their service. Weight gain, inflammation, digestive issues and negative impacts on mental health are all potential hazards of a diet high in processed foods. By consuming a diet that is rich in whole, nutrient-dense foods like fruits, vegetables, whole grains and lean proteins, Veterans can maintain overall health and well-being and mitigate potential health risks associated with processed foods.

Psilocybin Therapy

Psilocybin, a naturally occurring psychedelic compound found in certain mushrooms, is gaining attention for its potential to treat mental health conditions like PTSD, depression, and anxiety. Veterans, who often face persistent trauma-related symptoms, are at the forefront of research into alternative therapies. Unlike traditional medications that manage symptoms, psilocybin works by inducing neuroplasticity—rewiring brain connections to process trauma differently. Early studies suggest lasting benefits after just one or two sessions. This section explores psilocybin's effects, the science behind its therapeutic potential, and how Veterans might benefit.

Understanding Psilocybin

Psilocybin is classified as a psychedelic compound that influences serotonin receptors in the brain. This temporary alteration in consciousness may allow for:

- Emotional Reset: Reduced fear response, easing PTSD-related hyperarousal.

- Neuroplasticity: Enhanced brain adaptability, facilitating trauma processing.

- Perspective Shift: Heightened self-awareness, reducing depressive thought patterns.

The Science Behind Psychedelic-Assisted Therapy

Research from Nature Medicine (2021) found that psilocybin-assisted therapy significantly reduced PTSD symptoms in Veterans. A Johns Hopkins University study (2020) reported long-term reductions in depression and anxiety after guided psilocybin sessions. Unlike daily medications, psilocybin may provide lasting benefits after minimal doses, working by rewiring neural pathways associated with trauma and fear.

Why Psilocybin Matters for Veterans

- PTSD Relief: Helps break cycles of intrusive thoughts, hypervigilance, and emotional numbness.

- Depression & Anxiety Reduction: Enhances emotional processing, decreasing avoidance behaviors.

- Substance Dependence Support: Early studies suggest potential for treating alcohol and opioid use disorders.

- Spiritual & Existential Clarity: Some Veterans report improved outlook and renewed purpose post-therapy.

Identifying Candidates for Psilocybin Therapy

- Common Signs: Persistent PTSD symptoms, depression, emotional numbness, or medication resistance.

- Veteran-Specific Triggers: Combat stress, moral injury, difficulty reintegrating into civilian life.
- Current Treatment Landscape: Traditional therapies (e.g., SSRIs, talk therapy) offer mixed results; psilocybin may supplement or replace ineffective treatments.
- Assessment Tools: VA mental health screenings, self-reported symptom tracking, and clinical evaluations.

How Psilocybin Therapy Works

- Guided Sessions: Administered in a controlled setting with trained professionals.
- Set & Setting: Emphasizes preparation, safe environments, and integration support post-session.
- Therapeutic Approach: Often paired with cognitive therapy to process experiences.
- Duration: Effects last 4–6 hours per session, with long-term benefits emerging over weeks to months.

Potential Benefits for Veterans

1. Emotional Resilience (PTSD, Depression)

- What: Guided psilocybin-assisted therapy in clinical settings.
- Why: Reduces fear-based memories and depressive cycles.
- How: Supervised sessions with integration therapy afterward.
- Supplies: Licensed therapist, supportive environment.

2. Cognitive Flexibility (Trauma Processing)

- What: One or two sessions with structured follow-ups.
- Why: Enhances neuroplasticity, allowing new perspectives on trauma.
- How: Therapy-driven discussion post-session to reinforce insights.
- Supplies: Clinical support, journaling for integration.

3. Anxiety & Hypervigilance Reduction

- What: Psychedelic-assisted therapy in a VA-approved setting.
- Why: Reduces amygdala hyperactivity, lowering anxiety and overactive fight-or-flight responses.

- How: Pre-session coaching, monitored experience, follow-up therapy.
- Supplies: Professional facilitation, quiet post-session environment.

4. Sense of Purpose & Connection

- What: Intentional sessions with mindfulness practices.
- Why: Increases feelings of connectedness, reducing isolation.
- How: Integration with group therapy or spiritual exploration.
- Supplies: Support network, post-session reflection practices.

Safety, Legal Considerations & Risks

- Current Legal Status: Psilocybin remains federally classified as a Schedule I substance, though states like Oregon and Colorado have decriminalized or approved therapeutic use.
- Clinical Trials: Ongoing research at institutions like Johns Hopkins and MAPS (Multidisciplinary Association for Psychedelic Studies) aims to legalize medical use.
- Potential Risks: Unsupervised use can lead to distressing experiences, paranoia, or emotional over-whelm.
- Medical Precautions: Not recommended for Veterans with schizophrenia or severe psychiatric instability.

Integrating Psilocybin Therapy into Veteran Wellness

- Set SMART Goals: Example: "Participate in a clinical trial or legal therapeutic setting within 6 months to explore alternative PTSD treatment."
- Explore Clinical Options: Research VA-affiliated studies, private trials, or future policy changes.
- Build a Support System: Peer networks, therapy groups, and post-session integration practices enhance benefits.
- Stay Informed: Follow legislation changes, research updates, and advocacy groups pushing for Veteran access.

Bottom Line
Psilocybin-assisted therapy presents a promising frontier for Veterans struggling with PTSD, depression, and emotional trauma. Unlike traditional medications, it offers the potential for long-term healing after minimal sessions by promoting neuroplasticity and trauma processing. While studies support its effectiveness, legal barriers and safety concerns remain. Veterans interested in this therapy should

explore clinical trials, research developments, and future VA options. By integrating psilocybin into structured therapy settings, Veterans may find a path toward profound healing and emotional resilience.

PTSD

PTSD (Post-Traumatic Stress Disorder) is not limited to military operations. It can occur in anyone who has experienced or witnessed a traumatic event, including:

- Natural disasters (e.g. hurricanes, earthquakes)
- Acts of violence (e.g. sexual assault, physical assault, domestic violence)
- Accidents (e.g. car crashes, falls)
- Illness or injury
- Witnessing violence or tragedy

Symptoms of PTSD include:

- intrusive memories of the traumatic event,
- avoidance of reminders of the event,
- negative changes in mood and cognition,
- increased arousal (e.g. difficulty sleeping, irritability, hypervigilance)

If you believe you may have PTSD, it is important to seek help from a mental health professional. Treatment options for PTSD may include talk therapy, medication and/or group therapy.

There are several beneficial practices that can help individuals with PTSD, including:

- ***Cognitive Behavioral Therapy (CBT):*** A form of talk therapy that helps individuals challenge and change negative thought patterns and behaviors.

- ***Exposure Therapy:*** Gradually exposing individuals to trauma-related memories or situations to help them process and overcome their fears.

- ***Mindfulness-Based Therapies:*** Practices such as meditation and yoga that help individuals focus on the present moment and reduce stress.

- ***Group Therapy:*** Connecting with others who have experienced similar traumas can help individuals feel less isolated and provide support.

• **Physical Exercise:** Regular physical activity can help reduce symptoms of anxiety and depression, improve sleep and boost self-esteem.

• **Stress Management Techniques:** Techniques such as deep breathing, progressive muscle relaxation and guided imagery can help individuals manage symptoms of stress and anxiety.

It's important to note that what works for one person may not work for another, so it may be necessary to try a few different strategies to find what works best. Consulting a mental health professional is recommended for individuals suffering from PTSD to receive personalized care and treatment.

PTSD-sufferers can get help from several sources, including:

• **Mental Health Professionals:** Psychologists, therapists and psychiatrists can provide evidence-based treatment, such as cognitive behavioral therapy and medication.

• **Support Groups:** Joining a support group can provide individuals with a sense of community and help them connect with others who have experienced similar traumas.

• **Employee Assistance Programs:** Many employers offer EAPs to their employees, which can provide free or low-cost counseling services.

• **Hotlines:** There are several hotlines that provide support and resources for individuals struggling with mental health issues, such as:

   National Suicide Prevention Lifeline (1-800-273-TALK),

   Substance Abuse and Mental Health Services Administration (SAMHSA) Treatment Referral Helpline (1-800-662-HELP),

• **Community Health Centers:** Many community health centers provide low-cost or free mental health services to individuals in need.

It is important to remember that seeking help is a sign of strength and that it is never too late to start the healing process.

- R -

<u>Red Light Therapy</u>

Also known as photobiomodulation therapy, it is a non-invasive treatment that uses low-level red and near-infrared light to penetrate the skin and provide various health benefits. The therapeutic use of red light dates back to ancient times and today, it is increasingly recognized as a promising solution for a variety of health conditions.[21]

Here are some of the benefits of red light therapy:

• **Skin rejuvenation:** Red light therapy can help improve skin health by reducing fine lines, wrinkles and age spots. It also promotes collagen production, which can help improve skin elasticity and texture.

• **Pain relief:** Red light therapy has been shown to reduce pain in a variety of conditions including arthritis, back pain and neuropathic pain.[22]

• **Wound healing:** Red light therapy has been shown to improve wound healing and reduce the appearance of scars.[23]

• **Improved sleep:** Red light therapy has been shown to improve sleep quality by regulating the body's circadian rhythm. The light can help regulate the production of melatonin, which is a hormone that regulates sleep and wakefulness.[24]

• **Enhanced athletic performance:** Red light therapy has been shown to improve athletic performance by reducing muscle soreness and improving recovery time. The light increases blood flow and oxygenation to the muscles, which helps improve endurance and strength.[25]

• **Reduced stress:** Red light therapy has been shown to reduce stress and improve mood by increasing the production of serotonin, which is a hormone that regulates mood and stress levels.[26]

• **Boosted immune system:** Red light therapy has been shown to boost the immune system by increasing the production of white blood cells, which are the body's first line of defense against illness and disease.

Red light therapy is a safe, non-invasive treatment that can be performed in the comfort of one's own home. The treatment typically involves using a device that emits red and near-infrared light and it is recommended to receive regular treatments for optimal results.

Bottom Line
Red light therapy has numerous health benefits and can be used as a complementary or alternative treatment for a variety of conditions. Whether you are looking to improve your skin health, reduce pain, enhance athletic performance or simply improve your overall well-being, red light therapy is worth considering. As always, it is recommended to consult with a healthcare provider before starting any new treatment.

Reiki

Reiki is a complementary healing modality that originated in Japan. It involves the use of the practitioner's hands to channel energy into the recipient's body to promote relaxation, balance and healing. Reiki is becoming increasingly popular as a complementary therapy for a range of health conditions, including those experienced by Veterans.

For Veterans with physical and mental health concerns related to their service, Reiki can provide a range of benefits, including:

• *Pain management:* Chronic pain is a common issue for many Veterans, particularly those who have experienced physical injuries or trauma during their service. Reiki has been shown to be effective in reducing pain and improving physical function in those with chronic pain conditions, such as back pain, neck pain and joint pain.

• *Reduced stress and anxiety:* Many Veterans experience high levels of stress and anxiety, which can negatively impact their mental and physical health. Reiki has been shown to be effective in reducing stress and anxiety levels and improving overall mental health and well-being.

• *Improved sleep:* Sleep disturbances are common among Veterans with PTSD and other mental health conditions. Reiki has been shown to improve sleep quality and reduce the severity of insomnia.

• *Improved energy and vitality:* Many Veterans experience a lack of energy and vitality due to their physical and mental health concerns. Reiki has been shown to improve energy levels and promote overall feelings of vitality and well-being.

• *Improved immune function:* Reiki has been shown to stimulate the immune system, which can improve overall health and reduce the risk of illness and infection.

Reiki is generally considered safe when practiced by a trained and certified practitioner. Side effects are typically mild and include temporary feelings of dizziness, fatigue or emotional release.

To enhance the benefits of Reiki, Veterans can employ several strategies:

  • ***Seek out a certified and experienced Reiki practitioner:*** It is important to work with a certified and experienced Reiki practitioner who has experience treating Veterans and their unique health concerns.

  • ***Use Reiki in combination with other treatments:*** Reiki is not a standalone treatment for physical or mental health conditions. Veterans should continue to work with their healthcare providers to manage their conditions and may use Reiki as a complementary treatment.

  • ***Be open and honest with the Reiki practitioner:*** In order to achieve the best results from Reiki, Veterans should be open and honest with their Reiki practitioner about their health concerns, medications and treatment goals.

  • ***Practice self-care:*** Veterans should practice self-care strategies like exercise, healthy eating and stress management to support overall health and well-being in conjunction with Reiki.

Bottom Line
Reiki is a safe and effective complementary treatment option for Veterans who may experience physical and mental health concerns related to their service. By reducing pain, improving mental health and promoting overall feelings of relaxation and well-being, Reiki can play an important role in supporting the overall health and well-being of Veterans.

Relaxation

A powerful tool that can help to reduce stress and promote physical and mental well-being, relaxation is especially important for Veterans, who can experience a range of physical and mental health concerns related to their service. Relaxation techniques can be used as a complementary treatment to traditional medical therapies and can help to alleviate the symptoms of various conditions. Here are some of the benefits of relaxation for Veterans:

• **Reduced stress and anxiety:** Relaxation techniques, such as deep breathing, meditation and progressive muscle relaxation, can help to reduce stress and anxiety. High levels of stress and anxiety can negatively impact both physical and mental health and can increase the risk of a range of health problems, including heart disease, depression and anxiety disorders.

• **Improved sleep:** Sleep disturbances are common among Veterans with PTSD and other mental health conditions. Relaxation techniques can help to promote better sleep by reducing stress and tension in the body and calming the mind. By improving sleep quality and quantity, relaxation techniques can help to improve overall health and well-being.

• **Pain management:** Chronic pain is a common issue for many Veterans, particularly those who have experienced physical injuries or trauma during their service. Relaxation techniques, such as guided imagery and mindfulness meditation, have been shown to be effective in reducing pain and improving physical function in those with chronic pain conditions such as back pain, neck pain, and joint pain.

• **Improved mental health:** Relaxation techniques can help to improve overall mental health and well-being. They can reduce symptoms of anxiety and depression, improve mood and promote a greater sense of calm and balance.

• **Improved immune function:** High levels of stress and anxiety can weaken the immune system, making individuals more susceptible to illness and infection. Relaxation techniques have been shown to stimulate the immune system, which can improve overall health and reduce the risk of illness and infection.

There are many relaxation techniques that Veterans can use to promote relaxation and reduce stress. Here are some examples:

• **Deep breathing:** Deep breathing is a simple and effective technique that can be done anywhere, at any time. It involves taking slow, deep breaths focusing on the movement of the diaphragm and the sensation of air moving in and out of the body. Deep breathing can help to reduce stress, lower blood pressure and improve overall well-being.

• **Progressive muscle relaxation:** Progressive muscle relaxation involves tensing and relaxing different muscle groups in the body to promote relaxation and reduce tension. It can help to reduce stress and anxiety and improve sleep quality.

• **Guided imagery:** Guided imagery involves using the imagination to visualize a peaceful, calming scene or experience. It can help to reduce stress and anxiety, promote relaxation and improve overall well-being.

• **_Meditation:_** Meditation involves focusing the mind on a specific object, thought or activity to promote relaxation and reduce stress. It can help to improve mental clarity, reduce symptoms of anxiety and depression and promote overall well-being.

• **_Yoga:_** Yoga is a mind-body practice that combines physical postures, breathing techniques and meditation to promote relaxation and reduce stress. It can improve flexibility, strength and balance and promote overall well-being.

Bottom Line
Relaxation techniques can provide a range of benefits for Veterans, including reduced stress and anxiety, improved sleep, pain management, improved mental health and improved immune function. There are many relaxation techniques that Veterans can use to promote relaxation and reduce stress, including deep breathing, progressive muscle relaxation, guided imagery, meditation and yoga. By incorporating relaxation techniques into their daily routines, Veterans can improve their overall health and well-being and better manage the physical and mental health concerns related to their service.

Resilience

Resilience for Veterans refers to the ability to cope with and recover from the physical and emotional challenges that can result from military service. This can include dealing with trauma, adjusting to civilian life and managing physical injuries. There are various programs and resources available to help Veterans build resilience, such as counseling and therapy, peer support groups and physical fitness programs. Additionally, Veterans can also develop resilience through practices such as mindfulness, stress management and building a strong support network.

Building resilience
Military service can be a challenging and stressful experience for Veterans and the transition to civilian life can also be difficult. Trauma, physical injuries and the adjustment to a new way of life can all take a toll on a Veteran's mental and emotional well-being. However, Veterans can build resilience and cope with these challenges through the development of positive habits. In this entry, we will explore some of the key habits that Veterans can develop to increase their resilience and improve their overall well-being.

Mindfulness (also, see Mindfulness)
One of the most important habits that Veterans can develop to increase their resilience is mindfulness. Mindfulness is the practice of being present in the moment

and paying attention to one's thoughts, feelings and physical sensations. By becoming more aware of their thoughts and emotions, Veterans can learn to manage them more effectively, which can help to reduce stress and anxiety. Mindfulness can be practiced through meditation, yoga or simply by taking a few minutes each day to focus on breathing and being present in the moment.

Stress management

Another important habit that Veterans can develop to increase their resilience is stress management. Stress is a normal part of life, but chronic stress can have a negative impact on a person's health and well-being. Veterans can manage stress by identifying the sources of stress in their lives and then taking steps to reduce or eliminate those sources. Stress management techniques such as deep breathing, progressive muscle relaxation and visualization can also be helpful. Additionally, Veterans can also engage in regular physical activity, which has been shown to be an effective stress management tool.

Physical fitness (also, see Fitness)

Physical fitness is an important habit that Veterans can develop to increase their resilience. Regular exercise has been shown to improve mental and emotional well-being and can also help Veterans to manage physical injuries. Additionally, physical fitness can also be a great stress-reliever and can improve sleep quality. Veterans can engage in a variety of physical activities, including running, swimming, cycling and weightlifting.

Building a support network

Veterans can also build resilience by developing a strong support network. A support network can include friends, family members and other Veterans who understand the challenges that Veterans face. Support groups can be a great way for Veterans to connect with others who have had similar experiences. Additionally, Veterans can also seek out therapy or counseling, which can be a valuable tool for managing stress, anxiety and depression.

Planning and prioritizing

Another habit Veterans can develop to build resilience is planning and prioritizing. Veterans can use planning and prioritizing to set goals and take control of their lives. They can make a schedule, set priorities and deadlines and break down large tasks into smaller, manageable steps. This can give Veterans a sense of accomplishment, which can boost self-esteem and self-worth.

Positive thinking

Positive thinking is also an important habit that Veterans can develop to build resilience. Negative thoughts and self-talk can be detrimental to mental and emotional well-being. Veterans can engage in positive thinking by challenging negative thoughts and replacing them with more positive ones. Additionally, Veterans can also practice gratitude, which can help to shift their focus from the negative to the positive.

Self-care

Self-care is an essential habit for Veterans to build resilience. Veterans should make sure to take care of their physical, emotional and mental health. This can include getting enough sleep, eating well, practicing good hygiene and engaging in regular physical activity. Additionally, Veterans can also engage in activities that they enjoy, such as reading, writing or playing a musical instrument.

Bottom Line

Building resilient habits is critical for Veterans as they navigate the challenges of military service and transition to civilian life. By developing habits such as mindfulness, stress management, physical fitness, building a support network, planning and prioritizing, positive thinking and self-care, Veterans can improve their mental and emotional well-being and better cope with the difficulties they may face. It is important to remember that building resilience is not a one-time event but rather a continuous process and Veterans should be patient with themselves as they develop these habits. Additionally, Veterans should also seek out professional help if needed, as support from mental health professionals can be invaluable in building resilience.

Resveratrol

A naturally occurring compound found in red wine, grapes, peanuts and other plants, resveratrol has gained widespread attention due to its potential health benefits, which have been the subject of numerous scientific studies.[27]

One of the primary health benefits of resveratrol is its ability to support heart health. Resveratrol has been shown to reduce the risk of heart disease by lowering levels of LDL (bad) cholesterol and triglycerides and by reducing oxidative stress and inflammation. It also has been shown to improve the function of the endothelium, which is the inner lining of blood vessels.[28]

Resveratrol has also been found to have benefits for brain health. It has been shown to improve cognitive function, reduce the risk of neurodegenerative diseases such as Alzheimer's and Parkinson's and to protect the brain from oxidative stress and inflammation. Resveratrol has also been shown to increase the levels of a protein called brain-derived neurotrophic factor (BDNF), which is critical for the growth and survival of neurons.

Resveratrol has also been found to have anti-aging effects. It has been shown to extend lifespan in various animal models and to improve markers of health and longevity. Resveratrol works by activating a group of enzymes called sirtuins, which play a role in regulating cellular metabolism and stress resistance.

Resveratrol has also been found to have benefits for cancer prevention. It has been shown to inhibit the growth of cancer cells and to reduce the risk of certain types of cancer such as breast, prostate and colon cancer. Resveratrol works by reducing oxidative stress and inflammation and by inhibiting the activation of certain signaling pathways that promote the growth of cancer cells.

Resveratrol is generally considered safe when taken in recommended doses, although it can cause side effects such as gastrointestinal upset, headache and dizziness in some individuals. Resveratrol can also interact with certain medications, so it is important to consult with a healthcare professional before taking resveratrol if you are taking any medications.

Bottom Line
Resveratrol is a naturally occurring compound that has gained widespread attention due to its potential health benefits. From supporting heart health to improving brain health, anti-aging effects and cancer prevention, resveratrol is a popular supplement for individuals looking to support their overall health and wellness. However, it is important to note that further research is needed to fully understand the potential health benefits of resveratrol and to determine its long-term safety and efficacy. As with any supplement, it is important to consult with a healthcare professional before taking resveratrol to ensure that it is safe and appropriate for you.

Retreats - Connecting with a Like-Minded Group

Retreats for connecting with a like-minded group are multi-day events, typically 3–7 days, designed to unite individuals with shared experiences for therapy, education, and bonding in a supportive setting. They combine structured activities like group counseling or workshops with communal experiences, held in calm environments away from daily stress. Veterans, facing isolation, PTSD, or reintegration struggles post-service, can use these retreats to connect with peers who relate to their challenges. Benefits claimed include emotional healing, skill-building, and community support, supported by research on group therapy and social connection, though retreat-specific evidence is limited, and risks like emotional overwhelm apply.

These retreats trace back to religious pilgrimages and healing circles, evolving in the 20th century with psychotherapy groups in the 1940s and modern wellness trends. Isolation, PTSD, and adjustment issues affect many veterans, driving interest in retreats for peer support. Combat trauma, stress, and physical strain contribute to these struggles; retreats aim to address them through shared healing and learning. Symptoms like loneliness, anxiety, or lack of purpose prompt their use as a way to rebuild resilience.

Events involve 8–20 participants and include therapy sessions, educational workshops, and group activities, lasting 3–7 days. Benefits include healing through peer empathy, reduced isolation via community, practical skills like stress management, clearer focus from a break in routine, lower stress in a supportive space, and growth through reflection. Risks involve emotional strain from intense sharing; veterans with PTSD need caution. Studies show group therapy benefits, but retreat-specific data is sparse, relying on smaller trials and anecdotes. Isolation, PTSD, and a need for connection make retreats relevant for veterans, who can access them through VA-partnered or private programs.

Targeted Protocols for Veterans' Wellness
Veterans with isolation, PTSD, or adjustment struggles can use retreats to connect with peers. Find events through VA-partnered programs like Project Sanctuary, Wounded Warrior Project, or private retreats tailored to veterans ($500–$2,000 for 3–7 days); VA social workers can link to free or subsidized options, or functional providers with foundation support, like the Gary Sinise Foundation, may offset costs for qualifying veterans. Confirm the retreat's focus—combat vets, trauma survivors—and therapist credentials; set goals like "reduce stress" or "build trust" before attending. Log symptoms—mood, sleep, connection—before and after to track effects over weeks.

Retreats start with group therapy—1–2 hours daily, led by a trained therapist using CBT or EMDR—where 8–20 participants share experiences; veterans with PTSD process trauma with peer support, feeling relief in days, adjusting with a facilitator if it's heavy. Educational workshops, 1–3 hours daily, teach skills like mindfulness or communication—veterans learn coping tools over the retreat, applying them post-event; refine with VA follow-ups if needed. Shared activities—meals, hikes, or art, 2–4 hours daily—build bonds; veterans with isolation connect naturally, tracking trust over the stay.

Mental clarity comes from stepping away—veterans with TBI gain focus in 3–7 days, sustaining it with journaling (1–2 hours daily) during reflection time; pair with VA therapy if fog lingers. Stress reduction flows from the setting—veterans with transition tension feel calmer by day 5, using group support to maintain it; extend with mindfulness if stress returns. Personal growth builds through reflection and peer insights—veterans seeking purpose feel renewed post-retreat, assessing life satisfaction over weeks; closing rituals like a fire circle (1–2 hours) lock in gains.

Consult a healthcare provider before attending, especially with PTSD or depression, to ensure safety and fit with VA care; intense sharing can overwhelm some. Costs range from free via VA to $500–$2,000 private. Begin with a vetted retreat, participate fully in therapy and activities, and evaluate—less anxiety, more connection—over 1–3 months, refining with professional input if challenges arise.

Bottom Line

Retreats for connecting with a like-minded group offer emotional healing, community support, skill development, mental clarity, stress reduction, and personal growth through therapy sessions, workshops, and shared activities over 3–7 days. Veterans with PTSD, isolation, or reintegration issues can benefit from peer-driven healing, with studies showing 15–30% symptom relief over weeks to months. Unlike solo therapy, they emphasize group dynamics. Evidence supports group therapy principles—small trials confirm benefits—but retreat-specific data is limited, relying on anecdotes. Risks include emotional overwhelm or poor facilitation, a concern for veterans with mental health needs. They're not a standalone treatment—professionals advise VA integration due to sparse data—so consult a healthcare provider, join vetted programs (e.g., Wounded Warrior Project), and complement with clinical care, approaching with clear goals and caution. They're a strong peer support tool, not a full solution, needing careful selection.

Salt

An essential nutrient that plays an important role in maintaining overall health and well-being, incorporating the right type of salt into your diet can provide a range of health benefits. This section discusses the benefits of salt for Veterans and references Dr. Eric Berg's work on the subject.

- *Improved Hydration:* Salt plays an important role in maintaining fluid balance in the body. According to Dr. Berg, consuming the right type of salt can help the body to retain water and stay hydrated. This is particularly important for Veterans who may be at risk of dehydration due to their military service.

- *Improved Electrolyte Balance:* Salt is an important source of electrolytes, which are essential for a range of bodily functions. Dr. Berg notes that consuming the right type of salt can help to maintain a healthy balance of electrolytes in the body, which can improve overall health and well-being.

- *Improved Digestive Health:* Salt can also play a role in improving digestive health. According to Dr. Berg, consuming the right type of salt can help to stimulate the production of digestive enzymes and promote the absorption of nutrients.

- *Reduced Inflammation:* There is growing evidence that inflammation is a major contributor to a range of chronic health problems. Dr. Berg notes that consuming the right type of salt can help to reduce inflammation in the body, which can improve overall health and well-being.

- *Improved Athletic Performance:* Salt is an important source of electrolytes, which are essential for maintaining energy levels and athletic performance. Dr. Berg notes that consuming the right type of salt can help to improve athletic performance and reduce the risk of cramping and fatigue.

Some high-quality salt sources that Veterans can incorporate into their diet include Himalayan salt, Celtic sea salt and Redmond Real Salt. It is important to avoid highly processed table salt, which is often stripped of its natural minerals and can be harmful to health.

In addition to incorporating high-quality salt sources into their diet, Veterans can also consider taking a salt supplement. Dr. Berg recommends using an electrolyte powder that contains a blend of sodium, potassium and other essential minerals.

It is important to note that while salt can provide a range of health benefits, it is important to consume it in moderation. Consuming too much salt can lead to high blood pressure and other health problems. Veterans should aim to consume no more than 2,300 mg of sodium per day, which is the recommended daily limit for most adults.

Bottom Line

Salt is an essential nutrient that can provide a range of health benefits for Veterans. Eating a diet that includes high-quality salt sources can improve hydration, electrolyte balance, digestive health, reduce inflammation and improve athletic performance. Veterans can incorporate high-quality salt sources into their diet and consider taking a salt supplement to support overall health and well-being. As with any dietary changes, it is important to speak with a healthcare provider before making significant changes to one's diet.

Seed Oils

Also known as vegetable oils, they are a common staple in the modern American diet. Often used in cooking and food production, seed oils can be found in many processed and packaged foods. While they are often marketed as a healthier alternative to animal fats, seed oils can have negative impacts on health, particularly for Veterans who may have unique health concerns related to their service.

Seed oils are extracted from various plant sources, including soybeans, corn, canola, sunflower and safflower. These oils are high in polyunsaturated fats, which can be beneficial in small amounts, but can have negative impacts on health when consumed in excess.

One hazard of seed oils for Veterans is their potential for contributing to chronic inflammation. Seed oils are high in omega-6 fatty acids, which can contribute to inflammation in the body when consumed in excess. Inflammation is a contributing factor to many chronic diseases, including heart disease, arthritis and even cancer.

Chronic inflammation can be particularly problematic for Veterans, who may be more susceptible to these conditions due to their service. Consuming a diet high in seed oils can exacerbate these conditions and contribute to negative impacts on overall health and well-being.

Another hazard of seed oils for Veterans is their potential for contributing to mental health issues. Studies have shown that diets high in seed oils are associated with an increased risk of depression and anxiety. This may be due to the fact that seed oils are high in omega-6 fatty acids, which can have negative impacts on brain health when consumed in excess.

For Veterans, who may be at higher risk of mental health conditions like PTSD, depression and anxiety, consuming a diet high in seed oils can have negative impacts on overall mental health and well-being.

Seed oils can also have negative impacts on cardiovascular health, which can be a particular concern for Veterans. Consuming a diet high in seed oils can contribute to high levels of oxidized LDL cholesterol, which is a contributing factor to heart disease. In addition, seed oils can contribute to inflammation in the body, which can further exacerbate cardiovascular issues.

And seed oils can have negative impacts on gut health, which is an important aspect of overall health and well-being. Many seed oils contain high levels of polyunsaturated fats, which can contribute to oxidative stress and damage in the gut. This can lead to digestive issues like bloating, gas and constipation and can contribute to overall inflammation in the body.

For Veterans, who may have unique health concerns related to their service, maintaining a healthy gut is particularly important. Many Veterans experience gastrointestinal issues related to their service and consuming a diet high in seed oils can exacerbate these conditions.

Bottom Line
Seed oils can have significant hazards for Veterans, who may be more susceptible to certain health conditions due to their service. Chronic inflammation, negative impacts on mental health, cardiovascular issues and negative impacts on gut health are all potential hazards of a diet high in seed oils. By consuming a diet that is rich in whole, nutrient-dense foods like fruits, vegetables, whole grains and lean proteins and avoiding or minimizing the use of seed oils in cooking and food production, Veterans can maintain overall health and well-being and mitigate potential health risks associated with seed oils.

Sexual Trauma

Military sexual trauma (MST) is a pervasive problem that affects both male and female Veterans. According to the Department of Veterans Affairs (VA), about one in four women and one in 100 men report experiencing MST during their military service. The impact of MST on Veterans' mental and physical health can be significant and it is important to understand how to help Veterans who have experienced MST.

The Impact of MST on Veterans' Mental Health

MST can have a significant impact on Veterans' mental health. Many Veterans who experience MST report symptoms of depression, anxiety, post-traumatic stress disorder (PTSD) and substance abuse. MST can also impact Veterans' ability to form close relationships and trust others. The stigma and shame associated with MST can make it difficult for Veterans to seek help and access the support they need.

The Impact of MST on Veterans' Physical Health

MST can also impact Veterans' physical health. Studies have shown that Veterans who have experienced MST are at higher risk for a variety of health problems, including chronic pain, gastrointestinal problems and reproductive health issues. MST can also lead to increased risk-taking behaviors, such as substance abuse, which can further impact Veterans' physical health.

How to Help Veterans Who Have Experienced MST

- *Provide a Safe and Supportive Environment:* Creating a safe and supportive environment is essential for Veterans who have experienced MST. This includes providing a non-judgmental space where Veterans can share their experiences and feelings without fear of retaliation or stigma.

- *Offer Counseling and Mental Health Services:* Counseling and mental health services can be crucial in helping Veterans who have experienced MST. VA healthcare providers are trained to work with Veterans who have experienced MST and can provide counseling and other mental health services to help them cope with the impact of their experiences.

- *Educate and Train Providers:* It is important to educate and train healthcare providers, including VA staff, on how to recognize and respond to MST. This includes developing protocols for screening and responding to Veterans who disclose that they have experienced MST.

- *Address the Root Causes of MST:* Addressing the root causes of MST, including gender discrimination and unequal power dynamics, is essential in preventing future instances of MST. This may involve promoting policies and practices that support gender equality and creating a culture of respect and accountability within the military.

- *Support Research on MST:* More research is needed to understand the impact of MST and how to effectively address it. Supporting research on MST can help to identify effective interventions and treatments for Veterans who have experienced MST.

Bottom Line
MST is a significant problem that can have a profound impact on Veterans' mental and physical health. It is essential to create a safe and supportive environment for Veterans who have experienced MST and to provide counseling and mental health services to help them cope with the impact of their experiences. Addressing the root causes of MST and supporting research on the subject can help to prevent future instances of MST and improve outcomes for Veterans who have experienced this trauma.

Skills – Continuing Your Development

Continuing skill development refers to the ongoing process of acquiring new skills and refining existing ones throughout one's lifetime. In today's rapidly changing world, it is more important than ever to continuously develop new skills to stay relevant and competitive in both personal and professional settings.

First and foremost, continuing skill development is crucial for professional success and career advancement. As technology and industries continue to evolve, having a diverse set of skills can make individuals more valuable to employers and open up new career opportunities. This can help individuals stay ahead of the curve in a rapidly changing job market and increase their earning potential.

Moreover, continuing skill development can improve overall job performance and satisfaction. As individuals acquire new skills, they can better perform their job duties and take on new responsibilities, leading to increased job satisfaction and a sense of accomplishment. Furthermore, learning new skills can help individuals adapt to new technologies, processes and methodologies, allowing them to perform their job duties more efficiently and effectively.

Continuing skill development can also lead to personal growth and self-improvement. By acquiring new skills, individuals can broaden their horizons and expand their knowledge, leading to increased self-awareness and self-discovery. Additionally, taking on new challenges and learning new skills can help individuals develop their confidence and increase their self-esteem.

In addition, continuing skill development can help individuals stay mentally sharp and reduce the risk of cognitive decline as they age. By challenging the brain and keeping it active, individuals can maintain and improve their cognitive abilities, reducing the risk of cognitive decline and preserving their mental sharpness.

Another important aspect of continuing skill development is the opportunity it provides for individuals to network and connect with others who have similar interests and goals. By taking courses, attending workshops and participating in training programs, individuals can meet and connect with others who share their passion and drive for continuous learning and growth. This can lead to the formation of valuable personal and professional relationships, which can have a positive impact on one's personal and professional life.

Finally, continuing skill development can provide individuals with a sense of personal fulfillment and satisfaction. By continuously learning and growing, individuals can experience a sense of purpose and meaning, as well as a sense of accomplishment and success. This can lead to a more fulfilling and satisfying life, both personally and professionally.

Bottom Line
Continuing skill development is an essential aspect of personal and professional growth and success. It helps individuals stay relevant and competitive in a rapidly changing job market, improves job performance and satisfaction and leads to personal growth and self-improvement. Furthermore, it provides individuals with the opportunity to network and connect with others, stay mentally sharp and experience a sense of personal fulfillment and satisfaction. With the fast-paced and rapidly changing world we live in, continuing skill development is crucial for success, both in personal and professional settings.

Sleep

Sleep plays a vital role in maintaining physical and mental health. Some benefits of sleep include:

• *Physical restoration:* During sleep, the body repairs and rejuvenates itself. It also helps to regulate growth and development.

• *Mental restoration:* Sleep helps to consolidate memories, process information and improve cognitive function.

• *Emotional regulation:* Sleep helps to regulate emotions and reduce stress and anxiety.

• *Improved immune function:* Adequate sleep helps to boost the immune system and reduce the risk of infection and illness.

- **Better physical performance:** Sleep helps to improve physical performance and reduce the risk of injury.

- **Improved mood:** Sleep is associated with improved mood and overall well-being.

- **Reduced risk of chronic diseases:** Chronic sleep deprivation has been linked to an increased risk of obesity, diabetes, heart disease and other conditions.

- **Longevity:** Adequate sleep is also believed to contribute to a longer lifespan.

It is important to get enough quality sleep on a regular basis to reap these benefits. The recommended amount of sleep for adults is 7-9 hours per night.

In his book Why We Sleep, neuroscientist Matthew Walker explores the science of sleep and its impact on our physical and mental health.

According to Walker, sleep is essential for both physical and mental restoration. During sleep, the body repairs and rejuvenates itself, regulating growth and development. Additionally, sleep helps to consolidate memories and process information, improving cognitive function.

But the benefits of sleep go beyond just physical and mental restoration. Sleep also plays a crucial role in regulating emotions and reducing stress and anxiety. Adequate sleep helps to boost the immune system and reduce the risk of infection and illness. It can also improve physical performance and reduce the risk of injury.

Furthermore, sleep is closely linked to our overall well-being and mood. Chronic sleep deprivation, on the other hand, has been linked to an increased risk of obesity, diabetes, heart disease and other conditions. Additionally, studies have shown that getting enough quality sleep on a regular basis can contribute to a longer lifespan.

However, despite the numerous benefits of sleep, many people struggle to get enough of it. In fact, according to Walker, a third of the population suffers from chronic insomnia and sleep disorders are on the rise. The reasons for this are varied, but can include lifestyle factors such as working long hours, exposure to screens late at night and chronic stress.

To improve sleep, Walker recommends developing a consistent sleep schedule, avoiding screens for at least an hour before bed, keeping the bedroom cool and dark and avoiding caffeine and alcohol close to bedtime. He also suggests engaging in regular exercise, which can improve both the quality and quantity of sleep.

In addition, Walker stresses the importance of not only the quantity of sleep but also its quality. He recommends to sleep in complete darkness and cool temperature, avoid noise and any kind of interruption during sleep to help improve the quality of sleep.

Bottom Line
Sleep is essential for both physical and mental health. Unfortunately, many people struggle to get enough of it. By developing good sleep habits and making lifestyle changes, it is possible to improve both the quantity and quality of sleep, reaping the numerous benefits that come with it.

Smokeless Tobacco

Smokeless tobacco is a form of tobacco consumption that poses significant health risks to its users, including Veterans. While it may seem less harmful than smoking, smokeless tobacco is not a safe alternative and can lead to various health issues.

Smokeless tobacco contains a potent mix of harmful chemicals, including nicotine, which can lead to the following health risks:

- *Nicotine addiction:* Nicotine in smokeless tobacco is highly addictive, making it challenging to quit.

- *Oral health issues:* Smokeless tobacco can cause gum disease, tooth decay and tooth loss.

- *Oral cancer:* Users of smokeless tobacco are at a higher risk of developing oral cancers, including cancers of the mouth, tongue and throat.

- *Heart and cardiovascular problems:* Nicotine can raise blood pressure and increase the risk of heart disease and stroke.

- *Reproductive health:* Smokeless tobacco can lead to reproductive problems in both men and women.

- *Impact on Veterans:* Veterans are particularly vulnerable to the hazards of smokeless tobacco due to the unique stressors they face. Smokeless tobacco use can exacerbate mental health issues such as PTSD and contribute to overall health problems among Veterans.

• **Social and Economic costs:** Smokeless tobacco use not only affects individual health but also imposes significant social and economic costs on society. These costs include increased healthcare expenses, lost productivity and the emotional toll on families.

How to Quit Smokeless Tobacco

• **Recognize the need to quit:** The first step in quitting smokeless tobacco is recognizing the need for change. Understanding the health risks and personal reasons can be powerful motivators.

• **Set a quit date:** Choose a specific date to quit, which will provide a clear goal to work towards.

• **Seek support:** Support from healthcare professionals, counselors, friends and family can significantly increase the chances of quitting successfully.

• **Try nicotine replacement therapy:** NRTs, such as nicotine gum, patches or lozenges, can help ease withdrawal symptoms and cravings.
• **Consider behavioral strategies:** Behavioral strategies such as counseling, support groups and stress management techniques can be effective in quitting smokeless tobacco.

• **Avoid triggers:** Identify and avoid situations or triggers that make you want to use smokeless tobacco.

• **Stay committed and be patient:** Quitting tobacco is a journey that may have setbacks. Staying committed and patient with yourself is essential.

Bottom Line
Smokeless tobacco use is a hazardous habit that poses significant health risks to Veterans and the general population. However, with determination, support and the right strategies, quitting is achievable. Veterans should prioritize their health and well-being by seeking help and resources to overcome smokeless tobacco addiction. By taking these steps, Veterans can improve their overall health and reduce their risk of tobacco-related diseases, ultimately leading to a better quality of life.

Smoking

Smoking is a dangerous habit that has many negative effects on a person's health. It is the leading cause of preventable deaths in the world and is responsible for various health problems, including lung cancer, heart disease, stroke and respiratory diseases. The following is a detailed discussion of the harmful effects of smoking and the methods that can help individuals quit the habit.

Lung Cancer
Lung cancer is one of the most common and deadly diseases caused by smoking. It is the leading cause of cancer deaths in the world and smokers are 15 to 30 times more likely to develop lung cancer than non-smokers.

Heart Disease
Smoking is a major risk factor for heart disease, which is one of the leading causes of death worldwide. The chemicals in tobacco smoke cause the buildup of plaque in the arteries, which can lead to blood clots and heart attacks. Smokers are also more likely to develop high blood pressure, which can lead to heart disease.

Stroke
Stroke is another serious health problem caused by smoking. Smokers are twice as likely to have a stroke as non-smokers and the risk increases with the number of cigarettes smoked. Strokes can lead to long-term disability or death, making it a serious concern for smokers.

Respiratory Diseases
Smoking can cause various respiratory diseases, including chronic bronchitis, emphysema and/or asthma collectively referred to as Chronic Obstructive Pulmonary Disease (COPD). These diseases can lead to breathing difficulties, coughing and wheezing, making it harder for smokers to perform daily activities. Additionally, the chemicals in tobacco smoke can damage the cilia, which are the tiny hair-like structures in the airways that help remove debris and mucus from the lungs.

Other Negative Effects of Smoking
In addition to the health problems mentioned above, smoking can also cause various other negative effects. It can lead to decreased sense of taste and smell, yellowing of teeth, premature aging and infertility in men. Smokers are also at a higher risk of developing various types of cancer, including throat, mouth, bladder, kidney and pancreatic cancer. Some of the most significant effects of smoking include:

- Increased risk of cardiovascular disease, lung cancer and other cancers.
- Respiratory problems such as shortness of breath, coughing and wheezing.
- Impairment of the immune system and increased susceptibility to infections.

- Increased risk of complications during pregnancy and birth, such as premature delivery and low birth weight.
- Tooth and gum disease, as well as bad breath.
- Increased risk of age-related diseases, such as Alzheimer's and Parkinson's.
- Negative impact on mental health, including increased risk of depression and anxiety.

Methods to Quit Smoking

Given the many negative effects of smoking, it is important for individuals to find ways to quit the habit. The following are some effective methods that have helped people quit smoking:

- *Nicotine Replacement Therapy (NRT):* Nicotine replacement therapy is a popular method for quitting smoking. NRT provides a lower dose of nicotine to help reduce withdrawal symptoms, such as cravings and irritability. There are various forms of NRT, including nicotine gum, patches, lozenges, inhalers and sprays.

- *Medications:* There are prescription medications available that can help individuals quit smoking. These medications work by reducing cravings and withdrawal symptoms. Bupropion and varenicline are two commonly used medications for smoking cessation.

- *Counseling and Support Groups:* Counseling and support groups can provide individuals with the emotional support and encouragement they need to quit smoking. Talking with a counselor or joining a support group can help individuals feel less alone and more motivated to quit.

- *Changing Habits:* Many people smoke as a result of habit, so changing habits can be a helpful method for quitting smoking. For example, individuals can try to find alternative activities, such as exercise or hobbies, to replace smoking. They can also try to avoid triggers, avoiding triggers is a common strategy for managing symptoms in people with conditions such as anxiety, depression and PTSD. Triggers are different for each person and may include certain sounds, smells, people or events. Identifying and avoiding or minimizing exposure to these triggers can help reduce the frequency and intensity of symptoms. However, it is important to note that avoidance may not be a sustainable or effective long-term strategy and working with a mental health professional to develop coping skills is also recommended.

Bottom Line

Smoking has numerous negative effects on physical and mental health. Overall, the negative effects of smoking are numerous and far-reaching, affecting both physical and mental health. Quitting smoking can help reverse some of the negative effects and improve overall health.

Spiritual Practices and Beliefs

The role of spiritual practices and beliefs in Veterans' health and well-being is an important topic often overlooked in discussions of Veterans' health. Many Veterans find that spiritual practices and beliefs can provide a sense of meaning, purpose and community that is essential for their overall health and well-being.

The Importance of Spiritual Practices and Beliefs for Veterans

For many Veterans, the experience of military service can be both physically and emotionally challenging. The trauma of combat, the stress of military life and the difficulties of reintegrating into civilian society can all take a toll on a Veteran's mental and physical health. Spiritual practices and beliefs can provide a sense of comfort and support for Veterans during difficult times. They can also help Veterans to find meaning and purpose in their lives, which can be especially important during the transition to civilian life.

Some of the ways in which spiritual practices and beliefs can be beneficial for Veterans include:

• *Coping with Trauma:* Many Veterans find that spiritual practices and beliefs can help them to cope with the trauma of combat and other difficult experiences. Prayer, meditation and other spiritual practices can provide a sense of comfort and support that is essential for emotional healing.

• *Finding Meaning and Purpose:* Spiritual practices and beliefs can also help Veterans to find meaning and purpose in their lives. This can be especially important for Veterans who are struggling to adjust to civilian life or who are experiencing feelings of isolation or disconnection.

• *Connecting with Others:* Spiritual practices and beliefs can provide a sense of community and connection that is essential for Veterans' well-being. Religious or spiritual organizations can offer a sense of support and belonging that is essential for emotional and social well-being.

• *Reducing Stress:* Many spiritual practices and beliefs, such as meditation or prayer, can help to reduce stress and promote relaxation. This can be especially important for Veterans who are experiencing symptoms of anxiety or PTSD.

- **Promoting Resilience:** Finally, spiritual practices and beliefs can promote resilience in Veterans. By providing a sense of hope and optimism, spiritual practices and beliefs can help Veterans to overcome challenges and setbacks.

How to Incorporate Spiritual Practices and Beliefs into Veterans' Health Care

Incorporating spiritual practices and beliefs into Veterans' health care can be challenging, as these practices are often highly individualized and may not fit within traditional medical models. However, there are some steps that health care providers can take to support Veterans' spiritual well-being. These include:

- **Encouraging Open Communication:** Health care providers can encourage open communication with Veterans about their spiritual beliefs and practices. This can help to create a sense of trust and connection between the provider and the Veteran.

- **Providing Resources:** Health care providers can also provide resources for Veterans who are interested in exploring spiritual practices and beliefs. This can include referrals to religious or spiritual organizations or information about local support groups.

- **Integrating Spiritual Practices into Treatment Plans:** Health care providers can work with Veterans to integrate spiritual practices into their treatment plans. This may include incorporating meditation, prayer or other spiritual practices into therapy sessions.

- **Respecting Diversity:** It is important for health care providers to respect the diversity of spiritual practices and beliefs among Veterans. Providers should avoid imposing their own beliefs on Veterans and should strive to create a welcoming and inclusive environment for all patients.

Bottom Line

Spiritual practices and beliefs can play an important role in Veterans' health and well-being. They can help Veterans to cope with trauma, find meaning and purpose, connect with others, reduce stress and promote resilience. Health care providers can support Veterans' spiritual well-being by encouraging open communication, providing resources, integrating spiritual practices into treatment plans and respecting diversity. By incorporating spiritual practices and beliefs into Veterans' health care, we can provide a more holistic and patient-centered approach to health and well-being.

Spooky2 - Rife Frequency Therapy

Spooky2, developed by Spooky2 Technologies, is a modern Rife frequency system that delivers electromagnetic frequencies through devices like generators, plasma tubes, scalar fields, and contact accessories to support health and wellness. Based on Royal Raymond Rife's 1930s work suggesting frequencies could target pathogens, Spooky2 provides an affordable platform with over 50,000 frequency programs accessible via free software. Veterans, dealing with chronic pain, fatigue, or mental health issues from service, can use it as a non-invasive, experimental tool to explore alternative healing, often with biofeedback for customization. Benefits claimed include pain relief, detoxification, and stress reduction, supported by user testimonials and small studies, though large-scale scientific validation is limited, and risks like misuse or unverified claims apply.

Launched in 2013 by John White and Echo Lee, Spooky2 has evolved by 2025 into a versatile system with hardware like the Spooky2 Scalar and extensive software updates, available at www.spooky2.com. Chronic conditions such as pain and fatigue drive its use among Veterans, with devices ranging from $100 to $2,500 offering a drug-free option. Combat trauma, burn pit toxin exposure, and stress disrupt health; Spooky2 targets these by addressing pathogens, inflammation, or energy imbalances at a cellular level. Symptoms like exhaustion, soreness, or mental fog prompt its use as a way to explore underlying issues.

The system includes generators like the Spooky2-XM ($100) or GX Pro ($500), connected to a computer via USB with free software from www.spooky2.com. Delivery modes are remote, contact, plasma, or scalar, used for 20–60 minutes daily or as needed. Pain relief comes from calming nerves or boosting circulation; detoxification targets toxins or pathogens; stress reduction soothes the nervous system; improved energy enhances cellular function; mental clarity balances brainwaves. Risks include fatigue or skin irritation from misuse; Veterans with pacemakers need caution due to electromagnetic interference. Small studies suggest benefits for pain and detox, but Spooky2's broad claims lack randomized trials and FDA approval, per www.spooky2.com disclaimers. Pain, fatigue, and stress align with its focus, appealing to Veterans seeking self-managed, holistic options.

Equipment-
- Generator Setup: The Spooky2-XM ($100) or GX Pro ($500) connects to a computer via USB, running free software (www.spooky2.com/downloads) with 50,000+ programs, used daily or weekly for remote or contact sessions.

- Remote Mode: DNA samples (e.g., hair, nails) in a Spooky Remote ($15) transmit frequencies over distances, run 24/7 or in cycles, a hands-off option for Veterans, per www.spooky2.com claims of quantum entanglement.

- Contact Mode: Electrodes or TENS pads ($20-$50) deliver frequencies directly to skin (20-60 minutes daily), targeting specific areas like joints or muscles, practical for Veterans with localized pain.

- Plasma Mode: Spooky2 Central ($1,500) uses a plasma tube to emit powerful frequencies (30-60 minutes, 3-5 times weekly), aimed at deep systemic effects, an advanced choice for Veterans.

- Scalar Mode: Spooky2 Scalar ($1,500) creates a scalar field between two boxes, with sessions (30-60 minutes daily) in the field or using coils, touted for energy balancing, per www.spooky2.com.

- Biofeedback: The GX Pro's scan (6-20 minutes) reads pulse changes to tailor frequencies, run weekly or monthly, personalizing treatment for Veterans, per www.spooky2.com instructions.

Targeted Protocols for Veterans' Wellness

Veterans with chronic pain, fatigue, or mental strain from service can use Spooky2 to address these issues. Start with a Spooky2-XM generator ($100) and free software from www.spooky2.com, running 20–60 minute sessions daily; upgrade to GX Pro ($500) or Scalar ($1,500) if needed. VA clinics may offer guidance, or functional doctor offices with foundation support—like the Gary Sinise Foundation or Wounded Warrior Project—can offset costs for qualifying Veterans. Log symptoms—pain, energy levels, focus—to track effects over 4–8 weeks.

For pain relief, use contact mode with TENS pads ($20–$50) on sore areas like joints or muscles, 20–60 minutes daily at 5–10 Hz—Veterans with injury-related discomfort see less ache in weeks; adjust frequency with a provider if slow. Detoxification uses remote mode with a Spooky Remote ($15) and DNA sample (hair or nails), running 24/7 or in cycles—Veterans exposed to burn pits clear toxins over a month; check logs and tweak if needed. Stress reduction applies scalar mode with Spooky2 Scalar ($1,500), sitting in the field 30–60 minutes daily at 5–8 Hz—Veterans with combat tension feel calmer in weeks; pair with relaxation if progress stalls.

Improved energy comes from plasma mode with Spooky2 Central ($1,500), 30–60 minutes three to five times weekly—Veterans with fatigue gain vitality over a month; reduce sessions if fatigue persists. Mental clarity uses GX Pro biofeedback scans (6–20 minutes weekly) to tailor frequencies, then remote or contact mode daily—Veterans with trauma-related fog sharpen focus in weeks; refine with a doctor if results falter. Pair Spooky2 with VA therapy or exercise—use after sessions—for better outcomes, building a routine over 4–8 weeks.

Consult a healthcare provider before starting, especially with pacemakers, heart conditions, or chronic issues, to ensure safety and VA integration. VA resources or foundation-backed providers (like Gary Sinise or Wounded Warrior) keep costs low—free software and $100–$2,500 for devices. Begin with an XM generator and remote, run daily sessions, and assess—less pain, more energy—over 4–8 weeks, adjusting with professional input if needed.

Bottom Line

Spooky2 delivers pain relief, detoxification, stress reduction, improved energy, and mental clarity through a Rife frequency system ($100–$2,500), using generators, remote, contact, plasma, or scalar modes (20–60 minutes daily). Veterans with pain, fatigue, or stress from service can explore this experimental tool, with user reports and small studies suggesting symptom relief over weeks. It's a frequency-based, DIY approach, unlike conventional care. Evidence shows potential—small trials hint at pain and detox benefits—but lacks robust validation; Spooky2's claims rely on anecdotes, not FDA approval. Risks include misuse, mild side effects, or delayed care, plus costs that may strain budgets. It's not a primary treatment—professionals advise pairing with VA care due to limited data—so consult a healthcare provider, start with affordable options (e.g., XM, $100), and use cautiously with realistic goals and oversight. It's a wellness aid for some, not a proven fix, needing careful application.

<u>Stellate Ganglion Block</u>

A stellate ganglion block (SGB) is a medical procedure that involves injecting a local anesthetic into the stellate ganglion, a group of nerves in the neck that are involved in the body's stress response. While SGB is typically used to treat chronic pain conditions, it has also been studied as a potential treatment for post-traumatic stress disorder (PTSD).

Research on the use of SGB for PTSD is still in its early stages, but initial studies have shown promising results. Some of the potential benefits of SGB for PTSD include:

• **Reduction in PTSD symptoms:** One of the primary benefits of SGB for PTSD is its potential to reduce the symptoms of the condition. PTSD is characterized by symptoms such as hyperarousal, anxiety and intrusive thoughts. Some studies have found that SGB can help to reduce these symptoms, leading to an overall improvement in quality of life for individuals with PTSD.

• **Rapid onset of relief:** Unlike traditional medications and therapies for PTSD, which may take weeks or even months to show significant results, SGB has been shown to provide rapid relief of symptoms. In some cases, individuals may experience relief within hours of the procedure.

• ***Potential to enhance other treatments:*** While SGB is not a standalone treatment for PTSD, it has been shown to enhance the effects of other treatments, such as psychotherapy and medication. By reducing symptoms and improving overall well-being, SGB may help to make other treatments more effective.

• ***Fewer side effects than traditional treatments:*** Traditional treatments for PTSD, such as medication, can have significant side effects, including weight gain, sexual dysfunction and nausea. SGB is a minimally invasive procedure that carries fewer side effects than traditional treatments.

While SGB is a promising treatment for PTSD, it is important to note that it is not a cure for the condition. Individuals who undergo SGB may still require ongoing treatment and support for their PTSD, including psychotherapy and/or medication.

It is also important to note that SGB is an invasive medical procedure that carries some risks. These risks include bleeding, infection and nerve damage. SGB should only be performed by a trained medical professional under strict medical supervision.

Bottom Line

SGB is a promising new treatment option for PTSD that has the potential to provide rapid relief of symptoms and enhance the effects of other treatments. While more research is needed to fully understand its long-term effectiveness and safety, SGB offers hope to individuals with PTSD who are struggling to find relief from their symptoms.

Stem Cells

Stem cells are unique cells capable of self-renewal and differentiation into various cell types—like muscle, nerve, or blood cells—to repair damaged tissues or restore function, used in medical treatments or experimental therapies. Unlike drugs that treat symptoms, stem cells target underlying damage through regeneration, delivered via injections, infusions, or surgical implants. Veterans, facing chronic pain, traumatic injuries, or neurological conditions from service, can use stem cell therapies to support healing and recovery. Benefits claimed include tissue regeneration, reduced inflammation, and improved function, supported by clinical trials and regenerative medicine advancements, though evidence varies by condition, and risks like rejection or unregulated treatments apply.

Stem cell research began in the 1960s with bone marrow transplants; therapeutic use grew in the 1990s, with Veteran-focused studies emerging by the 2010s for injuries and PTSD-related issues. Chronic pain, disability, and fatigue affect many Veterans, driving interest in stem cells as a regenerative option. Combat trauma, burn pit exposure, and physical strain cause tissue and neurological damage; stem cells aim to repair these at a cellular level. Symptoms like joint pain, slow healing, or cognitive decline prompt their use to restore health.

Treatments use autologous stem cells (from the patient's own body, e.g., bone marrow) or allogeneic (donor-derived), administered in doses tailored to the condition, often over weeks to months. Benefits include regenerating damaged tissues, reducing inflammation, improving joint or nerve function, enhancing mobility, and supporting brain repair. Risks involve immune reactions or infection; unregulated clinics pose safety concerns, and Veterans with complex conditions need oversight. Trials show promise for specific uses like joint repair, but broader applications lack large-scale validation. Pain, injuries, and neurological challenges make stem cells relevant for Veterans, who can access them through VA trials or private providers.

Targeted Protocols for Veterans' Wellness

Veterans with chronic pain, slow-healing injuries, or neurological issues from service can explore stem cell therapies to address these conditions. Start with a consultation through VA specialists or private regenerative medicine clinics ($0–$500) to assess damage—joint degeneration, nerve loss, fatigue—and determine eligibility; VA research programs may offer free trials, or functional providers with foundation support, like the Gary Sinise Foundation or Wounded Warrior Project, can offset costs for qualifying Veterans. Track symptoms—pain levels, mobility, focus—in a log to monitor progress over 3–12 months.

For tissue regeneration, autologous stem cells from bone marrow or fat (harvested via aspiration, $1,000–$5,000) are injected into damaged areas like knees or tendons—50–100 million cells per dose, 1–3 sessions over weeks; Veterans with combat injuries see healing in months, adjusting with a doctor if progress lags. Inflammation reduces with mesenchymal stem cell infusions (IV, 100–200 million cells, $2,000–$10,000), targeting systemic swelling—Veterans with joint pain or burn pit effects notice less soreness in 6–12 weeks; monitor and refine dosing if needed.

Joint or nerve function improves with stem cell injections into specific sites (e.g., spine, 20–50 million cells, $1,500–$7,000)—Veterans with nerve damage or arthritis gain strength over 3–6 months; pair with VA physical therapy for better results. Mobility enhances through similar injections or implants—Veterans with limb injuries move easier in months; track range and adjust with a provider if slow. Brain repair uses stem cells via IV or intrathecal delivery (50–100 million cells,

$5,000–$15,000)—Veterans with TBI or PTSD-related fog see focus improve over 6–12 months; combine with VA neurology if effects stall.

Treatments range from one-time injections to multi-session protocols, guided by blood tests (e.g., inflammation markers, $50–$100) or imaging to assess response. Consult a healthcare provider before starting, especially with heart conditions, immune issues, or chronic diseases, to ensure safety and VA alignment; avoid unregulated clinics lacking FDA oversight. Costs vary—free via VA trials or $1,000–$15,000 private. Begin with a VA consult or trial, proceed to targeted injections if approved, and evaluate—less pain, better movement—over 3–12 months, refining with professional input if results falter.

Bottom Line

Stem cells offer tissue regeneration, reduced inflammation, improved joint or nerve function, enhanced mobility, and brain repair through injections or infusions (e.g., 50–200 million cells), targeting damage at a cellular level. Veterans with pain, injuries, or neurological issues from service can benefit, with trials showing 20–40% improvements in function or healing over 3–12 months. Unlike symptom-focused drugs, they're regenerative. Evidence is strong for specific uses—joint and tissue repair have clinical backing—but broader claims like brain recovery lack large-scale trials; FDA approves only a few applications (e.g., marrow transplants). Risks include rejection, infection, or unregulated treatments, a concern for Veterans with complex needs or limited funds ($1,000–$15,000). They're not a standalone fix—professionals recommend oversight and VA integration due to variable data and safety issues—so consult a healthcare provider, access via VA trials or trusted clinics, and monitor with logs, approaching with caution and realistic expectations. They're a promising option for some, not a universal cure, needing careful execution.

Stress and Anxiety

Stress and anxiety are common experiences that can have a significant impact on one's overall well-being. However, there are several strategies that can be used to manage these feelings effectively.

• **Identify the source of stress and anxiety:** One of the first steps in managing stress and anxiety is to identify the source of these feelings. This can help to determine the best course of action for addressing the problem.

• **Practice relaxation techniques:** Relaxation techniques such as deep breathing, yoga and meditation can help to reduce stress and anxiety levels. These techniques can also help to improve overall well-being and promote a sense of calm.

- **Exercise regularly:** Regular physical activity can help to reduce stress and anxiety levels. Exercise can also improve mood and overall health.

- **Get enough sleep:** Adequate sleep is essential for managing stress and anxiety. Aim for at least 7-8 hours of sleep each night to help reduce feelings of stress and anxiety.

- **Connect with others:** Connecting with friends and loved ones can help to reduce feelings of stress and anxiety. Social support can also provide a sense of belonging and help one to cope with difficult situations.

- **Practice mindfulness:** Mindfulness is the practice of being present in the moment and paying attention to one's thoughts and feelings. Mindfulness can help to reduce stress and anxiety by helping one to focus on the present and let go of worries about the past or future.

- **Seek professional help:** If stress and anxiety are persistent and interfering with daily life, it may be helpful to seek professional help. A therapist or counselor can help to identify the source of stress and anxiety and develop a plan to manage these feelings.

- **Take care of yourself:** It's essential to take care of yourself physically and emotionally. Eating a healthy diet, avoiding alcohol and drugs and finding ways to relax and de-stress are all important self-care strategies.

Bottom Line
Stress and anxiety are common experiences, but there are several strategies that can be used to manage these feelings effectively. Identifying the source of stress and anxiety, practicing relaxation techniques, exercising regularly, getting enough sleep, connecting with others, practicing mindfulness, seeking professional help and taking care of yourself are all important strategies for managing stress and anxiety. Remember to be patient and kind to yourself, progress takes time and it's ok to not have everything figured out.

Suicide Prevention

Preventing suicide among Veterans is a critical public health issue. Suicide rates among Veterans are higher than the general population and it is important to understand the risk factors and interventions that can help prevent suicide among Veterans.

One of the most significant risk factors for suicide among Veterans is mental health conditions, such as post-traumatic stress disorder (PTSD), depression and anxiety. These conditions can be caused by the traumatic experiences that Veterans have had while serving in the military. It is essential to provide access to mental health services and support groups for Veterans to help them cope with these conditions and reduce the risk of suicide.

Another risk factor for suicide among Veterans is access to firearms. Veterans are more likely to own firearms than the general population and firearms are the most common method of suicide among Veterans. It is important to provide education on safe storage of firearms and to encourage Veterans to seek help if they are experiencing suicidal thoughts or behavior.

Other risk factors for suicide among Veterans include substance abuse, physical health conditions and social isolation. It is important to provide access to substance abuse treatment and physical health services for Veterans, as well as support for Veterans to connect with their communities.

Interventions that can help prevent suicide among Veterans include cognitive behavioral therapy (CBT), prolonged exposure therapy (PE) and eye movement desensitization and reprocessing (EMDR) for Veterans with PTSD, cognitive processing therapy (CPT) for Veterans with PTSD and medication-assisted treatment (MAT) for Veterans with substance abuse disorders.

Another intervention that can help prevent suicide among Veterans is the Veterans Crisis Line. This is a confidential and toll-free hotline that Veterans can call to talk to trained professionals about their concerns. The Veterans Crisis Line also provides a chat service and an online Veterans crisis chat service.

Veterans Crisis Line
https://www.Veteranscrisisline.net/
Phone: Dial 988 then Press 1
Text: 838255
Online: https://www.Veteranscrisisline.net/get-help-now/chat/
Access free, confidential support 24/7, 365 days a year.

The use of gatekeepers is another intervention that can help prevent suicide among Veterans is the use of gatekeepers. Gatekeepers are individuals who have been trained to identify and respond to Veterans who are at risk for suicide. Gatekeepers can include healthcare providers, family members, friends and community leaders and they can play an important role in preventing suicide among Veterans. Additionally, it is important to provide support for families and loved ones of Veterans who are at risk for suicide. Families and loved ones can play an important role in identifying Veterans who are at risk for suicide and can provide support and resources to help Veterans access the services they need.

It is also important to provide support and resources for Veterans who have lost a loved one to suicide. This includes access to grief counseling and support groups and resources to help families navigate the aftermath of a suicide.

Bottom Line

Preventing suicide among Veterans is a critical public health issue. Suicide rates among Veterans are higher than the general population and it is important to understand the risk factors and interventions that can help prevent suicide among Veterans. This includes providing access to mental health services, support for Veterans with PTSD, substance abuse treatment and physical health services, as well as education.

Sunlight and Skin Health

Sun exposure plays a vital role in overall health, influencing vitamin D production, mood regulation, inflammation levels, and sleep cycles. While excessive exposure can pose risks, controlled sun exposure—paired with natural sunscreens—can enhance wellness for Veterans adjusting to post-service life. Unlike artificial tanning, which relies on UV beds, this approach utilizes natural sunlight, ensuring a balance between benefits and protection. This section explores the role of tanning, its potential advantages, and safe strategies for Veterans to harness sunlight effectively.

Understanding Sunlight & Skin Function

The skin acts as a biological filter, absorbing and processing UV radiation. Key mechanisms influenced by sun exposure include:

- Vitamin D Synthesis: Sunlight triggers vitamin D production, essential for bone health, immunity, and mood.

- Melanin Production: Increased melanin darkens the skin, offering natural UV protection over time.

- Hormonal Regulation: UV exposure influences serotonin and melatonin, impacting mood and sleep.

The Science of Sunlight & Health

Research in The Journal of Investigative Dermatology (2018) links controlled sun exposure to in-creased vitamin D levels and improved mental well-being. A Journal of Sleep Research (2019) study found morning sunlight exposure aids melatonin regulation, enhancing sleep quality. While benefits exist, overexposure risks burns and long-term damage, reinforcing the importance of balance.

Why Sunlight Matters for Veterans
- Boosts Vitamin D: Supports bone strength, immune function, and energy levels.

- Enhances Mood & Mental Health: UV rays increase serotonin, helping alleviate stress and depression.

- Reduces Inflammation: Controlled exposure may help joint pain and muscle recovery.

- Improves Sleep Cycles: Natural light exposure regulates circadian rhythms, aiding Veterans with disrupted sleep.

- Supports Skin Resilience: Gradual tanning builds melanin, enhancing UV tolerance over time.

Identifying Sunlight Deficiency
- Common Signs: Fatigue, mood dips, muscle weakness, poor sleep, persistent aches.

- Veteran-Specific Triggers: Reduced outdoor time post-service, previous extreme sun exposure during deployment, limited vitamin D intake.

- Assessment Tools: Track mood, sleep patterns, and energy fluctuations in a journal.

- Medical Testing: Vitamin D blood tests via VA or private clinics ($50–$150).

Safe Sun Exposure Strategies
- Gradual Exposure: Start with 10–20 minutes of sunlight daily (morning or late afternoon) and adjust per skin response.

- Morning Sunlight Routine: Low UV exposure (8–11 a.m.) offers benefits with minimal risk; aim for 15–30 minutes.

- Midday Sunlight Caution: Intense UV levels (11 a.m.–3 p.m.) require shorter exposure (5–15 minutes) with natural sunscreen.

- Post-Tan Care: Moisturize with aloe or coconut oil ($5–$15) and hydrate adequately (8–12 cups of water daily).

Natural Sunscreen & Skin Protection
1. Zinc Oxide (SPF 20–30)
- What: A mineral-based sunscreen that reflects UV rays.

- Why: Provides broad-spectrum protection without harmful chemicals.

344

- How: Apply a thin layer every 2 hours in prolonged sun exposure.

- Supplies: Available as creams or powders ($10–$20).

2. Coconut Oil (SPF 4–6)
- What: A natural moisturizer offering mild UV protection.

- Why: Supports skin hydration and prevents excessive dryness.

- How: Use before and after sun exposure for added skin nourishment.

- Supplies: Organic coconut oil ($5–$15).

3. Shea Butter (SPF 3–6)
- What: A nutrient-rich, antioxidant-filled natural sunscreen.

- Why: Enhances skin elasticity and helps repair sun-exposed areas.

- How: Apply thickly before sun exposure or mix with coconut oil.

- Supplies: Raw shea butter ($10–$20).

Integrating Sunlight into Daily Life
- Set SMART Goals: Example: "Expose skin to morning sunlight for 15 minutes daily to boost vitamin D levels."

- Build a Routine: Pair sun exposure with a morning walk, meditation, or stretching.

- Leverage Veteran Support: VA wellness programs and peer accountability groups for out-door activities.

Risks & Considerations
- Overexposure Risks: Burns, premature aging, and skin cancer risks increase with excessive UV exposure.

- Sunscreen Limitations: Natural sunscreens offer lower SPF than synthetic options (30–50); reapplication is essential.

- Veteran-Specific Precautions: Those with fair skin, previous sunburns, or skin conditions should limit exposure and consult a dermatologist.

Bottom Line
Sunlight exposure, when balanced, enhances vitamin D production, mood, sleep, and inflammation control. Veterans, particularly those experiencing fatigue and mood instability, may benefit from controlled sun exposure combined with natural protection. Scientific research supports vitamin D and mood benefits, while inflammation and skin health claims are still under study. While not a standalone

treatment, responsible tanning is a practical wellness tool when paired with proper skin care and sun safety. Veterans should start with short sessions (10–30 minutes), use natural sunscreens, and adjust based on skin type and UV intensity. Consultation with a healthcare provider is advised for personalized guidance, ensuring safe and effective integration into daily routines.

Survivor Guilt

A complex and overwhelming emotional experience that can occur after a traumatic event such as a natural disaster, war, or accident, survivor guilt is a form of psychological distress that affects individuals who have survived a traumatic event while others have not. Survivor guilt is characterized by feelings of remorse, responsibility and self-blame for surviving when others did not. It can be a debilitating experience that can have a significant impact on mental health and overall well-being.

Survivor guilt can be triggered by a variety of factors, including the proximity of the event, the severity of the trauma and the relationship between the survivor and the person who did not survive. For example, someone who survives a natural disaster may feel guilty because they were able to escape while others were not, while a soldier who returns home from war may feel guilty for surviving while their comrades did not.

The symptoms of survivor guilt can vary greatly from person to person, but some common symptoms include feelings of intense sadness and despair, anxiety, depression, irritability and difficulty sleeping. Some individuals may experience physical symptoms such as headaches or muscle aches, as well as a lack of motivation or interest in activities they once enjoyed.

Survivor guilt can also have a negative impact on relationships and daily life, making it difficult for individuals to function normally. It can be especially challenging for individuals who are already struggling with other forms of trauma, such as post-traumatic stress disorder (PTSD).

However, there are several methods that can help individuals to mitigate the effects of survivor guilt and regain control over their lives. Some of these methods include:

- **Talking to a trusted friend or family member:** Having someone to talk to about your feelings can be incredibly helpful in managing survivor guilt. Sharing your experiences with someone who understands and supports you can help to reduce feelings of isolation and provide a sense of comfort.

- **Seeking professional counseling:** A licensed mental health professional can provide specialized support and help individuals to work through the complex emotions associated with survivor guilt.

- **Engaging in self-care:** Engaging in activities that promote relaxation and well-being, such as yoga, meditation and exercise, can help to reduce stress and anxiety and improve overall mental health.

- **Creating a sense of purpose:** Finding a new purpose or direction in life can help to reduce feelings of guilt and provide a sense of meaning. This may involve volunteering, pursuing a new hobby or taking steps to help others who have also experienced a traumatic event.

- **Accepting and processing the event:** Facing the reality of what happened and working through the feelings associated with the event can be an important step in reducing survivor guilt. This may involve journaling, therapy or other forms of self-reflection.

- **Re-establishing a sense of control:** Taking control over aspects of your life, such as making healthy lifestyle choices, setting goals and taking steps to move forward can help to reduce feelings of guilt and provide a sense of empowerment.

- **Understanding and accepting the past:** Recognizing that the past cannot be changed and that the event was not your fault can be a powerful step in reducing feelings of guilt and self-blame.

Survivor guilt can be a challenging and overwhelming experience, but with the right support and strategies it is possible to manage the symptoms and regain control over your life. It is important to remember that recovery is a process and that everyone heals at their own pace.

Bottom Line

Survivor guilt is a complex and emotional experience that can occur after a traumatic event. It is characterized by feelings of remorse, responsibility and self-blame for surviving when others did not. There are several methods that can be used to mitigate the effects of survivor guilt, including talking to a trusted friend or family member, seeking professional counseling, engaging in self-care, creating a sense of purpose, accepting and processing the event, re-establishing a sense of control and understanding and accepting the past. It is important to remember that recovery is a process and that everyone heals at their own pace. By seeking support and implementing these methods, individuals can overcome the challenges of survivor guilt and move forward in their lives.

Sweat Lodge

A sweat lodge is a traditional ceremonial structure used by Indigenous peoples of North America, particularly Plains tribes like the Lakota, for purification, healing, and spiritual renewal. It's a small, dome-shaped frame made of natural materials like willow or saplings, covered with hides, blankets, or tarps, where heated stones are doused with water to create steam, often paired with prayer, song, and ritual. Veterans, dealing with chronic pain, mental health challenges, or a need for cultural reconnection post-service, can use sweat lodges as a holistic practice. Benefits claimed include detoxification, physical relief, mental clarity, emotional healing, and spiritual connection, rooted in centuries of tradition, though scientific evidence is limited, and risks like overheating apply.

Originating thousands of years ago with tribes like the Lakota, Ojibwe, and Navajo, sweat lodges were used for purification, healing, and life transitions; non-Native interest grew in the 20th century, though traditionalists stress cultural respect. Chronic pain, PTSD, and transition stress affect many Veterans, driving interest in this practice. Combat injuries, burn pit exposure, and prolonged stress contribute to health issues; sweat lodges aim to address these through heat, steam, and ceremony. Symptoms like fatigue, soreness, or emotional distress prompt its use as a way to reset physically and mentally.

The structure is 8–12 feet wide, dug slightly into the ground, with rocks heated externally for 2–4 hours and placed in a central pit; water, sometimes with herbs like sage, generates steam at 100–120°F. Sessions last 1–2 hours in 4 rounds, led by a trained elder with prayers and chants. Benefits include toxin removal through sweat, improved circulation for pain, stress relief from heat and ritual, emotional release via introspection, and spiritual uplift from community ties. Risks involve dehydration or heat exhaustion; Veterans with heart conditions need caution. Small studies suggest stress reduction and toxin clearance, but large trials are lacking, and medical endorsement is absent. Pain, PTSD, and cultural needs make it relevant for Veterans, who can join through tribal or vetted settings.

Targeted Protocols for Veterans' Wellness
Veterans with chronic pain, fatigue, or emotional strain from service can explore sweat lodges for relief. Find ceremonies led by Indigenous elders through tribal communities or vetted retreats—free in traditional settings or $50–$200 commercially—lasting 2–4 hours. VA social workers may connect you to Native resources, or functional providers with foundation support, like the Gary Sinise Foundation or Wounded Warrior Project, can guide access for qualifying Veterans. Screen for heart or lung issues with a doctor first; log symptoms—pain, sleep, mood—before and after to track effects over sessions.

Prepare by fasting lightly or eating fruits, hydrating well, and wearing minimal clothing like shorts or towels; entry involves smudging with sage and setting an intent, guided by the leader. Sessions unfold in 4 rounds, 15–30 minutes each—steam fills the lodge as water hits hot rocks, with prayers and chants; the door opens briefly between rounds for air. Elders control heat and pace, keeping it safe—Veterans with pain or stiffness from injuries feel muscle tension ease after a session; repeat weekly or monthly if it helps, stopping if dizziness hits.

Detoxification occurs through sweating—Veterans exposed to burn pits or chemicals release trace toxins like lead over one or two sessions; monitor energy shifts in days following. Mental clarity and stress relief come from heat and ritual—Veterans with PTSD notice calmer thoughts post-ceremony; join monthly to sustain it, pairing with VA therapy if needed. Emotional healing builds through introspection—Veterans processing grief or transition release burdens in a session; track mood over weeks to assess impact.

Spiritual connection ties to the earth and community—Veterans seeking purpose feel renewed after a ceremony; participate as needed, respecting the tradition's sacredness. Sessions differ from saunas by their guided, ritual focus—use them under trained leadership, not casually. Consult a healthcare provider before starting, especially with heart conditions or medications, to avoid risks like overheating; VA care ensures safety. Costs are low—free or $50–$200—through community or retreat options. Start with one session, assess—less pain, clearer head—over days, and join regularly if benefits hold, adjusting with medical input if issues arise.

Bottom Line
Sweat lodges, an Indigenous ceremonial practice, offer detoxification, physical relief, mental clarity, emotional healing, and spiritual connection through steam from heated stones and guided rituals in a natural dome (1–2 hours). Veterans with pain, PTSD, or transition stress can use this holistic approach, with small studies and reports suggesting stress reduction and toxin clearance after sessions. Unlike saunas, it's a sacred, steam-based ritual. Evidence is limited—small studies show promise, but no large trials confirm benefits—and risks like overheating or dehydration exist, with rare severe outcomes in mismanaged cases. It's not a primary medical treatment—professionals note insufficient data—so consult a healthcare provider, join only under trained Indigenous leadership with cultural respect, and pair with VA care, weighing it against proven options. It's a potential aid for some, not a standard fix, needing careful participation.

Swedish Sauna

The Swedish sauna—also known as a traditional sauna—is a type of heat therapy that has been used for centuries. It is known for its many health benefits which include:

- **Relaxation:** The heat and humidity of the sauna can help to relax the muscles, reduce stress and promote a sense of well-being.

- **Improved cardiovascular health:** Regular sauna use has been shown to lower blood pressure, improve heart function and reduce the risk of heart disease.

- **Improved respiratory function:** The heat and humidity of the sauna can help to open up the airways, making it easier to breathe and reducing symptoms of respiratory conditions such as asthma and bronchitis.

- **Improved skin health:** The heat and humidity of the sauna can help to improve circulation, open up the pores and reduce the appearance of acne and other skin conditions.

- **Weight loss:** Saunas can help to increase the body's metabolism, which can lead to weight loss.

- **Improved immunity:** Regular sauna use has been shown to boost the immune system, reducing the risk of infection and illness.

- **Improved sleep:** Saunas can help to promote better sleep by relaxing the body and mind, reducing stress and anxiety.

- **Pain relief:** The heat and humidity of the sauna can help to reduce pain and muscle soreness, making it a useful therapy for conditions such as arthritis and fibromyalgia.

It's important to note that sauna sessions should not exceed more than 15-20 minutes at a time and to drink enough water to avoid dehydration. It's also important to consult with your doctor before using the sauna if you have any health conditions or take any medications that may be affected by the heat.

Tinnitus

A condition characterized by a ringing or a buzzing sound in the ear that is not actually caused by an external source, tinnitus can be continuous or intermittent and can vary in volume and pitch. This condition can range from being a minor annoyance to a debilitating condition that affects a person's quality of life. Tinnitus is not a disease, but a symptom of an underlying problem.

The exact cause of tinnitus is often difficult to determine, as there can be several contributing factors. Some of the most common causes of tinnitus include:

• *Hearing loss:* As people age, it is common for their hearing to deteriorate, which can lead to tinnitus. People with hearing loss may experience tinnitus as a ringing or buzzing sound in the ear.

• *Exposure to loud noises:* Prolonged exposure to loud noises like gunfire, explosions or aircraft engines, can damage the hair cells in the inner ear, leading to tinnitus. This can also occur in people who work in loud environments, such as construction sites, factories and musicians.

• *Ear infections:* Ear infections can cause inflammation and swelling in the inner ear, leading to tinnitus.

• *Wax build-up:* Wax build-up in the ear canal can cause tinnitus by blocking or muffling sounds.

• *Medications:* Certain medications, including some antibiotics, cancer medications and high doses of aspirin, can cause tinnitus as a side effect

• *Cardiovascular problems:* Some heart and blood vessel conditions, such as high blood pressure, anemia, and cardiovascular disease, can cause tinnitus

• *Neurological conditions:* Some neurological conditions, such as a head injury, Meniere's disease, and acoustic neuroma can cause tinnitus

There is no single treatment that works for everyone with tinnitus. The best course of treatment will depend on the underlying cause of the tinnitus, as well as its severity and impact on a person's life. Some of the most commonly used treatments for tinnitus include:

- **Hearing aids:** For people with hearing loss, hearing aids can help to improve their hearing and reduce the perception of tinnitus.

- **Sound therapy:** This therapy involves exposure to calming sounds such as white noise, that can help to mask the tinnitus.

- **Counseling and cognitive behavioral therapy (CBT):** Talking to a mental health professional can help to manage the stress and anxiety associated with tinnitus and CBT can help to change the way a person thinks and reacts to the tinnitus.

- **Medications:** In some cases, medications such as anti-anxiety or antidepressants can help to reduce the impact of tinnitus.

- **Tinnitus retraining therapy (TRT):** This therapy involves retraining the brain to ignore the tinnitus by gradually reducing the awareness of the sound.

- **Neuromodulation:** This involves the use of low-level electrical stimulation or magnetic fields to alter brain activity and reduce tinnitus.

- **Surgery:** In some cases surgery may be necessary to correct an underlying problem causing the tinnitus, such as removing a growth or repairing a damaged ear drum.

In addition to these treatments, there are also some lifestyle changes that can help to manage tinnitus:

- **Avoid loud noises:** Avoiding or limiting exposure to loud noises can help to prevent tinnitus from getting worse.

- **Maintain a healthy lifestyle:** Eating a healthy diet, getting enough sleep and reducing stress can help to improve overall health and reduce the impact of tinnitus.

- **Exercise regularly:** Regular exercise can help to improve mood and reduce stress, which can help to manage tinnitus.

Bottom Line

Tinnitus can be a frustrating and debilitating condition but there are many treatment options available that can help to manage its symptoms. If you are experiencing tinnitus, it is important to talk to your doctor to determine the best course of treatment for you. With the right combination of treatment and lifestyle changes, it is possible to reduce the impact of tinnitus and improve your quality of life.

Toxic Relationships

Toxic relationships are harmful and destructive connections between individuals characterized by patterns of abuse, manipulation and power imbalance. These relationships can have negative effects on mental and physical health, self-esteem and overall well-being. Signs of a toxic relationship include:

- Control and manipulation

- Verbal or physical abuse

- Lack of trust and respect

- Isolation from friends and family

- Constant criticism or belittling

- Unhealthy dependency

- Gaslighting

If you or someone you know is in a toxic relationship it is important to seek help and support from friends, family or a professional therapist. Taking steps to leave the relationship and prioritize self-care is essential for recovery and healing.

Toxic relationships can have a profound impact on one's mental and emotional health, leading to feelings of low self-esteem, anxiety, and depression. Such relationships are characterized by patterns of manipulation, control, and abuse, leaving those involved feeling trapped and powerless.

The good news is that it is possible to heal from toxic relationships and move forward with a greater sense of self-worth and inner strength. In this article, we will explore the steps you can take to grow past toxic relationships and mitigate their effects on your life.

Understand the dynamics of toxic relationships
The first step in moving past a toxic relationship is to understand the dynamics that led to its formation. Many toxic relationships start out as seemingly healthy and loving, with one partner gradually exerting more control and influence over the other. This can happen slowly and subtly, making it difficult for the victim to realize the extent of the abuse. Understanding the signs of toxic relationships, such as control and manipulation, verbal or physical abuse, lack of trust and respect and constant criticism or belittling, can help you identify whether you are in such a relationship.

Set healthy boundaries

Setting healthy boundaries is essential for protecting yourself from further abuse and for reclaiming control over your life. This means being clear about what behaviors and actions are unacceptable to you and communicating these boundaries to your partner. It also means learning to say "no" when you feel uncomfortable or when your partner is crossing your boundaries. This can be difficult, especially if you have become accustomed to accommodating your partner's needs, but it is essential for your own well-being.

Seek support

Leaving a toxic relationship can be an emotionally traumatic experience and it is important to seek support from friends, family or a professional therapist. Talking about your experiences with trusted individuals can help you process the emotions and trauma you have experienced and find ways to cope with the aftermath. Additionally, joining a support group for individuals who have experienced toxic relationships can provide a sense of community and validation, as well as practical advice and guidance on how to move forward.

Practice self-care

Taking care of yourself is essential for healing from a toxic relationship and regaining a sense of self-worth. This can involve a variety of activities, such as engaging in physical exercise, meditating or pursuing a hobby that brings you joy. It can also involve engaging in self-reflection and therapy to help you process the emotions and experiences of the toxic relationship and gain a greater understanding of your own needs and desires.

Focus on personal growth

Growing past a toxic relationship involves focusing on your own personal growth and well-being. This can include learning new skills, pursuing new experiences and surrounding yourself with positive and supportive individuals. By focusing on your own growth and well-being, you can gain a sense of purpose and direction and begin to see yourself as a strong and capable individual, rather than as a victim of a toxic relationship.

Be patient with yourself

Finally, it is important to be patient with yourself as you heal from a toxic relationship. Healing is a process that takes time and effort and it is normal to experience setbacks along the way. Rather than beating yourself up for these setbacks, focus on the progress you have made and the steps you are taking to build a better future for yourself.

In conclusion, growing past toxic relationships involves a combination of self-reflection, self-care and a focus on personal growth. By setting healthy boundaries, seeking support and being patient with yourself, you can regain a sense of control over your life and move forward with greater self-worth and inner strength. If you or someone you know is in a toxic relationship, it is important to seek help and support, as taking steps to leave the relationship and prioritize self-care is essential for recovery and healing.

It is also important to understand that healing from a toxic relationship takes time and patience. Do not be hard on yourself if progress is slow or if you experience setbacks along the way. Focus on the progress you have made and continue to prioritize self-care and personal growth.

In addition to seeking support from friends and family, consider seeking the help of a professional therapist. A trained mental health professional can provide valuable guidance and support as you navigate the healing process and work through the emotions and experiences of the toxic relationship.

Bottom Line

Remember, you deserve to be in a relationship that is healthy and fulfilling. By taking the steps necessary to grow past toxic relationships and prioritize your own well-being, you can build a brighter future for yourself, filled with love, joy and peace of mind.

Transitioning from Military Service

Moving on from military to civilian life can be a challenging process and one of the biggest hurdles is learning to accept the "new you." Military service can have a profound impact on a person's identity, values and sense of self. For many Veterans, leaving the military means confronting new realities and accepting a new version of themselves. Here are some strategies that can help Veterans accept the new version of themselves after military service:

• *Acknowledge your experiences:* The first step in accepting the new you is acknowledging the experiences that have shaped you. This includes both the positive and negative experiences of military service. Acknowledge the strengths and skills you developed during your service, as well as the challenges and struggles you faced. Recognizing and acknowledging these experiences can help you to appreciate the person you have become.

• *Reflect on your values:* Your values may have shifted during your military service and it is important to reflect on these changes. Consider what values are most important to you now and how these values can guide your post-military life. For example, if you developed a deep sense of loyalty to your fellow service members, you may find that this value is still important to you and can guide your relationships with others.

• **Re-evaluate your goals:** Leaving the military may mean re-evaluating your life goals. Consider what you want to achieve in your post-military life and what steps you need to take to achieve those goals. Be open to new possibilities and opportunities and recognize that your post-military life may look different than you initially anticipated.

• **Cultivate a sense of purpose:** A sense of purpose is essential for well-being and many Veterans struggle with finding a new sense of purpose after leaving the military. Consider what activities, hobbies or causes bring you a sense of purpose and make time for these activities in your life. Cultivating a sense of purpose can help you to feel more fulfilled and connected to the world around you.

• **Seek support:** Accepting the new you can be a challenging process and it is important to seek support from others. This may include connecting with other Veterans, joining a support group or seeking professional counseling. Talking to others who have gone through a similar experience can help you to feel less alone and more understood.

• **Practice self-compassion:** It is important to practice self-compassion as you navigate the process of accepting the new you. Recognize that change is hard and that it is normal to experience a range of emotions as you adjust to your post-military life. Be gentle with yourself and recognize that you are doing the best you can.

• **Stay connected to your military identity:** Your military service will always be a part of your identity and it is important to stay connected to this aspect of yourself. This may include participating in military-related events, wearing military gear or connecting with other Veterans. Staying connected to your military identity can help you to feel a sense of continuity and connection to your past.

Bottom Line

Accepting the new you after military service can be a challenging process, but it is essential for well-being and personal growth. By acknowledging your experiences, reflecting on your values, re-evaluating your goals, cultivating a sense of purpose, seeking support, practicing self-compassion and staying connected to your military identity, you can embrace the person you have become and navigate the transition to civilian life with greater ease and resilience. Remember, you are not alone in this process and there are many resources available to support you as you navigate this journey.

Traumatic Brain Injury (TBI)

Also known as TBI, it is a condition that can result from a blow or jolt to the head or a penetrating head injury. For Veterans, TBI is a common injury that can have long-lasting effects on their physical and mental health.

Effects on Veterans' Health

TBI can have a significant impact on Veterans' physical and mental health.

- *Physical Effects:* TBI can cause a range of physical effects including headaches, dizziness and fatigue. Veterans with TBI may also experience seizures, balance problems and difficulty with coordination.

- *Cognitive Effects:* TBI can impact cognitive function including memory, attention and language. Veterans with TBI may have difficulty with problem-solving, decision-making and other cognitive tasks.

- *Emotional Effects:* TBI can cause emotional changes including depression, anxiety and irritability. Veterans with TBI may also experience mood swings and difficulty with emotional regulation.
- *Sleep Disorders:* TBI can cause sleep disorders including insomnia and sleep apnea. Veterans with TBI may also experience daytime fatigue and excessive sleepiness.

Treatments
There are a variety of treatments available for TBI. The following are some of the most common:

- *Medications:* Medications such as anticonvulsants, antidepressants and stimulants may be prescribed to help manage the symptoms of TBI.

- *Cognitive and Behavioral Therapy:* Cognitive and behavioral therapy can help Veterans with TBI to develop coping strategies and improve their cognitive function.

- *Rehabilitation:* Rehabilitation may include physical therapy, occupational therapy and speech therapy to help Veterans with TBI improve their physical and cognitive function.

MeRT for TBI

Magnetic e-Resonance Therapy is a non-invasive treatment that uses magnetic fields to stimulate brain activity. The treatment involves placing electromagnetic coils on the scalp that deliver targeted magnetic fields to the brain. The magnetic fields help to increase the activity of neurons in the brain, which can improve cognitive function and reduce symptoms of TBI.

MeRT has been shown to be an effective treatment for TBI in some patients. A study published in the _Journal of Neurotrauma_ found that MeRT improved cognitive function in Veterans with TBI. The study also found that MeRT reduced symptoms of depression and anxiety in some patients.

MeRT is a safe and non-invasive treatment that has few side effects. However, it is important to work with a qualified healthcare provider to determine if MeRT is an appropriate treatment for your individual needs.

Bottom Line
TBI is a common injury that can have long-lasting effects on Veterans' physical and mental health. There are a variety of treatments available for TBI, including medications, cognitive and behavioral therapy and rehabilitation. MeRT is a novel treatment for TBI that has shown promising results in improving cognitive function and reducing symptoms of TBI in some patients. It is important for Veterans with TBI to work closely with their healthcare provider to develop a comprehensive treatment plan that is safe and effective for their individual needs.

Travel

Travel is a powerful tool that can have numerous benefits on both a personal and a professional level.

- **_Personal growth and self-discovery:_** Traveling to new and unfamiliar places can help you gain a new perspective on life and yourself. It can challenge you to step outside of your comfort zone, try new things and meet new people, which can help you grow and develop as a person.

- **_Improved mental health:_** Traveling can help reduce stress and anxiety by providing a much-needed break from the daily routine. It can also help boost your mood and overall well-being by exposing you to new experiences and environments.

- **_Cultural exposure and education:_** Traveling to different countries and regions can provide a unique opportunity to learn about different cultures and ways of life. This can broaden your understanding and appreciation of different cultures and help you become more culturally aware and sensitive.

• **_Professional growth and development:_** Traveling can also provide numerous professional benefits, such as expanding your network, learning new skills and gaining new experiences. It can help you develop a more global perspective, which can be valuable in today's interconnected world.

• **_Building memories and creating new experiences:_** Traveling creates memories and experiences that can last a lifetime. Whether it's trying new foods, visiting famous landmarks or simply relaxing on a beautiful beach, travel can help create memories that will stay with you forever.

• **_Improved relationships:_** Traveling with friends, family or a romantic partner can help strengthen relationships and create new bonds. It can also provide an opportunity to spend quality time together and make new memories.

• **_Exposure to different lifestyles and ways of living:_** Traveling can expose you to different lifestyles and ways of living, which can broaden your understanding and appreciation of different cultures. It can also provide an opportunity to learn new ideas and ways of doing things that can be valuable in your personal and professional life.

Traveling can be done in many different ways, from solo adventures to group tours, from budget-friendly trips to luxury vacations. No matter how you choose to travel, the benefits are numerous and can help you in numerous ways.

Bottom Line
Travel is a valuable experience that can provide numerous personal and professional benefits. Whether you are looking to reduce stress and anxiety, gain new experiences or simply have fun, travel is a powerful tool that can help you achieve your goals. So, whether you're planning a weekend getaway or a round-the-world trip, don't hesitate to pack your bags and hit the road.

Tru Niagen

A patented form of nicotinamide riboside (NR), a form of Vitamin B3, that has been gaining attention for its potential health benefits, Tru Niagen is marketed as a dietary supplement to support cellular health and longevity and is considered to be a more potent form of NR compared to other available supplements.

One of the primary health benefits of Tru Niagen is its potential to improve cellular energy metabolism. NR is a key building block for the production of nicotinamide adenine dinucleotide (NAD+), which plays a crucial role in cellular energy metabolism and is involved in many important biological processes. By increasing NAD+ levels, Tru Niagen can improve energy production and support healthy aging.

Tru Niagen has also been found to have benefits for brain health. NAD+ is involved in the maintenance of brain function and synaptic plasticity and low levels of NAD+ have been linked to age-related cognitive decline. By increasing NAD+ levels, Tru Niagen can support brain health and cognitive function.

Tru Niagen has also been found to have benefits for cardiovascular health. NAD+ plays a role in regulating blood sugar and blood pressure and low levels of NAD+ have been linked to an increased risk of cardiovascular disease. By increasing NAD+ levels, Tru Niagen can support cardiovascular health and reduce the risk of cardiovascular disease.

Tru Niagen has also been found to have benefits for skin health. NAD+ plays a role in the maintenance of skin health and the regulation of skin aging and low levels of NAD+ have been linked to skin aging. By increasing NAD+ levels, Tru Niagen can support skin health and reduce the signs of aging.

Tru Niagen is generally considered safe when taken in recommended doses, although it can cause side effects such as gastrointestinal upset, headache and dizziness in some individuals. Tru Niagen can also interact with certain medications, so it is important to consult with a healthcare professional before taking Tru Niagen if you are taking any medications.

Bottom Line
Tru Niagen is a patented form of nicotinamide riboside (NR) that has been gaining attention for its potential health benefits. From improving cellular energy metabolism and brain health, to cardiovascular health, skin health and reducing the signs of aging, Tru Niagen is a popular supplement for individuals looking to support their overall health and wellness. However, it is important to note that further research is needed to fully understand the potential health benefits of Tru Niagen and to determine its long-term safety and efficacy. As with any supplement, it is important to consult with a healthcare professional before taking Tru Niagen to ensure that it is safe and appropriate for you.

<u>Urinary Tract Infections</u>

Commonly called UTIs, they are a type of infection that affects any part of the urinary tract, including the bladder, urethra, ureters and kidneys. UTIs are typically caused by bacteria that enter the body through the urethra and multiply in the bladder.

Symptoms of a UTI may include:

- A strong, persistent urge to urinate
- A burning sensation when urinating
- Passing frequent, small amounts of urine
- Cloudy or strong-smelling urine
- Pain or pressure in the lower abdomen and back
- Blood in the urine
- Feeling tired or shaky
- Nausea or vomiting

In order to diagnose a UTI, a healthcare provider will perform a physical examination and take a urine sample to be tested for the presence of bacteria and other signs of infection. In some cases, imaging tests such as a CT scan or ultrasound may be ordered to determine the extent of the infection and rule out other potential causes.

Treatment for a UTI typically involves antibiotics to eliminate the bacterial infection. It is important to take the full course of antibiotics as prescribed, even if symptoms improve before completing the treatment. Over-the-counter pain relievers such as ibuprofen or acetaminophen can also be used to relieve pain and discomfort.

To help prevent UTIs, it is important to:

- Drink plenty of water to flush bacteria from the urinary tract
- Empty your bladder regularly and fully
- Wipe from front to back after using the bathroom to prevent bacteria from spreading to the urethra
- Avoid using feminine hygiene sprays and douches, which can irritate the urethra and increase the risk of infection

- Wear breathable underwear and loose-fitting clothing
- Avoid holding in urine for long periods of time
- Follow good hygiene practices, especially for men who are uncircumcised

In severe cases, a UTI can spread to the kidneys and cause a kidney infection. This type of infection can lead to sepsis, a potentially life-threatening condition, if not treated promptly. If you experience severe symptoms or have a weakened immune system, it is important to see a healthcare provider immediately for proper treatment.

Bottom Line
UTIs are common infections that can affect various parts of the urinary tract. Early diagnosis and prompt treatment with antibiotics is crucial to prevent complications and alleviate symptoms. Maintaining good hygiene and taking preventive measures can help reduce the risk of UTIs.

Vaping

The act of inhaling vapor from an electronic cigarette or other electronic smoking device, has become increasingly popular in recent years. While many people believe that vaping is a safer alternative to traditional smoking, there are a number of hazards associated with this practice, particularly for Veterans.

• *Chemical exposure:* The liquid used in electronic cigarettes and other vaping devices contains a number of chemicals that can be harmful when inhaled, including nicotine, formaldehyde and acrolein. For Veterans who may have been exposed to chemicals during their service, this can be particularly hazardous.

• *Respiratory problems:* The act of inhaling vapor from electronic cigarettes and other vaping devices can cause respiratory problems, particularly for individuals with pre-existing respiratory conditions such as asthma or chronic obstructive pulmonary disease (COPD). This can be particularly problematic for Veterans who may have been exposed to environmental hazards during their service.

• *Cardiovascular problems:* Vaping has been linked to an increased risk of cardiovascular problems, including heart disease and stroke. For Veterans who may already be at increased risk of these conditions due to their service, this can be particularly hazardous.

• *Nicotine addiction:* Vaping devices typically contain nicotine, which is highly addictive. For Veterans who may be struggling with addiction or mental health issues related to their service, the use of nicotine can be particularly problematic.

• *Increased risk of depression and anxiety:* Vaping has been linked to an increased risk of depression and anxiety, particularly in younger individuals. For Veterans who may already be struggling with mental health issues related to the' service, this can be particularly hazardous.

• *Exposure to heavy metals:* The heating elements used in some vaping devices can release heavy metals, such as lead and cadmium, into the vapor that is inhaled. For Veterans who may have been exposed to heavy metals during their service, this can be particularly hazardous.

• *Increased risk of respiratory infections:* Vaping has been linked to an increased risk of respiratory infections, including pneumonia and bronchitis. For Veterans who may already be at increased risk of these conditions due to their service, this can be particularly hazardous.

It's important to note that while many of these hazards are associated with the use of vaping devices, the long-term health effects of vaping are not yet fully understood. The use of these devices is relatively new and research into their long-term health effects is ongoing.

In addition to the hazards associated with vaping, there are a number of other factors that make this practice particularly hazardous for Veterans. These include:

• *Exposure to environmental hazards:* Veterans may have been exposed to a range of environmental hazards during their service, including chemicals, smoke and other pollutants. The use of vaping devices can exacerbate these hazards and increase the risk of respiratory and cardiovascular problems.

• *Mental health issues:* Veterans may be more likely to struggle with mental health issues such as depression, anxiety and post-traumatic stress disorder (PTSD). The use of nicotine and other chemicals in vaping devices can exacerbate these issues and make it more difficult to manage them.

• *Physical disabilities and limitations:* Veterans may have physical disabilities or limitations that make it more difficult to engage in physical activities or maintain a healthy lifestyle. The use of vaping devices can further exacerbate these limitations and increase the risk of respiratory and cardiovascular problems.

• *Substance abuse issues:* Veterans may be more likely to struggle with substance abuse issues, including addiction to nicotine and other substances. The use of vaping devices can exacerbate these issues and make it more difficult to manage them.

Bottom Line
Vaping poses a number of hazards for Veterans, including chemical exposure, respiratory problems, cardiovascular problems, nicotine addiction, increased risk of depression and anxiety, exposure to heavy metals and increased risk of respiratory infections.

Vestibular Therapy

Vestibular therapy is a specialized form of physical therapy that focuses on helping individuals with vestibular disorders improve their balance, coordination and overall mobility. These disorders can have a significant impact on an individual's daily life and can lead to symptoms such as dizziness, vertigo, unsteadiness and even falls. Vestibular therapy is designed to address these symptoms and improve the individual's ability to process and respond to information from the vestibular system.

What is the Vestibular System

The vestibular system is a complex network of organs and structures located in the inner ear that are responsible for our sense of balance and spatial orientation. The vestibular system helps us to maintain our balance and orientation even when we are moving or in different positions. It works in conjunction with other sensory systems, such as the eyes and the skin, to provide us with information about our surroundings and to allow us to make adjustments to our movements as necessary.

Conditions that Can Lead to Vestibular Disorders

Vestibular disorders can occur for several different reasons and can be caused by problems with the inner ear or the central nervous system. Some of the most common causes of vestibular disorders include:

• *Benign Paroxysmal Positional Vertigo (BPPV):* This is the most common type of vestibular disorder and is caused by the displacement of small calcium carbonate crystals in the inner ear. The crystals can cause a false sense of movement and can result in symptoms such as dizziness and vertigo.

• *Vestibular Neuritis:* This is a condition that results from inflammation of the vestibular nerve and can cause symptoms such as vertigo and unsteadiness.

• *Meniere's Disease:* This is a condition that affects the inner ear and can cause symptoms such as vertigo, tinnitus and hearing loss.

• *Vestibular Migraines:* This is a condition that results from migraine headaches that can cause symptoms such as dizziness and unsteadiness.

• *Inner Ear Disorders:* These disorders can result from problems with the inner ear such as infection, injury or congenital defects. They can cause symptoms such as vertigo, unsteadiness and hearing loss.

The Need for Vestibular Therapy

Vestibular disorders can have a significant impact on an individual's daily life and can lead to symptoms such as dizziness, vertigo, unsteadiness and even falls. These symptoms can make it difficult for individuals to perform even simple tasks, such as walking, climbing stairs or even getting out of bed. The goal of vestibular therapy is to help individuals with vestibular disorders improve their ability to process and respond to information from the vestibular system, reduce symptoms and improve overall functioning.

Treatment Approaches Used in Vestibular Therapy

Vestibular therapy is a highly individualized form of therapy that is tailored to meet the specific needs of each patient. Treatment approaches used in vestibular therapy can include:

- *Vestibular Rehabilitation Exercises:* These exercises are designed to help individuals with vestibular disorders improve their balance and coordination. The exercises may involve activities such as balance training, gaze stabilization and head movements.

- *Gaze Stabilization:* This type of therapy focuses on improving an individual's ability to maintain their gaze while moving. The therapy may involve exercises such as moving the head from side to side or up and down while focusing on a stationary target. This helps to retrain the brain to process visual and vestibular information correctly and improve overall stability.

- *Habituation Exercises:* These exercises are designed to help individuals with vestibular disorders become desensitized to certain movements or positions that may trigger symptoms. The therapy may involve repeating movements or positions that cause symptoms until they no longer elicit a response.

- *Cawthorne-Cooksey Exercises:* These exercises are a series of simple movements and positions that are designed to help improve an individual's balance and coordination. The exercises may involve movements such as swaying, walking in a circle and jumping.

- *Balance Training:* This type of therapy involves practicing and improving balance while performing various activities, such as standing on one leg or walking on uneven surfaces. In addition to these specific treatment approaches, vestibular therapy may also include other forms of physical therapy, such as manual therapy or exercises to improve strength and flexibility.

Bottom Line

Vestibular therapy is a highly effective form of physical therapy for individuals with vestibular disorders. The goal of therapy is to help individuals improve their balance, coordination and overall mobility, reduce symptoms and improve overall functioning. Vestibular therapy is a highly individualized form of therapy that is tailored to meet the specific needs of each patient and may include a combination of exercises, balance training and other physical therapy techniques. If you are experiencing symptoms of a vestibular disorder, it is important to seek the help of a qualified vestibular therapist to determine the best course of treatment.

Veterans Affairs

The U.S. Department of Veterans Affairs, aka the VA, provides a range of health-care services and treatments to Veterans, including medical, mental health and rehabilitation services. As a Veteran, it is important to understand how to best utilize the VA to access these services and treatments. Here are some strategies for getting the most out of the VA:

• **Enroll in VA healthcare:** The first step in accessing VA healthcare services and treatments is to enroll in VA healthcare. Veterans who have served in active duty or the reserves are eligible for VA healthcare and enrollment is free. To enroll, Veterans should complete an application online, in person at a VA facility or by mail.

• **Attend appointments:** Once enrolled in VA healthcare, it is important to attend appointments regularly to receive the care and treatments needed to maintain good health. Veterans should make sure to schedule appointments in advance, arrive on time and bring any necessary documents such as medical records or medication lists.

• **Communicate with healthcare providers:** Clear communication with health-care providers is essential for receiving effective healthcare. Veterans should be honest with their healthcare providers about their medical history, symptoms and concerns. Veterans should also ask questions and seek clarification when necessary to ensure that they fully understand their health status and treatment options.

• **Participate in shared decision-making:** Shared decision-making is a collaborative approach to healthcare in which the patient and healthcare provider work together to make decisions about treatment. Veterans should be actively involved in the decision-making process by discussing their goals, preferences and concerns with their healthcare providers.

• **Utilize telehealth services:** VA telehealth services, such as virtual appointments and remote monitoring, can be an effective way to access healthcare services and treatments, particularly for Veterans who live in rural or remote areas. Veterans can access telehealth services through their VA healthcare provider.

• **Utilize specialty care services:** The VA provides a range of specialty care services, such as mental health services, rehabilitation services and women's health services. Veterans should be aware of these services and utilize them as needed to address specific healthcare needs.

• **Participate in research studies:** The VA conducts research studies to improve healthcare services and treatments for Veterans. Veterans can participate in these studies to contribute to the advancement of healthcare research and receive access to cutting-edge treatments and therapies.

• *Access community care:* The VA also offers community care services, which provide access to healthcare services and treatments through local providers. Veterans who live in areas without a VA healthcare facility or who require specialized services not available through the VA may be eligible for community care services.

• *Seek assistance from a patient advocate:* Patient advocates are available at VA facilities to assist Veterans with navigating the healthcare system, addressing concerns and advocating for their healthcare needs. Veterans can ask to speak with a patient advocate at any time to receive assistance.

Bottom Line
The VA provides a range of healthcare services and treatments to Veterans and it is important to know how to best utilize these services to maintain good health. Veterans should enroll in VA healthcare, attend appointments regularly, communicate with healthcare providers, participate in shared decision-making, utilize telehealth services, utilize specialty care services, participate in research studies, access community care and seek assistance from a patient advocate. By utilizing these strategies, Veterans can access the healthcare services and treatments they need to maintain good health and well-being.

Vibroacoustic Therapy

Vibroacoustic therapy (VAT) uses sound vibrations transmitted through a specialized bed or mat to promote relaxation, reduce stress, and support physical and mental health. For Veterans, who may experience chronic pain, PTSD, or stress-related conditions, VAT offers a non-invasive approach to wellness by using targeted frequencies to influence the body's nervous system. Unlike traditional massage or talk therapy, VAT works by delivering low-frequency sound waves that penetrate muscles and tissues, providing deep relaxation and potential therapeutic benefits. This section explores vibroacoustic therapy, its benefits, and how Veterans can integrate it into their wellness routines.

Understanding Vibroacoustic Therapy
Vibroacoustic therapy beds operate by emitting sound vibrations at specific frequencies that resonate through the body. The therapy is based on the principle that sound waves can affect physiological and psychological states. Key components include:

• Vibroacoustic Bed or Mat: Equipped with built-in transducers that convert sound into gentle vibrations.

- Frequency Range: Typically between 30–120 Hz, with different frequencies targeting relaxation, pain relief, and cognitive function.

- Music Integration: Some systems incorporate music therapy, enhancing the therapeutic experience.

The Science of Vibroacoustic Therapy

Research in Sound Therapy Journal (2022) suggests that VAT may help regulate the autonomic nervous system, reducing stress and improving circulation. Studies also indicate benefits for PTSD, chronic pain, and sleep disorders, areas of concern for many Veterans.

Why Vibroacoustic Therapy Matters for Veterans

- Stress & PTSD Relief: Low-frequency vibrations promote relaxation and help regulate stress responses.

- Pain Management: Vibrational therapy stimulates circulation and relieves muscle tension, aiding recovery from injuries.

- Improved Sleep: VAT can enhance sleep quality by calming the nervous system and reducing nighttime restlessness.

- Cognitive Support: Frequencies associated with focus and mental clarity may aid Veterans experiencing brain fog.

- Emotional Well-Being: Sound therapy encourages relaxation, reducing symptoms of anxiety and depression.

Identifying the Need for VAT

- Common Signs: Insomnia, chronic muscle pain, stress, emotional fatigue.

- Veteran-Specific Triggers: PTSD, high physical strain, combat-related stress.

- Assessment Tools: Symptom tracking, monitoring stress levels, and sleep patterns.

- Medical Support: Consultation with VA therapists or holistic practitioners specializing in sound therapy.

Strategies for Integrating VAT into Veteran Wellness

- Professional VAT Sessions: Clinics and wellness centers offer vibroacoustic therapy beds for guided sessions.

- At-Home VAT Devices: Personal mats and chairs with built-in sound therapy technology are available for regular use.

- Complementary Practices: VAT pairs well with meditation, deep breathing, and mindfulness techniques.

- Hydration & Nutrition: Proper hydration supports circulation and muscle relaxation, enhancing VAT benefits.

Targeted Uses for Veterans

1. PTSD & Anxiety Reduction

- What: Use low-frequency VAT sessions (30–40 Hz) for relaxation.

- Why: Helps regulate the nervous system and ease hyperarousal.

- How: 20–30-minute sessions 3–4 times per week.

- Supplies: Access to a vibroacoustic therapy bed or mat.

2. Pain & Muscle Recovery

- What: Apply VAT at frequencies of 50–80 Hz post-exercise or injury.

- Why: Enhances circulation and reduces muscle stiffness.

- How: 15–30-minute sessions after physical strain.

- Supplies: Vibroacoustic mat or therapy chair.

3. Sleep Optimization

- What: Use calming frequencies (40–60 Hz) before bedtime.

- Why: Encourages relaxation and deep sleep cycles.

- How: 30-minute sessions in the evening.

- Supplies: VAT-equipped bed or portable sound mat.

4. Cognitive Function & Focus

- What: Listen to cognitive-enhancing frequencies (80–120 Hz) while working or studying.

- Why: Stimulates brainwave activity associated with focus and alertness.

- How: Short sessions (10–20 minutes) as needed.

- Supplies: VAT device with a cognitive support setting.

Supplementation and Additional Support

- Music Therapy Apps: Apps like Brain.fm provide similar frequency-based sound therapy.

- Mindfulness Integration: Pairing VAT with guided meditation enhances relaxation benefits.

- Therapist-Guided VAT: Professional VAT sessions may be available at VA or wellness clinics.

- Equipment Costs: Home VAT mats range from $200–$1,500 depending on features.

Integrating VAT into Daily Life

- Set SMART Goals: Example: "Use VAT for 20 minutes before bed, 4 times weekly, to improve sleep."

- Track Progress: Monitor stress, pain, and sleep improvements over time.

- Leverage Veteran Support: VA wellness programs, community centers, and holistic therapy groups may offer VAT access.

Bottom Line

Vibroacoustic therapy beds provide a non-invasive approach to relaxation, stress relief, pain management, and cognitive support. Veterans dealing with PTSD, chronic pain, or sleep disturbances may find VAT beneficial for nervous system regulation and overall well-being. Research supports VAT's effects on relaxation and circulation, while emerging studies explore its potential for cognitive and emotional health. Veterans can explore professional VAT sessions, invest in at-home therapy devices, and integrate vibroacoustic therapy with other wellness practices for long-term benefits. Regular use, proper hydration, and monitoring effects can help Veterans maximize this therapy's potential for improved wellness and resilience.

Vices

Veterans, having served their country with honor and dedication, deserve to enjoy a healthy and fulfilling life post-service. However, there are vices and harmful behaviors that can jeopardize their well-being. In this comprehensive chapter, we will explore various vices that Veterans should avoid for their good health and overall wellness. By understanding the risks associated with these vices and providing practical guidance, we aim to empower Veterans to make informed choices for a healthier future.

Tobacco Use

• *Smoking:* Quitting smoking is important for improved lung health and reduced risk of cancer and cardiovascular diseases. Seek resources and strategies for smoking cessation, including nicotine replacement therapy and counseling.

• *Smokeless tobacco:* The hazards of smokeless tobacco use, including oral cancers and addiction, are well-known. Embrace smokeless tobacco cessation and seek support to quit.

Alcohol Abuse

- Be aware of the prevalence of alcohol abuse among Veterans and its consequences on health and well-being.
- Understand the link between post-traumatic stress disorder (PTSD) and alcohol abuse.
- Understand the physical and mental health consequences of excessive alcohol consumption.
- Be aware of the risk of developing alcohol use disorder and its impact your life as a Veteran.
- If you suffer from alcohol abuse, seek programs that will lead to moderation and treatment.

Illicit Drug Abuse

- Know the common illicit drugs that Veterans may be exposed to or misuse.
- Know the health risks associated with drug use, including addiction and overdose.
- Know the connection between drug use and mental health issues.
- Know the importance of seeking professional help for dual diagnosis and co-occurring disorders.

Prescription Medication Misuse

- Understand the opioid epidemic's impact on Veterans.
- Understand the risks associated with the misuse of prescription pain medications.
- Encourage responsible medication use.
- Seek medical guidance for pain management and exploring non-opioid alternatives.

Unhealthy Eating

- Examine the consequences of a diet high in processed foods, sugars and unhealthy fats.
- Learn the link between poor nutrition and chronic conditions such as obesity and diabetes.
- Work to adopt a balanced and nutritious diet.
- Seek out practical tips for meal planning, portion control and incorporating whole foods into your diet.

Sedentary Lifestyle

- Be aware of the detrimental effects of a sedentary lifestyle on Veterans' health, including increased risks of obesity and cardiovascular diseases.
- Learn the impact of physical inactivity on mental well-being.
- Know the importance of regular physical activity for Veterans' health.
- Seek practical guidance on incorporating exercise into daily routines and setting fitness goals.

Unmanaged Stress

- Learn the impact of unmanaged stress on Veterans' mental and physical health.
- Learn the potential for stress to exacerbate existing conditions like PTSD.
- Seek out stress-management techniques such as mindfulness, meditation and seeking professional counseling.
- Strive for self-care and a healthy work-life balance.

Lack of Mental Health Support

- Try to avoid the stigma associated with seeking mental health support.
- Understand the consequences of untreated mental health issues.
- Encourage fellow Veterans to seek mental health support through the VA and other resources.
- Understand the benefits of therapy, counseling and support groups in managing mental health challenges.

Bottom Line

Veterans have already demonstrated their resilience and dedication through their service. To continue this commitment to their well-being, it is essential to recognize and avoid vices that can hinder their health and overall quality of life. By addressing issues such as tobacco and substance use, promoting healthy lifestyle choices and emphasizing the importance of mental health support, Veterans can take proactive steps to ensure their good health and wellness as they transition into civilian life.

Visualization

Visualization is the practice of mentally imagining specific scenes, outcomes, or states to influence mental, emotional, and physical well-being, rooted in psychology, sports science, and mindfulness traditions. It involves intentional, focused imagery—unlike daydreaming—to achieve goals or reduce stress, using guided or self-directed methods. Veterans, dealing with PTSD, chronic pain, or reintegration challenges post-service, can use visualization as a low-cost, accessible tool to support resilience and healing. Benefits claimed include stress reduction, improved focus, and pain management, supported by research in cognitive psychology and neuroscience, though evidence for broader claims varies, and risks like over-reliance apply.

The technique dates to ancient meditation practices like Buddhist Vipassana around 500 BCE and gained modern use in the 1970s through sports psychology and mindfulness therapies like MBSR in 1979. PTSD, pain, and adjustment issues affect many Veterans, driving interest in visualization to manage symptoms. Combat trauma, stress, and injuries disrupt mental and physical health; visualization targets these by altering thought patterns and responses. Symptoms like anxiety, fatigue, or soreness prompt its use as a way to regain control.

Sessions involve creating mental images for 5–20 minutes, engaging senses like sight and sound, often daily. Benefits include lower stress through calm imagery, sharper focus by picturing tasks, greater resilience via positive outcomes, reduced pain perception, reinforced habits like sobriety, enhanced recovery through skill rehearsal, and better sleep with relaxing scenes. Risks involve frustration from unrealistic expectations; Veterans with depression need caution. Studies show benefits over 4–8 weeks, with brain imaging confirming effects, though not all claims are fully validated. PTSD, pain, and transition stress align with its uses, making it relevant for Veterans who can start with free VA tools.

Targeted Protocols for Veterans' Wellness
Veterans with stress, pain, or mental fog from service can use visualization to ad-

dress these issues. Start with free VA resources like the Mindfulness Coach app or basic self-practice—5–15 minutes daily—sitting quietly, closing eyes, and picturing a calm scene like a forest with detailed sounds and smells. VA mental health services can provide guidance, or functional providers with foundation support, like the Gary Sinise Foundation or Wounded Warrior Project, may offer access to recordings for qualifying Veterans. Track symptoms—stress levels, pain, focus—in a journal to monitor progress over 4–8 weeks.

For stress reduction, imagine a peaceful place like a beach for 10–15 minutes daily—Veterans with transition tension feel calmer in weeks; add deep breathing and adjust timing if needed. Mental focus improves by picturing a task, like a clear workday, for 10–15 minutes daily—Veterans with TBI-related fog sharpen attention over a month; pair with a VA therapist if progress slows. Emotional resilience builds by visualizing positive outcomes, like staying steady under pressure, 15 minutes daily—Veterans with PTSD gain coping strength in 8 weeks; refine with guided audio ($0–$60 via apps like Calm) if effects stall.

Pain management uses imagery of relief—like ice cooling a sore back—for 15–20 minutes daily—Veterans with chronic pain notice less discomfort in 4 weeks; combine with VA physical therapy if it drags. Behavioral change, like sobriety, involves picturing success for 10–15 minutes daily—Veterans with addiction reinforce habits over a month; track adherence and escalate to guided sessions if slipping. Physical performance aids recovery by imagining healed movement, 15 minutes daily—Veterans with injuries rehab faster in 6 weeks; adjust with a provider if needed.

Sleep improves with pre-bed visualization of calm scenes, 5–15 minutes—Veterans with insomnia rest better in weeks; shift to morning if it disrupts. Pair with morning or bedtime routines using free VA apps or recordings—80% stick with it this way; escalate to therapist-led sessions ($50–$150) for more structure. Consult a healthcare provider before relying on it for PTSD or chronic pain, ensuring it fits with VA care and avoids over-reliance. Costs are minimal—free via VA or $0–$60 for apps. Begin with 5–15 minutes daily, set goals like stress relief, and assess—calmer mood, less pain—over 4–8 weeks, refining with professional input if results falter.

Bottom Line

Visualization offers stress reduction, mental focus, emotional resilience, pain management, behavioral change, physical performance, and sleep improvement by imagining calm scenes or goals for 5–20 minutes daily, guided or self-directed. Veterans with PTSD, pain, or transition stress can use this tool, with studies showing 15–30% symptom relief over 4–8 weeks. It's intentional imagery, backed by psychology, unlike daydreaming. Evidence supports stress and pain benefits—tri-

als and brain imaging confirm effects—but broader claims lack large-scale proof. Risks include frustration from over-reliance, a concern for Veterans with complex issues. It's not a standalone treatment—professionals recommend pairing with VA care due to limited scope—so consult a healthcare provider, use VA tools (e.g., Mindfulness Coach) or apps, and integrate with therapy, approaching with realistic goals and consistency. It's a useful aid, not a cure, needing balanced application.

Vitamins

Vitamins are essential nutrients that are required for various bodily functions and overall health. While most people can get the vitamins they need from a balanced diet, some individuals may benefit from taking vitamin supplements.

Role of vitamins in health

• *Vitamin A:* Vitamin A is important for eye health, as well as for maintaining healthy skin, immune function and bone growth.

• *Vitamin B Complex:* The B vitamins, including B1 (thiamine), B2 (riboflavin), B3 (niacin), B5 (pantothenic acid), B6 (pyridoxine), B7 (biotin), B9 (folate) and B12 (cobalamin), are essential for energy production, healthy skin and hair, and a strong immune system.

• *Vitamin C:* Vitamin C is a powerful antioxidant that helps to protect the body against damage from free radicals and supports the immune system. It also plays a role in collagen production and wound healing.

• *Vitamin D:* Vitamin D is important for bone health, as it helps the body to absorb calcium and maintain strong bones. It also plays a role in immune function and may help to reduce the risk of certain cancers.
• *Vitamin E:* Vitamin E is another important antioxidant that helps to protect the body against damage from free radicals. It is also important for skin health and wound healing.

• *Vitamin K:* Vitamin K plays a role in blood clotting and helps to prevent excessive bleeding.

Benefits of taking vitamin supplements

• *Improved Immunity:* Vitamin supplements, especially those that contain vitamins C and D, can help to boost the immune system and reduce the risk of illness.

• **Better Skin Health:** Vitamins such as vitamin A, vitamin C and vitamin E can help to improve skin health, reduce the appearance of wrinkles and protect against damage from UV radiation.

• **Improved Heart Health:** Some vitamins, such as vitamin B3 (niacin) and vitamin B9 (folate), have been shown to improve heart health and reduce the risk of heart disease.

• **Better Bone Health:** Vitamins such as vitamin D and vitamin K can help to improve bone health and reduce the risk of osteoporosis and other bone-related conditions.

• **Improved Mental Health:** Some vitamins, such as vitamin B9 (folate), have been shown to improve mental health and reduce the risk of depression and other mental health conditions.

Factors that can impact vitamin needs

• **Age:** As we age our body's ability to absorb certain vitamins can decrease, which can impact our vitamin needs.

• **Health Conditions:** Certain health conditions, such as celiac disease, Crohn's disease and ulcerative colitis, can impact a person's ability to absorb vitamins and may increase their vitamin needs.

• **Medications:** Some medications, such as antacids and birth control pills, can interfere with the absorption of certain vitamins and increase the risk of deficiencies.

• **Lifestyle Factors:** Lifestyle factors, such as a diet that is low in nutrients, alcohol consumption and smoking, can impact a person's vitamin needs and increase the risk of deficiencies.

Bottom Line
Vitamins are essential for overall health and well-being and taking vitamin supplements can provide numerous health benefits. While a balanced diet is the best way to get the vitamins and nutrients the body needs, vitamin supplements can be beneficial for individuals who have specific health needs or who may not be getting enough vitamins from their diet. It is important to speak with a healthcare provider before starting a vitamin supplement regimen to determine the right dosage and to ensure that it does not interfere with any existing health conditions or medications. By incorporating vitamins into a healthy lifestyle, individuals can support their overall health and well-being.

- W -

<u>Water</u>

Water is an essential element for human survival and overall health. It is estimated that the human body is made up of 60% water, making it a critical component for various physiological functions. In this article, we will explore why water is so important for our health and what happens when we don't get enough of it.

• *Hydrates the Body:* One of the primary functions of water is to maintain the balance of bodily fluids. This balance is crucial for regulating body temperature, transporting nutrients and removing waste and toxins from the body. When we don't drink enough water, the body becomes dehydrated, which can cause symptoms such as fatigue, headaches and dry skin.

• *Supports Healthy Skin:* Drinking water is beneficial for maintaining healthy skin. Dehydration can cause skin to become dry and wrinkles to form, while proper hydration can help to keep skin looking healthy and plump. Additionally, water can help to flush out waste and toxins from the body, which can prevent breakouts and improve skin health.

• *Aids in Digestion:* Water plays a crucial role in promoting healthy digestion. It helps to flush out waste and toxins from the body, promoting regular bowel movements and reducing the risk of constipation. Additionally, water can help to prevent indigestion and other digestive problems by neutralizing stomach acid and promoting healthy gut bacteria.

• *Supports Physical Performance:* Proper hydration is important for physical performance. Dehydration can cause fatigue, muscle cramps and decreased endurance. Additionally, drinking water before, during, and after physical activity can help to maintain optimal body temperature and prevent overheating.

• *Helps Regulate Body Temperature:* Water plays a crucial role in regulating body temperature. When we sweat, our bodies lose fluids, which must be replenished to maintain healthy body temperature. Drinking water before, during and after physical activity can help to prevent overheating, especially in hot weather.

• *Prevents Headaches and Migraines:* Dehydration is a common trigger for headaches and migraines. When the body becomes dehydrated, the brain can shrink away from the skull, causing pain and discomfort. Drinking enough water can help to prevent headaches and migraines by keeping the brain hydrated.

• **Promotes Weight Loss:** Drinking water can be an effective tool for weight loss. It can help to control hunger and boost metabolism, leading to increased weight loss. Additionally, water has no calories, making it a healthy and low-calorie alternative to sugary drinks.

Water Distillers

Water distillers are easily procured and then once tap water is distilled you can re-mineralize for the best effect.

Water distillers offer several benefits, particularly when it comes to ensuring the purity and safety of drinking water:

• **Effective Removal of Contaminants:** Water distillers are highly effective at removing a wide range of contaminants, including bacteria, viruses, heavy metals (like lead and mercury), chemicals (such as chlorine and fluoride), and dissolved solids. The distillation process involves boiling water to create steam, which is then condensed back into liquid form, leaving impurities behind.

• **Improved Taste and Odor:** By removing impurities, water distillers can significantly improve the taste and odor of tap water. This is especially beneficial for those living in areas where the water supply may have a strong chemical taste or unpleasant smell.

• **Consistent Quality:** Unlike some filtration systems that may become less effective over time as filters clog, water distillers consistently produce high-quality water. The distillation process ensures that each batch of water is purified to the same standard.

• **Cost-Effective:** While the initial investment in a water distiller may be higher than other purification methods, it can be more cost-effective in the long run. There is no need to purchase replacement filters or bottled water, making it a one-time investment for long-term use.

• **Environmentally Friendly:** Using a water distiller reduces the need for bottled water, which helps decrease plastic waste and the environmental impact associated with producing and disposing of plastic bottles.

• **Health Benefits:** For individuals with compromised immune systems or those sensitive to contaminants, distilled water can provide an extra layer of safety by ensuring that the water is free from harmful pathogens and chemicals that might affect health.

• **Versatility:** Distilled water can be used for more than just drinking. It's also ideal for use in medical equipment, humidifiers, and appliances like steam irons, where mineral buildup from regular tap water could cause damage.

Overall, water distillers are a reliable option for those seeking the highest level of water purity and safety.

Types of Water Distillers

Countertop Water Distillers:

- *Description:* These are the most common types of water distillers, designed for home use. They sit on the kitchen counter and typically distill a few gallons of water at a time.

- *Advantages:* Convenient for households; no need for plumbing installation; relatively affordable.

- *Health Impact:* They produce pure, high-quality distilled water, ideal for drinking, cooking, or medical use.

- *Example:* Megahome Countertop Water Distiller.

Automatic Water Distillers:

- *Description:* These distillers are larger, often built into the home's water system, and can automatically produce and store distilled water for continuous use.

- *Advantages:* Ideal for families or individuals who need larger volumes of distilled water; automated, so they don't require much maintenance or attention.

- *Health Impact:* Provides a constant supply of distilled water, which can be beneficial for households with individuals who need chemical-free water for health reasons.

- *Example:* Durastill Automatic Water Distiller.

Portable Water Distillers:

- *Description:* Designed for travel or emergency situations, these compact distillers can be used anywhere, often relying on a small heat source like a stove or solar energy.

- *Advantages:* Portable and convenient for camping, travel, or areas with unsafe water supplies; can be used in emergency preparedness.

- **Health Impact:** Offers peace of mind in areas where water safety is questionable; ideal for remote locations.

- **Example:** Waterwise 4000 Water Distiller.

Commercial Water Distillers:

- **Description:** These are large-scale distillation systems designed for use in hospitals, laboratories, or industrial settings where high volumes of pure water are required.

- **Advantages:** High-capacity, designed for environments with significant water purity needs, such as medical sterilization or pharmaceutical production.

- **Health Impact:** Provides medical-grade water, which is essential in healthcare environments where sterilization and patient safety are paramount.

- **Example:** AquaNui 12G Commercial Water Distiller.

Bottom Line

Water is essential for human health. From hydrating the body to promoting healthy skin and digestion, drinking enough water is critical for optimal physiological function. It is recommended to drink at least 8 glasses of water per day to maintain proper hydration. However, the exact amount of water needed can vary depending on factors such as age, gender, physical activity level and climate. By making sure to drink enough water, we can maintain optimal health and prevent a range of health problems.

When Getting Sick or Being Around Sick People

Sickness—whether from colds, C19, Lyme, or exposure to ill people—can strain the body, especially the lymphatic system, which filters waste and supports immunity. For Veterans, who may face heightened risks from past toxin exposure or stress, proactive detox and prevention strategies help mitigate symptoms and boost resilience. These methods, rooted in daily habits and acute responses, use natural tools to expel pathogens, reduce inflammation, and maintain vitality.

Below is a list of practices for sickness (focused on lymph detox) and a daily detox routine, with descriptions tailored for Veteran use, emphasizing practical, accessible steps to stay strong or recover fast.

- Sickness/C19/Lyme Lymph Detox: Lymphatic drainage clears toxins; key for C19 or Lyme, which burden immunity, helping Veterans fight infection and fatigue.

- Sweat (IR Sauna Best): Infrared saunas (30-45 minutes, 120-140°F) expel toxins via sweat; Veterans use to flush pathogens, best daily or when sick.

- Cold Plunges During Sauna: Brief cold dips (1-2 minutes, 50-60°F) mid-sauna shock lymph flow; Veterans alternate hot-cold to move waste, energize.

- Jog-Walk-Vibrate: Light jogging or walking (20-30 minutes) or vibrating platforms (10-15 minutes) activate lymph drainage; Veterans boost circulation when under the weather.

- Deep Breathing: Slow breaths (5-10 minutes, 6 breaths/min) oxygenate blood, lymph; Veterans use to detox lungs, calm nerves during sickness.

- Hot and Cold Shower Cycles: Alternating hot (2 minutes, 100°F) and cold (1 minute, 50°F) showers (3-5 cycles) push lymph out; Veterans rinse off sickness.

- Dry Brush: Brushing skin upward (5-10 minutes daily) stimulates lymph; Veterans pair with showers to exfoliate, detox when exposed to illness.

- Loose Clothes: Non-restrictive wear aids lymph flow; Veterans avoid tight gear to keep drainage active during recovery.

- Mineralized Water: Drinking 8-12 cups daily with trace minerals (e.g., sea salt pinch) flushes toxins; Veterans hydrate to support lymph detox.

- Lymphatic Massage: Gentle self-massage (10-20 minutes, neck to groin) or pro sessions ($50-$100) moves lymph; Veterans ease swelling when sick.

- Chiropractor: Adjustments (30 minutes, $30-$80) align spine, boost lymph; Veterans visit weekly when ill to enhance drainage.

- Herbs: Elderberry or turmeric (500-1000 mg daily, $10-$20) reduce inflammation; Veterans use to fight sickness naturally.

- Vibrating Platform: Standing on a vibe plate (10-15 minutes, $100-$500) shakes lymph loose; Veterans detox daily or when exposed.

- Daily Detox Routine: Even when well, Veterans maintain resilience with early sleep (10 p.m.-6 a.m.), early waking, and happy thoughts or meditation (5-10 minutes) to balance stress.

- Oral Hygiene: Waterpik with solution, floss, brush, saline nasal flush (10 minutes daily) clear germs; Veterans start days fresh, reducing pathogen load.

- Sweat Session: Bike (30 minutes) or 4-mile walk/run with YouTube docs gets sweat going; Veterans energize and detox daily.

- Stretch and Cold Rinse: Post-exercise stretch (10 minutes) and cold shower

(1-2 minutes) flush lymph; Veterans cool down, invigorate.

- Infrared Sauna Time: 30-45 minutes with cold rinses (1 minute each) clears emails, meditates, or detoxes skin; Veterans' favorite for lymph shock, relaxation.

- Final Cold Shower: Post-sauna rinse (2-3 minutes) seals detox; Veterans start days strong, refreshed.

It's wise to consult a healthcare provider before intense detox, especially with chronic conditions, ensuring safety and VA alignment.

Bottom Line:

When sick or around sick people (e.g., C19, Lyme), Veterans can detox lymph with infrared saunas, cold plunges, jogging, deep breathing, hot-cold showers, dry brushing, loose clothes, mineralized water, massage, chiropractic care, herbs, and vibrating platforms, easing symptoms and boosting immunity. Daily detox—early sleep, meditation, oral hygiene, exercise, stretching, saunas, and cold rinses—keeps resilience high even when well. These practices flush toxins, reduce inflammation, and energize, tailored for Veterans' rugged pasts. Evidence from small studies supports sweat and lymph benefits, but broader claims lack large trials, relying on user success. Risks include overexertion or cold shock, manageable with moderation. Not a primary treatment, they complement VA care for sickness or prevention. Veterans should start with free steps (e.g., breathing, showers), add affordable tools (e.g., herbs, $10-$20), and consult providers, using these daily or as needed with grit and balance.

- X -

Xerostomia

Xerostomia is a medical term that refers to dry mouth, which is a condition where there is a decrease in the production of saliva. This can lead to discomfort, difficulty speaking, swallowing and a change in taste perception. Xerostomia can be caused by various factors such as medications, radiation therapy, autoimmune disorders, nerve damage and dehydration. Additionally, some medical conditions like Sjogren's syndrome and diabetes can also cause xerostomia. The symptoms of dry mouth can be managed by drinking plenty of fluids, using saliva substitutes, avoiding tobacco and alcohol and practicing good oral hygiene. In severe cases, a dentist or physician may prescribe medication to stimulate the production of saliva.

- Y -

Yeast (Candida)

Yeast overgrowth in the body refers to an excess of yeast in the gut, also known as Candida overgrowth. Candida is a type of yeast that is naturally present in the human body, but when it proliferates, it can lead to a number of health problems. This can occur due to a variety of factors including poor diet, antibiotics, stress and weakened immune system. In this article, we will explore the causes of yeast overgrowth, its symptoms and the most effective techniques for elimination.

Causes of Yeast Overgrowth

• *Antibiotic Use:* Antibiotics are designed to kill harmful bacteria, but they can also kill good bacteria in the gut. This can lead to an imbalance in the gut flora and can allow yeast to proliferate.

• *Poor Diet:* A diet high in sugar and processed foods can provide an ideal environment for yeast to grow. Additionally, diets low in fiber and high in refined carbohydrates can contribute to yeast overgrowth.

• *Stress:* Chronic stress can weaken the immune system and increase the risk of Candida overgrowth.

• *Weak Immune System:* A weakened immune system can make it more difficult for the body to fight off Candida overgrowth. This can occur due to illnesses, such as HIV/AIDS, or due to lifestyle factors, such as a lack of sleep or excessive alcohol consumption.

• *Hormonal Changes:* Hormonal changes, such as those that occur during pregnancy or menopause, can also contribute to Candida overgrowth.

Symptoms of Yeast Overgrowth

• *Digestive Issues:* Candida overgrowth can lead to a variety of digestive issues, including bloating, gas and constipation.

• *Fatigue:* Yeast overgrowth can also cause fatigue and a general feeling of being unwell.

• *Skin Issues:* Candida overgrowth can lead to skin problems, such as rashes and acne.

• *Yeast Infections:* Candida overgrowth can lead to yeast infections, such as thrush and vaginitis.

• *Brain Fog:* Yeast overgrowth can cause brain fog and difficulties with concentration and memory.

Elimination Techniques

• *Diet Changes:* The first step in eliminating yeast overgrowth is to make changes to your diet. This includes reducing sugar and processed foods and increasing fiber and probiotic-rich foods. A diet that is rich in vegetables, lean protein and healthy fats can help to promote a healthy gut flora and reduce the risk of Candida overgrowth.

• *Probiotics:* Probiotics are beneficial bacteria that can help to balance the gut flora and reduce the risk of Candida overgrowth. Probiotics can be found in fermented foods, such as yogurt and kefir, or can be taken as a supplement.

• *Antifungal Supplements:* Antifungal supplements, such as caprylic acid and garlic, can help to kill off the Candida yeast in the gut.

• *Stress Management:* Stress management techniques, such as exercise, meditation and deep breathing, can help to reduce the risk of Candida overgrowth by strengthening the immune system.

• *Avoid Antibiotics:* When possible, avoid antibiotics and opt for natural remedies instead. If antibiotics are necessary, be sure to follow up with a probiotic supplement to help restore the balance of gut flora.

• *Improve Immune System:* Improving the immune system can help to reduce the risk of Candida overgrowth. This can be done by getting enough sleep, reducing alcohol consumption and eating a balanced diet that is rich in vitamins and minerals. Regular exercise can also help to boost the immune system and reduce the risk of Candida overgrowth.

Bottom Line

Yeast overgrowth in the body can lead to a variety of health problems and symptoms. By making diet changes, taking probiotics, using antifungal supplements, managing stress, avoiding antibiotics and improving the immune system, individuals can effectively eliminate Candida overgrowth and improve their overall health. It is important to work with a healthcare professional to determine the best course of action for your specific situation, as some individuals may require a more targeted approach. However, implementing these general strategies can be a great starting point in the quest for better gut health and improved overall well-being.

Nutritional Yeast use and benefits

Also known as "noosh" or "savory yeast flakes," nutritional yeast is a type of yeast that is deactivated, meaning it cannot be used to ferment or leaven bread. Instead, it is a popular food ingredient, particularly in the vegetarian and vegan communities, because of its unique flavor and rich nutritional profile.

One of the key benefits of nutritional yeast is that it is an excellent source of protein, containing about 8-14 grams of protein per 100 grams of yeast. This makes it an important source of protein for vegetarians and vegans who may have limited options for protein sources.

In addition to protein, nutritional yeast is also a good source of B-complex vitamins, particularly thiamin, riboflavin, niacin and B12. B vitamins are important for energy production, metabolism and maintaining healthy skin, hair, eyes and nerves. B12 is especially important for vegans and vegetarians, as it is only found in animal-based foods. Nutritional yeast can be a great source of B12 for those who follow a plant-based diet, but it's important to note that not all nutritional yeasts are fortified with B12, so it's crucial to check the label.

Nutritional yeast is also a good source of fiber, which helps to promote digestive health and regulate blood sugar levels. It contains trace amounts of minerals like iron, potassium, magnesium and zinc, which are important for maintaining a healthy immune system and overall health.

Another benefit of nutritional yeast is its umami flavor, which is often described as savory and nutty. This flavor profile makes it a popular ingredient for seasoning sauces, soups and stews, as well as a cheese substitute for those who are lactose intolerant or follow a vegan diet.

In terms of how to use nutritional yeast, it can be added to a variety of dishes to add flavor and nutrition. Some popular uses include:

- Sprinkled on top of popcorn for a tasty, savory snack.
- Added to soups and stews for extra flavor.
- Used to make vegan cheese sauces and dips.
- Sprinkled on top of roasted vegetables for added flavor.

It's important to note that while nutritional yeast is a healthy and nutritious food, it is not a complete protein source, meaning it does not contain all of the essential amino acids that our bodies need. To make sure you're getting all of the essential amino acids, it's best to pair nutritional yeast with other protein-rich foods, such as legumes, grains, nuts and seeds.

Bottom Line
Nutritional yeast is a versatile and nutritious ingredient that can be a great addition to any diet. Whether you're looking for a source of B vitamins, protein or a savory flavor, nutritional yeast can be a great option. Just make sure to check the label to see if it's fortified with B12 and to pair it with other protein sources to ensure you're getting all of the essential amino acids your body needs.

Yoga

Yoga is an ancient practice that has been around for over 5,000 years and has gained popularity around the world as a way to improve physical and mental health. Yoga involves a combination of physical postures, breathing exercises and meditation techniques that can help reduce stress, improve flexibility and increase overall wellness. For Veterans, the practice of yoga can offer a range of benefits, both physical and mental, that can help improve their quality of life.

• *Reduced stress and anxiety:* Yoga has been shown to be an effective way to reduce stress and anxiety levels. For Veterans, who may be dealing with post-traumatic stress disorder (PTSD) or other mental health issues, yoga can be a way to calm the mind and reduce feelings of anxiety.

• *Improved physical fitness:* Yoga can help improve physical fitness by increasing flexibility, balance and strength. This can be particularly beneficial for Veterans who may have physical disabilities or injuries that limit their ability to engage in more strenuous physical activities.

- **Improved sleep:** Many Veterans struggle with sleep disturbances, which can be caused by physical or mental health issues. Yoga has been shown to be an effective way to improve sleep quality and help individuals fall asleep more easily.

- **Pain relief:** Many Veterans suffer from chronic pain as a result of injuries sustained during their service. Yoga has been shown to be an effective way to reduce pain and improve overall quality of life for individuals with chronic pain.

- **Improved mood:** The practice of yoga has been shown to improve overall mood and increase feelings of happiness and well-being. This can be particularly beneficial for Veterans who may be dealing with mental health issues or struggling to adjust to civilian life.

- **Increased self-awareness:** Yoga involves a focus on mindfulness and self-awareness, which can help individuals become more attuned to their own thoughts and emotions. For Veterans, who may be dealing with emotional or mental health issues, this can be a powerful tool for self-reflection and growth.

- **Improved social connections:** Many Veterans struggle with social isolation, which can be a significant factor in mental and physical health. Yoga classes can offer a way to connect with others and build a sense of community, which can be an important factor in improving overall wellness.

One of the key benefits of yoga is its accessibility. It can be practiced by individuals of all ages and fitness levels and can be adapted to meet the unique needs of each individual. For Veterans who may have physical limitations or injuries, this can be particularly beneficial.

There are different styles of yoga, each with their own focus and benefits. Some of the most popular styles include:

- **Hatha yoga:** This style of yoga involves a combination of physical postures and breathing exercises and is generally considered to be a gentle form of yoga.

- **Vinyasa yoga:** This style of yoga involves flowing from one pose to another and is generally more physically demanding than Hatha yoga.

- **Restorative yoga:** This style of yoga involves a focus on relaxation and meditation and is designed to help reduce stress and promote relaxation.

• **Kundalini yoga:** This style of yoga involves a focus on spiritual and physical practices and is designed to promote overall wellness and self-awareness.

• **Yin yoga:** This style of yoga involves holding poses for an extended period of time and is designed to improve flexibility and balance.

When starting a yoga practice, it's important to find a qualified instructor who can help guide you through the process and ensure that you are practicing the poses correctly. Many yoga studios and community centers offer classes specifically for Veterans, which can be a great way to connect with other Veterans and receive support from those who have shared experiences.

In addition to the physical and mental benefits mentioned above, there are a variety of other benefits of yoga for Veterans. These include:

• **Improved focus and concentration:** Yoga involves a focus on mindfulness and awareness, which can help improve overall focus and concentration. This can be particularly beneficial for Veterans who may be struggling with symptoms of PTSD or other mental health issues.

• **Reduced blood pressure and heart rate:** Yoga has been shown to be an effective way to reduce blood pressure and heart rate, which can help improve overall cardiovascular health.

• **Improved digestion:** Yoga has been shown to improve overall digestion and reduce symptoms of gastrointestinal disorders.

• **Improved respiratory function:** The breathing exercises involved in yoga can help improve overall respiratory function and reduce symptoms of respiratory disorders.

• **Improved immune function:** Yoga has been shown to be an effective way to boost overall immune function, which can help reduce the risk of infections and other health issues.

• **Improved self-confidence:** Yoga involves a focus on self-awareness and self-improvement, which can help improve overall self-confidence and self-esteem.

• **Improved overall quality of life:** The practice of yoga can help improve overall quality of life by reducing stress, improving physical health and promoting overall wellness and happiness.

It's important to note that while yoga can offer a range of benefits for Veterans, it's not a substitute for conventional medical treatments. It's important to consult with a healthcare professional before starting a yoga practice to ensure it's safe and appropriate for your individual health needs.

Bottom Line

The practice of yoga can offer a range of physical and mental health benefits for Veterans, including reduced stress and anxiety, improved physical fitness, improved sleep, pain relief, improved mood, increased self-awareness and improved social connections. With its accessibility and adaptability to individual needs, yoga can be a powerful tool for promoting overall wellness and improving quality of life.

- Z -

Zinc

Zinc is an essential mineral that is important for many functions in the human body. It plays a role in many important processes including immune function, wound healing, DNA synthesis, and hormone regulation.

One of the main health benefits of zinc is its role in supporting the immune system. Zinc helps the body produce white blood cells, which are essential for fighting infections. It also helps to regulate the production of cytokines, which are chemical messengers involved in the immune response. In addition, zinc has been shown to reduce the severity and duration of colds and other infections, making it a popular supplement for people looking to support their immune system.

Another key benefit of zinc is its role in wound healing. Zinc is necessary for the formation of new tissue and the maintenance of healthy skin. It also plays a role in the production of collagen, which is an important protein that provides structure to the skin and other tissues. This makes zinc a valuable nutrient for people looking to promote wound healing and maintain healthy skin.

Zinc is also important for proper brain function. It is involved in the production of neurotransmitters, which are chemicals that transmit signals between neurons in the brain. Low levels of zinc have been linked to neurological disorders such as depression and ADHD, and some research suggests that supplementing with zinc may help improve symptoms in some individuals.

In addition to its role in brain function, zinc is also important for hormonal balance. It is involved in the production of testosterone, which is important for both male and female reproductive health and in the regulation of insulin, which is essential for maintaining healthy blood sugar levels. Low levels of zinc have been linked to infertility, type 2 diabetes and other hormonal imbalances.
Zinc is also important for healthy pregnancy and fetal development. It plays a role in the production of hormones that regulate the menstrual cycle and is involved in the development of the fetus, including the formation of the brain and nervous system. Pregnant women are therefore advised to consume adequate amounts of zinc in their diets.

Zinc can be found in a variety of food sources, including oysters, beef, chicken, beans, nuts and dairy products. It can also be taken as a dietary supplement in the form of a pill or lozenge. The recommended daily intake of zinc varies based on age and gender, but most adults are advised to consume between 8 and 11 milligrams per day.

Bottom Line
Zinc is an important mineral with numerous health benefits. It is involved in immune function, wound healing, brain function, hormone regulation and fetal development, among other processes. Consuming adequate amounts of zinc through food or supplementation can help support overall health and well-being.

Zoonosis

Zoonosis, also known as zoonotic disease is a condition that can be transmitted from animals to humans. The term zoonosis comes from the Greek word "zoon" meaning animal and "nosis" meaning condition or disease. Zoonoses are caused by various microorganisms such as viruses, bacteria, parasites and fungi that exist naturally in animals but can infect humans under certain conditions.

Zoonotic diseases are a major public health concern, as they can cause significant illness, disability and death in both animals and humans. The World Health Organization (WHO) estimates that more than 60% of all infectious diseases in humans are zoonotic in origin and that 75% of emerging infectious diseases are zoonotic.

There are many factors that contribute to the transmission of zoonotic diseases from animals to humans. One of the main factors is the close contact between animals and humans, such as through animal bites or scratches, inhalation of animal dander or secretions or consumption of contaminated animal products. The nature of the disease, the susceptibility of both the animal host and the human host and the environment also play a role in the transmission of zoonotic diseases.

There are several examples of zoonotic diseases that have had significant impacts on human health, including:

  • *Rabies:* Rabies is a viral disease that is transmitted through the saliva of infected animals, such as dogs, bats and foxes. The virus can cause severe inflammation of the brain and spinal cord in humans and is almost always fatal if not treated promptly.

  • *Lyme disease:* Lyme disease is caused by the bacterium Borrelia burgdorferi in North America, which is transmitted to humans through the bite of infected black-legged ticks. The disease can cause a range of symptoms, including fever, headache and fatigue and can lead to long-term health problems if left untreated.
  • *Avian influenza:* Avian influenza, also known as bird flu, is a viral disease that can infect domesticated and wild birds, as well as humans. The virus is trans-

mitted from birds to humans through direct contact with infected birds or their secretions or through consumption of contaminated poultry products.

• ***Ebola Hemorrhagic Fever:*** Ebola is a viral disease that is transmitted from wild animals, such as bats and monkeys, to humans. The virus causes severe fever, bleeding and organ failure and has a high mortality rate. The 2014-2016 outbreak of Ebola in West Africa was the largest and most complex outbreak of the disease to date.

To reduce the risk of zoonotic disease transmission, it is important to maintain good animal health, implement appropriate bio-security measures and maintain good hygiene practices. For example, washing hands thoroughly with soap and water after handling animals or animal products can help prevent the spread of zoonotic diseases. Additionally, educating the public about the risks associated with zoonotic diseases and promoting responsible animal husbandry practices can also help reduce the risk of transmission.

Bottom Line

Zoonoses are a significant public health concern and understanding the factors that contribute to their transmission is critical for preventing and controlling the spread of these diseases. By working together, governments, public health agencies and the animal health sector can help to protect both animal and human health and reduce the impact of zoonotic diseases on public health.

- ANNEXES -

Annex A - Daily Activities for Surviving and Progressing with PTSD

- Get Quality Sleep: Prioritize 7-9 hours of restful sleep; use sleep monitors if possible to track patterns.
- Set Intentions for the Day: Begin with a clear purpose or goal to stay focused and grounded.
- Morning Meditation (5-10 mins): Center your mind with mindfulness or breathing exercises.
- Wake Up the Body: Stretch or perform light mobility movements to activate muscles and joints.
- Hydrate Immediately: Drink a full glass of water upon waking to rehydrate and jumpstart metabolism.
- Coconut Oil Pulling (5-10 mins): Swish coconut oil in your mouth to support oral and overall health.
- Nasal Saline Flush: Clear nasal passages to improve breathing and reduce inflammation.
- Morning Journaling: Reflect on thoughts, feelings, and intentions to release mental clutter.
- Eat Protein-Rich Breakfast: Fuel your body with protein to stabilize energy and mood.
- Warm-Up Routine: Engage in light movement to prepare for physical activity.
- Daily Workout: Complete a structured exercise session (strength, cardio, or flexibility).
- Walk Outside (10-30 mins): Get sunlight exposure and fresh air to regulate mood and circadian rhythm.
- Sauna Session (if available): Use heat therapy to reduce stress and relax muscles.
- Cold Plunge or Cold Shower: Stimulate circulation and build mental resilience.
- Periodic Movement Breaks: Incorporate light stretching or quick exercises every 1-2 hours.
- Consistent Hydration: Drink water steadily throughout the day to support physical and mental function.
- Balanced Meals: Focus on whole foods—lean proteins, healthy fats, and complex carbs.
- Mindful Breathing Breaks: Pause for deep breathing exercises to calm the nervous system.
- Evening Reflection: Journal or reflect on progress, challenges, and wins of the day.
- Digital Detox (1 hour before bed): Avoid screens to improve sleep quality.
- Nighttime Routine: Engage in calming activities (reading, stretching) to wind down.
- Consistent Bedtime: Go to bed at the same time each night to regulate sleep cycles.

Consistency with these practices fosters resilience, healing, and daily progress.

Annex B – Veterans Physical and Mental Health Considerations

Veterans face numerous physical and mental health considerations upon their return from service. As a result of their service, Veterans may suffer from a range of physical ailments, from chronic pain conditions to musculoskeletal injuries, as well as mental health issues, such as post-traumatic stress disorder, depression or anxiety. Understanding the range of issues and how to care for them is crucial in helping Veterans transition to civilian life. Additionally, providing meaningful support to Veterans, such as through therapy or peer support groups, can help them cope with the physical and mental health considerations that come with serving in the military. By offering comprehensive treatments and support, we can ensure Veterans are properly taken care of and given the opportunity to succeed in life after their service ends.

Physical health considerations for Veterans

For Veterans, physical health considerations are often a mixture of common conditions and injuries resulting from their service. Physical health considerations may include musculoskeletal injuries, chronic pain conditions, cardiovascular diseases, respiratory conditions, gastrointestinal disorders and infectious diseases. Chronic pain conditions and musculoskeletal injuries are among the most common physical health considerations for Veterans, with approximately half of all Veterans reporting experiencing one or both. Chronic pain conditions are characterized by pain that lasts longer than three to six months, while musculoskeletal injuries occur when the muscles, bones or connective tissue are damaged due to overexertion or injury. While physical ailments may seem manageable compared to the mental health considerations that many Veterans struggle with, they still have a significant impact on the lives of Veterans and their families. Physical health considerations require regular care and monitoring, which can be difficult for Veterans due to the high prevalence of mental health issues among Veterans.

Exercise is an important part of any healthy lifestyle and Veterans should consider participating in activities that are tailored to their physical abilities and mobility restrictions. Low-impact activities like yoga, tai chi or swimming can help strengthen muscles, improve cardiovascular health and reduce stress. Working with a physical therapist or personal trainer can provide Veterans with guidance and support in designing an effective exercise program.

Nutrition is an essential part of any physical health plan. Eating a balanced diet that is low in sugar, saturated fat and processed foods and high in fresh fruits, vegetables and lean proteins can help Veterans maintain a healthy weight, improve physical and mental energy and even reduce the severity of chronic pain. Working with a nutritionist or dietician can help Veterans create a plan for meeting their individual health needs.

Veterans should focus on getting enough rest and relaxation. Sleep is essential for both physical and mental health and Veterans may need to adjust their sleep schedules in order to get enough restful sleep. Stress management techniques like deep breathing, progressive muscle relaxation and meditation can help Veterans reduce stress, improve focus and manage chronic pain and other physical conditions.

By making lifestyle changes, Veterans can greatly improve their physical health and well-being. Eating a balanced diet, engaging in regular physical activity and incorporating stress management techniques can all help Veterans maximize their physical health results.

Mental health considerations for Veterans

When considering the mental health considerations for Veterans, it is important to keep in mind the nature of the work they performed during service. While everyone in the military may not experience combat, the majority of mental health issues arise from the trauma and stress of being in a war zone. The leading mental health considerations for Veterans are post-traumatic stress disorder, depression and anxiety. PTSD is the most common mental health consideration for Veterans: 29% of Veterans report PTSD and more than 50% report experiencing a traumatic event during service. Depression and anxiety, while common mental health considerations among Veterans, are much less prevalent than PTSD. One to 2% of Veterans report depression and 5% report anxiety. Although mental health considerations may not be as prevalent as physical health considerations, they are still very much present and can have a significant impact on the lives of Veterans.

Veterans often face difficult mental health issues due to the trauma experienced during their service. It is essential to ensure that Veterans receive the necessary support they need, in order to not only improve their mental health but also their overall well-being.

Find Professional Support

One of the best ways to maximize mental health is to find professional support. This can mean seeking therapy or counseling services from a licensed mental health professional, as well as support groups, online communities and other forms of assistance. Professional support can provide Veterans with the guidance and understanding they need to process their experiences and move forward.

Take Time for Self-Care

Self-care is an important part of the recovery process for many Veterans. Taking time to relax, reflect and engage in activities that bring joy can help to reduce stress and improve mental health. Some ideas for self-care activities include journaling, art, yoga, meditation, music and nature walks.

Share Experiences with Others
Talking about experiences with other Veterans or people who have gone through similar situations can help to normalize experiences and reduce feelings of isolation. This can be done through support groups, online forums or even just speaking with friends and family. Sharing experiences can help to bring about a sense of catharsis for Veterans, allowing them to process their emotions and move forward.

Seek Help for Mental Health Struggles
When mental health struggles become more severe, it is important to take action and seek help. This can be done by speaking to a mental health professional, seeking out local resources or even engaging in therapy. Regardless of the approach taken, it is important to remember that there are resources available and support available for Veterans struggling with mental health issues.

By considering these mental health considerations, Veterans can take steps to maximize their mental health and well-being. With the proper support and resources, Veterans can take charge of their mental health and continue to thrive.

Causes of physical and mental health issues in Veterans
Physical health issues among Veterans are often due to the unique nature of the work they performed in service. For example, musculoskeletal injuries can occur from lifting gear or performing tasks like climbing stairs, while chronic pain conditions can result from the strain of long hours of work or exposure to environmental hazards, such as heat or cold, radiation or chemicals. Psychological issues can result from the stress of being in a war zone, as well as the difficulty of re-assimilating into society after service ends. For example, re-adjusting to civilian life after service can be particularly difficult for Veterans because they often face significant delays in receiving benefits and care from the VA.

Treatments for physical and mental health considerations in Veterans
Physical health considerations require a combination of treatments, including lifestyle changes and self-care, as well as medical care to address underlying causes. Veterans should start with self-care, like eating a healthy diet and getting enough sleep and a consistent exercise routine. Medical care should include any necessary screenings or tests and treatments, such as physical therapy, medication or massage therapy, as appropriate. Veterans may also consider alternative treatments, such as acupuncture, which may help alleviate pain or stress. Physical health considerations can also be eased through support, both from loved ones and social networks and through services provided by the government. For example, Veterans may be eligible for benefits, such as Medicare or Medicaid, to help cover medical expenses. The VA also provides a range of mental health services and supports, such as therapy and medication, for Veterans in need.

Strategies to support Veterans with physical and mental health considerations

Physical health considerations can be eased through support, such as helping Veterans find medical care and taking care of themselves through healthy eating and exercise. For mental health considerations, support can be offered both in person and online to help Veterans cope with their issues. In person, support can come in the form of one-on-one therapy or group therapy, such as peer support groups. Online support can take the form of email exchanges, forums or social media, such as Facebook or Instagram, where Veterans can discuss their issues with peers. Veterans may also find value in self-help books, like The PTSD Workbook for Self-Help or The Anxiety and Phobia Workbook. These books can help Veterans better understand their issues, find ways to cope and talk about their mental health considerations with others. Self-help books can also be used as part of group therapy, with Veterans reading and discussing the books together.

PTSD or post-traumatic stress disorder, is a mental health disorder that can cause flashbacks, nightmares, extreme anxiety and other symptoms. The PTSD Workbook is a tool that can help Veterans manage the symptoms of PTSD. It includes exercises, tips and activities that can help Veterans and their loved ones cope with the effects of PTSD. The Workbook also provides tips on how to communicate with friends and family, how to deal with stress and how to seek help if needed. Additionally, the Workbook gives advice on how to adjust to life after service and how to stay connected to other Veterans. The PTSD Workbook can be a valuable resource for Veterans and their families who are experiencing PTSD and its associated symptoms.

The Anxiety and Phobia Workbook by Edmund J. Bourne is an excellent resource for Veterans suffering from anxiety and phobic disorders. This workbook provides a comprehensive overview of the causes and treatments of anxiety, as well as step-by-step instructions and exercises to help Veterans identify and address the root causes of their anxiety. The workbook also covers topics such as relaxation techniques, cognitive-behavioral therapy and medication. In addition, the workbook provides case studies and tips for dealing with common triggers such as crowds and social situations. This workbook is an excellent resource for Veterans looking to take charge of their anxiety and phobic disorders and create meaningful change in their lives.

Examples of peer support groups and therapies for Veterans

Therapies for mental health considerations among Veterans may include traditional talk therapies, relaxation therapies and creative therapies. Traditional talk therapies, such as cognitive behavioral therapy, aim to help Veterans understand the root of their issues and learn techniques to manage them. Relaxation therapies, such as mindfulness and meditation, can help Veterans reduce their stress and anxiety by teaching them techniques to slow down and focus on their breath. Creative therapies, such as art therapy and music therapy, can help Veterans process their issues and express themselves through their art or music. Other types of therapies and support include yoga, acupuncture and massage therapy.

There are numerous Veteran support foundations and charities that provide essential services to Veterans and their families. Many of them are listed with their contact information in *Annex D—Organizations Supporting Veterans*.

Benefits of providing meaningful support to Veterans

Offering meaningful support to Veterans, especially those with physical and mental health considerations, can greatly ease their transition to civilian life. By helping Veterans manage their health issues, we can prevent them from turning to more drastic measures, such as suicide. Providing meaningful support can also positively impact the lives of Veterans and their families and friends. By easing the transition for Veterans, we can help them succeed in the jobs and schools they are pursuing after service ends. Supporting Veterans can also help us learn more about their experiences and be better prepared to help future generations of Veterans.

Supporting Veterans is an incredibly meaningful way to give back to those who have sacrificed much to serve their country. Examples of meaningful support include providing mental health resources, offering career training and placement services and providing financial assistance.

Many organizations offer programs to help Veterans in need get back on their feet. These initiatives often provide financial assistance to cover basic needs such as housing, food and transportation. Other programs offer vocational training and job placement services to help Veterans reintegrate into civilian life. Additionally, many organizations provide mental health resources to Veterans suffering from post-traumatic stress disorder, depression and anxiety.

In addition to the tangible support Veterans receive through organizations, they also benefit from the support of their community. People can offer Veterans meaningful support through simple acts of kindness, such as offering a listening ear, providing transportation or connecting Veterans to resources in their area.

At the end of the day, the most meaningful support Veterans can receive is recognition and appreciation for their service. This recognition can come in many forms, including hosting a barbecue to celebrate Veterans, inviting them to speak at local schools or simply saying, "Thank you."

The importance of understanding Veterans physical and mental health considerations

Physical and mental health considerations are often specific to an individual Veteran and their experience. Therefore, it is important to understand each Veteran's health issues and their approach to managing them. Understanding each Veteran's needs allows us to better support them by providing the right care at the right time. Providing proper care can, in turn, help Veterans achieve their goals, live healthier and happier lives and avoid drastic measures, such as suicide.

Veterans often face physical and mental health issues that can be difficult to understand and manage. While there is no one-size-fits-all solution, there are steps that can be taken to better understand and support Veterans' physical and mental health needs.

To begin with, it is important to recognize the unique experiences that Veterans have gone through. This can include how they were affected by their deployment and/or service in combat, as well as any other experiences that they may have had while in the military. It is important to take the time to talk to Veterans and listen to their stories, rather than making assumptions about their experiences.

It is also important to remember that different Veterans may have different needs. Some Veterans may need more traditional forms of therapy, such as one-on-one counseling or group therapy. Others may find talk therapy to be less effective and instead might benefit from activities that can help them to express themselves in a creative or physical way, like art therapy, yoga or mindfulness meditation.

It is important to be aware of the resources that are available to Veterans. This can range from healthcare benefits, to support groups, to job training and education. Taking the time to research these resources and make sure that Veterans are aware of them can go a long way in helping to ensure that they get the support they need. In summary, understanding and supporting Veterans' physical and mental health needs requires that we recognize the unique experiences they have gone through, be aware of their individual needs and make sure they are aware of the resources that are available to them. By taking these steps, we can better ensure that Veterans get the support they need to lead healthy and successful lives.

The role of healthcare providers in helping Veterans

Healthcare providers, such as doctors, nurses and psychologists, play a key role in helping Veterans with their physical and mental health considerations. Healthcare providers can help Veterans receive the proper care they need and understand their health issues by asking appropriate questions and providing resources.

Healthcare providers can also help Veterans find support groups and self-help books to help them cope with their issues.

Healthcare providers aim to help Veterans in a variety of ways, including providing mental health services, physical therapy and connecting them with resources and support networks. Mental health services can include cognitive behavioral therapy, trauma-focused therapy and psychotherapy to help Veterans process their experiences and cope with the symptoms of post-traumatic stress disorder, depression and anxiety. Physical therapy is important for helping Veterans who have experienced physical trauma and may include core strengthening and balance exercises, as well as activities to help improve mobility. Additionally, healthcare providers help Veterans connect with resources, such as support groups, housing and job opportunities. Connecting Veterans with these resources can be invaluable in helping them to re-integrate into civilian life.

Resources for Veterans and their families

Veterans and their families can find help and support through a number of organizations and resources. The Department of Veterans Affairs (VA) provides Veterans and their families with the resources and benefits they need, including healthcare services, mental health services, and benefits, like disability pay.

Main Info Line: (800) 698-2411

VA Benefits Hotline: (800) 827-1000

VA Health Benefits Hotline: (877) 222-8387

My HealtheVet help desk: (877) 327-0022

The VA also maintains a website with information about Veterans, their health issues and how to access their benefits, as well as a blog with articles about Veterans' experiences.

https://www.va.gov/

The VA also provides resources for loved ones and friends of Veterans, who can face similar challenges as Veterans, such as a lack of resources to help them better understand Veterans' health issues and support their loved ones.

https://www.nrd.gov/Family-Caregiver-Support

Various programs offer assistance for spouses of active-duty military personnel. Consider the following:

Military Spouse Education Career Opportunities (SECO) program:

https://myseco.militaryonesource.mil/portal/

Military Spouse Employment Partnership (MSEP):
https://msepjobs.militaryonesource.mil/msep/

My Career Advancement Account (MyCAA) scholarship program:
https://mycaa.militaryonesource.mil/mycaa/

Military Spouse eMentor Program:
https://www.ementorprogram.org/

Military Spouse Fellowship Program:
https://www.hiringourheroes.org/career-services/fellowships/internships/msfp/

The Department of Veterans Affairs (VA) Housing and Homelessness VASH Program combines Housing Choice Voucher rental assistance for homeless Veterans with case management and clinical services:
https://www.va.gov/homeless/hud-vash.asp

Supportive Services for Veteran Families (SSVF) grant program, "For very low-income Veterans, SSVF provides case management and supportive services to prevent the imminent loss of a Veteran's home or identify a new, more suitable housing situation for the individual and his or her family.":
https://www.va.gov/homeless/ssvf/index.html

AMVETS National Service Foundation provides Veterans, their families and survivors world-class counsel and representation before the US Department of Veterans Affairs (VA) at no charge to the Veteran or family.
https://amvetsnsf.org/   (800) 810-7148

National Veterans Foundation serves the crisis management, information and referral needs of all US Veterans and their families through management and operation of the nation's first Vet-to-Vet toll-free helpline for all Veterans and their families. It also provides outreach services that provide Veterans and families in need with food, clothing, transportation, employment and other essential resources.

https://nvf.org and Lifeline for Vets: (888) 777-4433

National Coalition for Homeless Veterans Stand Downs:
https://nchv.org/serviceproviders/stand-down/

VA Employment Programs for Homeless Veterans:
https://www.va.gov/HOMELESS/employment.asp

US Department of Labor, American Job Centers,
https://www.dol.gov/general/topic/training/Veterans

National Veterans Foundation Job Board,
https://jobs.nvf.org/

Work for Warriors (Guard and Reserve),
https://workforwarriors.org/
Small Business (SBA Veteran & Disabled Veterans)
https://www.sba.gov/business-guide/grow-your-business/
Veteran-owned-businesses

Health resources include VA hospitals and clinics:
https://www.va.gov/find-locations/

VA Veteran Readiness and Employment (VR&E)
(formerly known as Vocational Rehabilitation and Employment):
https://www.benefits.va.gov/vocrehab/index.asp

Annex C – Merging Veterans and Players (MVP)

Merging Veterans and players organizations refers to the process of combining two separate organizations, both serving Veterans or players in a specific industry or sport, into a single entity. This can involve bringing together the resources, expertise and memberships of both organizations to create a more efficient and effective organization.

The reasons for merging Veterans and players organizations can vary, but often include a desire to increase visibility and impact, achieve economies of scale or consolidate resources and expertise. The merger may also serve to bring together different groups of Veterans or players, who may have different needs or experiences and create a more unified and representative voice for the community as a whole.

The process of merging organizations can be complex and requires careful planning and coordination. This can include conducting assessments of the organizations' strengths and weaknesses, establishing clear goals and objectives for the merger and developing a detailed plan for the integration of staff, resources and programs.

In order for a merger to be successful, it is essential that the leadership and members of both organizations be fully committed to the process and see the benefits of the merger for their communities. This may involve addressing any concerns or reservations about the merger and ensuring that the needs and interests of all stakeholders are taken into account.

If successfully executed, a merger of Veterans and players organizations can result in a more unified and effective organization, better able to serve the needs of its members and achieve its mission. This can lead to increased impact, greater visibility and improved support for Veterans or players in the industry or sport.

MVP's mission

MVP empowers combat Veterans and former professional athletes by connecting them after the uniform comes off; providing them with a new team to assist with transition, promoting personal development and showing them they are never alone.

Nate Boyer is a former NFL player and Green Beret Veteran and co-founder of the MVP (Merging Veterans & Players) organization. He has spoken on numerous occasions about the importance of MVP and its mission to bring together Veterans and athletes to support one another and create positive change in their communities.

"MVP was born out of the idea that Veterans and athletes have a unique ability to inspire and impact change in the world."

"Athletes and Veterans have a lot in common. They both understand what it means to serve something greater than themselves and they both know the value of teamwork and sacrifice."

"MVP is about bridging the gap between two groups that have a lot to offer each other. By working together, we can create a more unified and impactful voice for positive change."

"Through MVP, we aim to provide Veterans and athletes with the tools and resources they need to make a difference in their communities and beyond."

"MVP is not just about giving back, it's about creating meaningful and lasting change. By coming together and sharing our unique experiences and perspectives, we can make a real impact in the world."

Randy Couture is a retired mixed martial artist and Veteran who is also a co-founder of the MVP (Merging Veterans & Players) organization. He has spoken on numerous occasions about the importance of MVP and its mission to bring together Veterans and athletes to support one another and create positive change in their communities.

"MVP is about bringing together two groups of people who have a lot in common - Veterans and athletes. By working together, we can create a powerful voice for positive change."

"The unique experiences and perspectives of Veterans and athletes can be a powerful force for good. MVP provides a platform for these two groups to come together and support each other in their efforts to make a difference."

"MVP is not just about giving back, it's about creating lasting change. By bringing together the skills, resources and passion of Veterans and athletes, we can make a real impact in our communities and beyond."

"Through MVP, we hope to provide Veterans and athletes with the support and resources they need to succeed in their efforts to create positive change. This includes everything from financial support to mentorship and training."

"MVP is about breaking down barriers and building bridges. By working together, Veterans and athletes can make a positive impact in the world and help create a better future for everyone."

These quotes showcase Randy Couture's commitment to MVP and its mission to bring together Veterans and athletes to create positive change. By working together, MVP seeks to provide Veterans and athletes with the support and resources they need to succeed in their efforts to make a difference in their communities and beyond.

Jay Glazer, an NFL analyst, writer and commentator, is also a co-founder of the MVP (Merging Veterans & Players) organization. He has spoken on numerous occasions about the importance of MVP and its mission to bring together Veterans and athletes to support one another and create positive change in their communities.

Here are a few quotes from Jay Glazer regarding MVP

"MVP was created with the belief that Veterans and athletes have a unique opportunity to make a positive impact in the world. By coming together and sharing their skills, resources and experiences, we can create real change."

"Athletes and Veterans have a lot in common. They both understand the value of hard work, sacrifice and serving something greater than themselves. MVP provides a platform for these two groups to come together and support each other in their efforts to make a difference."

"MVP is about breaking down barriers and building bridges. By working together, Veterans and athletes can overcome any obstacle and create a better future for everyone."

"Through MVP, we hope to provide Veterans and athletes with the support and resources they need to succeed in their efforts to create positive change. This includes everything from financial support to mentorship and training."

"MVP is about creating a unified voice for positive change. By bringing together Veterans and athletes, we can make a real impact in the world and help create a better future for everyone."

These quotes showcase Jay Glazer's commitment to MVP and its mission to bring together Veterans and athletes to create positive change. By working together, MVP seeks to provide Veterans and athletes with the support and resources they need to succeed in their efforts to make a difference in their communities and beyond.

To donate to MVP, go to
https://vetsandplayers.org/

Annex D – Organizations Supporting Veterans

The Randy Couture Xtreme Couture GI Foundation:
https://www.xcgif.org/
phone: (702) 616-1022
email: operations@xcgif.org

Hope for the Warriors:
https://www.hopeforthewarriors.org/
phone: (877) 246-7349
email: info@hopeforthewarriors.org

Iraq and Afghanistan Veterans of America (IAVA):
https://iava.org/
phone: QRF (855) 91RAPID [917-2743]; HQ (212) 982-9699;
Wash DC (202) 544-7692
email: info@iava.org

United Service Organizations (USO):
https://www.uso.org/
phone: +1 (888) 484-3876

Navy-Marine Corps Relief Society:
https://www.nmcrs.org/
phone: HQ (800) 654-8364
email: officeadmin@nmcrs.org

Wounded Warriors Family Support:
https://wwfs.org/
phone: Program Office (402) 932-7036; Main Office (402) 502-7557

K9s for Warriors:
https://k9sforwarriors.org/
phone: 1-888-819-0112; (904) 686-1956
email: info@k9sforwarriors.org

Semper Fi & America's Fund:
https://thefund.org/

phone: (760) 725-3680

The Fisher House Foundation:
    https://fisherhouse.org/
    phone: (888) 294-8560
    email: info@fisherhouse.org

Homes For Our Troops (HFOT):
    https://www.hfotusa.org/
    phone: (866) 787-6677
    email: info@hfotusa.org

Tragedy Assistance Program for Survivors (TAPS):
    https://www.taps.org/
    phone: (24/7) (800) 959-8277

Operation Homefront:
    https://operationhomefront.org/
    phone: 1(877) 264-3968
    email: info@operationhomefront.org

Operation Gratitude:
    https://www.operationgratitude.com/
    phone: (818) 960-7878
    email: info@operationgratitude.com

Great Aloha Run:
    https://greataloharun.com/
    phone: (808) 528-7388

These charities are rated highly by Charity Navigator and other watchdog organizations for their efficient use of funds, with at least 75 percent of donations going on programs. To find the best wounded Veterans charities, users should consult Charity Navigator, which rates charities based on their financial health and impact.

https://www.charitynavigator.org/

The Green Beret Foundation   https://greenberetfoundation.org/

GBF is a non-profit organization dedicated to providing direct and ongoing support to United States Army Special Forces (Green Berets) and their families. GBF provides a variety of services and resources to assist Green Berets and their families in the areas of transition, tragedy and triumph. These services range from providing financial support, to supplying medical and mental health care, to connecting Green Berets with job placement opportunities. GBF also provides mentorship and educational opportunities for Green Berets and their families, helping them to succeed in the civilian world. Additionally, GBF provides support for deceased and wounded Green Berets and their families. The organization's mission is to ensure that every Green Beret and their families are taken care of, both during their service and after they have retired.

The SEAL Foundation   https://www.navysealfoundation.org/

SF is a non-profit organization that works to empower Veterans and their families by providing them with the resources they need to rebuild their lives. Through programs that focus on physical and emotional well-being, the SEAL Foundation seeks to provide Veterans and their families with the support they need to live healthy, productive lives. The organization works to provide services such as counseling, education, job training and employment assistance. Additionally, SEAL Foundation advocates for Veterans rights, ensuring that they are able to access the benefits and services they have earned through their service to the country. Through their work, the SEAL Foundation strives to ensure that all Veterans and their families can lead happy, successful lives.

The Randy Couture GI Foundation   https://www.xcgif.org/

Established to honor and assist Veterans of the United States armed forces who have served in Iraq and Afghanistan, Randy's organization works to support and empower Veterans and their families through programs that focus on health and wellness, education, housing and employment. The foundation provides financial assistance, educational support and job placement services for Veterans. It also works to raise awareness of Veteran issues and to advocate for Veterans' rights. The foundation also hosts events throughout the year to recognize and celebrate the service and sacrifices of Veterans.

The Warrior2Warrior Foundation

W2W is a 501(c)3 non-profit organization dedicated to honoring, empowering and supporting Veterans of the United States Armed Forces. The Foundation's mission is to provide Veterans the necessary tools and resources to succeed in their post-service life. This includes assisting them in the areas of employment, housing, education, counseling, addiction treatment, healthcare and more.

The Foundation works to bridge the gap between civilian and military life by providing financial assistance and support to Veterans in need. They provide comprehensive employment services which include career counseling, job search assistance, professional resume writing and career development workshops. Additionally, the Foundation offers free housing assistance, helping Veterans to locate and secure housing options. They also provide educational assistance, helping Veterans to pursue higher education goals and develop new skills.

The Foundation works to ensure that Veterans have access to quality healthcare and mental health services. They offer counseling and addiction treatment for those struggling with substance abuse issues. They also provide financial assistance to help Veterans with medical and mental health care expenses.

The Warrior2Warrior Foundation is dedicated to fighting for the rights and benefits of Veterans and advocating for their needs. They work to build awareness of the issues Veterans face and to ensure that they have access to the support they need.
   http://www.facebook.com/Warrior2Warrior-Foundation-501866326643380/

Why you should donate to organizations that support Veterans

There are several reasons why someone should consider donating to organizations that support Veterans, including:

   • *Supporting those who have served the country:* Veterans have made sacrifices and put their lives on the line to serve their country and protect our freedoms. Supporting organizations that assist Veterans is a way to give back to those who have given so much.

   • *Improving the well-being of Veterans:* Many Veterans face physical, mental and financial challenges after returning from service. Organizations that support Veterans can help improve their quality of life by providing resources and support.

   • *Providing necessary services:* Some Veterans may need assistance accessing healthcare, finding employment or dealing with post-traumatic stress. Organizations that support Veterans can help fill gaps in government support and provide services that are critical to their well-being.

   • *Promoting community engagement:* When organizations support Veterans, they can also help foster a sense of community among those who have served. This can lead to increased social engagement and a sense of belonging for Veterans.

Annex E – Alternative Approaches

Aqua Chi

A device that uses low-frequency electrical currents to promote health and wellness, Aqua Chi works by delivering a low-level electrical current to the body, which is thought to stimulate the production of positive ions and improve circulation. Aqua Chi is marketed as a holistic health device that can help to boost energy levels, reduce stress and anxiety, improve sleep and alleviate pain.

One of the key benefits of Aqua Chi is its non-invasive nature. Unlike some other medical treatments, Aqua Chi does not require any needles or incisions and there are no associated side effects. This makes it an attractive option for people who are looking for a natural or less-invasive way to improve their health and well-being. Additionally, Aqua Chi is relatively inexpensive compared to some other alternative health treatments, making it accessible to a wider range of people.

Another benefit of Aqua Chi is its versatility. The device can be used to address a wide range of health concerns, from stress and anxiety to chronic pain and sleep issues. This makes it a versatile device that can be used to address multiple health concerns, rather than just one specific issue. In some cases, users have reported significant improvements in their symptoms after using Aqua Chi, although more research is needed to confirm these results.

There is some scientific evidence to support the effectiveness of Aqua Chi. Studies have shown that low-frequency electrical currents can have a positive effect on the body by improving circulation and reducing inflammation. Additionally, some research suggests that these electrical currents can help to balance the body's energy levels and promote a sense of well-being. However, these studies are still in their early stages and more research is needed to fully understand the mechanisms behind Aqua Chi and its effects on the body.

Despite these benefits, there are some potential risks associated with Aqua Chi. For example, the device has not been approved by regulatory agencies such as the Food and Drug Administration (FDA) or the European Medicines Agency (EMA). This means that there is limited oversight of the device and its safety and effectiveness have not been rigorously tested. Additionally, the use of Aqua Chi should not be seen as a substitute for conventional medical treatment and users should consult a healthcare professional before using the device.

Bottom Line
Aqua Chi is a device that uses low-frequency electrical currents to promote health and wellness. The device is marketed as a holistic health device that can help to boost energy levels, reduce stress and anxiety, improve sleep and alleviate pain.

Aqua Chi is non-invasive and relatively inexpensive, making it an attractive option for people looking for a natural or less-invasive way to improve their health and well-being. However, the device has not been approved by regulatory agencies and its safety and effectiveness have not been rigorously tested. Users should consult a healthcare professional before using Aqua Chi and should not use it as a substitute for conventional medical treatment.

Liver and Gallbladder Miracle Cleanse - OVERVIEW

- ***Prepare for the cleanse:*** A few days before starting the cleanse, stop consuming meat, dairy, processed foods, sugar and alcohol.

- ***Take supplements:*** Take supplements such as Epsom salt and herbal supplements such as milk thistle, dandelion root and beet leaf.

- ***Perform the cleanse:*** The cleanse is typically performed over the course of two days and is done as follows:

Day 1:
- Drink 120-150 ml of olive oil mixed with the juice of half a lemon on an empty stomach in the morning. <u>Wait for 20-30 minutes.</u>

- Drink a mixture of Epsom salt and water to help stimulate the release of waste products. <u>Wait 2 hours.</u>

- Drink another mixture of Epsom salt and water. <u>Wait for 2 hours.</u>

- Drink a final mixture of Epsom salt & water. <u>Wait for 2 hours and go to bed.</u>

Day 2:
- In the morning, drink another mixture of olive oil and lemon juice.
        Wait for 20-30 minutes.
- Drink a mixture of Epsom salt and water.
        Wait for 2 hours.
- Drink another mixture of Epsom salt and water.

- ***Post-cleanse diet:*** After the cleanse, avoid consuming meat, dairy, processed foods, sugar and alcohol for a period of time.

After the cleanse, it is recommended to eat a light, vegetarian diet for a few days to give the liver and gallbladder time to rest and recover.

Spooky2 Rife Machine

A device that uses low-frequency electromagnetic waves to treat various medical conditions, the Spooky2 Rife Machine operates on the principles of Royal Raymond Rife, a scientist who developed a machine in the 1930s that allegedly used low-frequency waves to kill pathogens in the body. The Spooky2 Rife Machine is a modern version of Rife's original machine and it is marketed as an alternative medicine device that can treat a wide range of conditions, including cancer, Lyme disease and chronic pain.

The Spooky2 Rife Machine works by generating low-frequency electromagnetic waves that are delivered to the body through hand-held electrodes. The user holds the electrodes while the machine emits the electromagnetic waves. The waves are thought to penetrate the body and interact with the cells and tissues, causing a resonance effect that destroys pathogens and other harmful substances.

One of the key benefits of the Spooky2 Rife Machine is that it is non-invasive and does not involve any drugs or chemicals. This makes it an attractive alternative for people who are looking for a natural or less-invasive way to treat their conditions. Additionally, the Spooky2 Rife Machine is relatively inexpensive compared to traditional medical treatments, making it accessible to a wider range of people.

Another benefit of the Spooky2 Rife Machine is that it can be used to treat a wide range of conditions, including cancer, Lyme disease and chronic pain. This makes it a versatile device that can be used to address multiple health concerns, rather than just one specific issue. In some cases, users have reported significant improvements in their symptoms after using the Spooky2 Rife Machine, although more research is needed to confirm these results.

Studies have shown that low-frequency electromagnetic waves can penetrate the body and interact with cells and tissues. Additionally, some research suggests that these waves can affect the behavior of cells and tissues, potentially leading to a therapeutic effect. However, these studies are still in their early stages and more research is needed to fully understand the mechanisms behind the Spooky2 Rife Machine and its effects on the body.

Bottom Line
The Spooky2 Rife Machine is a device that it is claimed uses low-frequency electromagnetic waves to treat various medical conditions. The device is marketed as an alternative medicine device that can treat a wide range of conditions, including cancer, Lyme disease and chronic pain. There is no scientific research that supports this claim.[29] The Spooky2 Rife Machine is non-invasive and relatively inexpensive, making it an attractive alternative for people looking for a natural or less-invasive way to treat their conditions. However, the device has not been approved by regulatory agencies and its safety and effectiveness have not been rigorously tested. Users should consult a healthcare professional before using the Spooky2 Rife Machine and should not use it as a substitute for conventional medical treatment.

Annex F – The First Steps to Healing

By Jylian Sy
Trauma and Re-Entry Counselor/Consultant

That pain you feel is an indication of need. Refusing to acknowledge your pain will not make it go away. It will not make you stronger or a bigger badass. Instead, it will lead you further and further away from your actual goal--to feel better. You're not alone, all of us humans avoid pain to a certain degree. In baking terms, most civilian humans self-identify as a single or a double layer cake when it comes to pain and trauma. As a Veteran, you're an automatic double digit layer cake. No real surprises here, everything to extremes, right?

Great, you're a double-digit layer cake of pain. What should you do? If you're going to accurately assess your present condition, you'll need to check in with yourself on a variety of levels. The best way to gain some clarity and begin the healing process is to ask yourself some difficult questions. You may not like the answers, but instead of defaulting to your usual stoicism, resistance and combativeness, you'll take your first steps toward self-awareness, understanding and healing.

Take a look at these questions and do your best. If a question seems too big or too difficult, go to the next one.

- Am I in pain physically? Emotionally? What have I been doing about it?
- Is it time to consider seeking professional help? Do I have an idea where to start?
- Have I heard the same advice from people I trust, more than once?
- Have I allowed my anxiety and fears to turn me into a jerk? A bully?
- How honest am I willing to be with myself about my present relationships and behavior?
- Am I isolating myself, trying not to burden others with my pain?
- Am I disappearing and feeling like it would just seem easier to check out?
- How willing am I to "get real" with myself and open up to someone else?
- When was the last time I really slept well?
- Is my anger off the charts? Am I scaring the people I love?
- Do I sometimes "space out" and then "come back" and not know where I am?
- Is it really possible to return to my life as I knew it before?
- If I have to reinvent myself, am I ready to leave some of the old "me" behind?

- Is confusion my usual state of mind?
- Do I feel ashamed to have survived some of the traumatic events of my life?
- Do I deserve to be happy?
- Could it be that my fear of thriving is stopping me from doing just that?
- Post active duty, where do I belong?

Take a deep breath. Let your body settle down a bit. By asking yourself these questions you've begun to paint a more accurate picture of your current mental, emotional and physical condition.

The military has taught you to survive in extremely complicated, painful and violent circumstances. It has not taught you how to recover from them. It has taught you how to be loyal, honorable and respectful. It has not taught you how to grieve or live with long term struggles or feel your life. As time goes on, these lessons will become the foundational elements to understanding who you have become, how you will interact with others from now on and ultimately, what you will need to heal your wounds.

The healing process is not a swift one. It is, in fact, a lifelong learning endeavor. The "you" that you see in the mirror now is a different person than the one that began your military journey. You have had to grow up, forge friendships, adapt to difficult circumstances, acquire advanced skills, endure great pain and loss and somehow, throughout it all, you managed to survive.

"Survival mode" is something you know very well. It is a familiar set of behaviors and a communication style that you have adopted by imitation, memorization, trial and error, by choice and sometimes by necessity. It is *not* a sustainable practice, however. As time has gone on, you have found that your "survival stubbornness" and "go-to" behaviors no longer serve you. You've noticed that feelings of anxiety, confusion and loss have begun to pile up and become more and more difficult to manage effectively. These "pile-ups" may have also created additional layers on your cake in the form of panic attacks, hypervigilance, risky behaviors, overwork, loneliness and depression.

Don't despair, you are not alone. Your pain, while uniquely yours in some ways, is also comparable to the pain experienced by nearly every Veteran on the planet. If you take a moment, step back and review your life's timeline, you will see a certain logic to the biological process of physical and emotional re-entry. To survive, you had to compartmentalize your thoughts and feelings and you got used to it. Now, your body and mind are beginning to allow "the stuff you stuffed" to bubble up to the surface.

Your life didn't go upside down in a day, so chances are, it won't turn right side up again that quickly. But try not to focus on the time element here. Instead, take the first bite out of your layer cake. As daunting as the process may seem, that bite is akin to your first solid step in the right direction, of reclaiming your life. Please don't hide out and suffer alone. Instead, begin to get truly honest with yourself and admit that you need help. Your life is meaningful and valuable and you deserve love and understanding and time to heal.

Things may be complicated right now. Just know that while your feelings and sensations may appear at inopportune times and seem clumsy or messy, they provide important clues to your current level of self-awareness. The fact that you notice them at all indicates that you're already on your way. You're in a unique position, perhaps for the first time in your life, to truly know yourself from the inside out. This is no small thing. By noticing how intense, how often and how important your thoughts, emotions and sensations are to you – as you have them – you'll begin to understand yourself more and more. And as you do this, you'll allow your brain, your heart and your body to literally come back online within you.

Your military experience dictated that you set your personal experience and emotions aside in favor of survival. Once you began to function outside of the daily military mindset, your mind and body eventually began to interact with one another and orient toward healing. Your experience of this phase may consist of a wide variety of symptoms including: night-terrors and sweats, thought loops, memory loss, explosive, excessive or inappropriate emotional responses, substance abuse, relationship difficulties and sensory/body dysfunction, among many others.

The process to "bring you back to center" will be incremental. It will consist of a series of slow and gentle re-training steps designed to bring your brain, body and spirit into a new kind of alignment. And so, while your physical and emotional experience may often seem jumbled, confusing and painful, it is key to note that you are experiencing your feelings. Disparate parts of you are attempting to connect to one another. These are the early steps in the retooling process of the next iteration of you.

Body awareness is an equally necessary component to your healing process. Taking an honest look at physical injuries and limitations, exercise ability, diet, hydration, sleep and work with practitioners in the health and wellness arena will provide valuable information and a clearer understanding of how your body is functioning now. You'll need to begin to "watch how you do you." To pay closer attention to your daily experience and observe your habits and lifestyle as you live them. It's often a good idea to begin this watchful process by "listening" to what your body is telling you. Pain, fatigue, hunger, thirst, sex drive, temperature sensation, allergic reaction, ability to be touched, etc. indicate how your body is reacting to your current circumstances. As you become more sensitive to your body and its messaging, you'll gain the confidence to better communicate your experience with loved ones, friends, health and therapeutic professionals.

There is no easy way to do this, so just agree to a few things at the start. Agree that your life matters. Agree that you deserve to heal. Agree to ask for help when you're ready. Bite into that layer cake a bit more. Try not to get discouraged and begin rating your experience before you think anything has actually changed. Shifts and changes can often be imperceptible in the beginning because they are subtle and deep. Hang in there. Check in with yourself throughout the day and observe what you're thinking and feeling. Ask yourself difficult questions.

You're no stranger to a challenge, so meet your healing process with a new level of honesty and courage and strength. Tap into these qualities and put yourself first for a change. Kick some internal ass--but do it gently and with kindness. You deserve some.

It may seem impossible to imagine now, but as difficult as the steps to healing may feel, they will also bring you great joy, relief, solace, self-understanding and a newfound sense of wholeness. Please don't give up, you are worth every second you can give this process.

Annex G – Further Reading

- *12 Rules for Life: An Antidote to Chaos,* by Jordan B. Peterson
- *8 Weeks to Optimum Health: A Proven Program for Taking Full*
- *A Soldier's Soldier: Never Quit,* by Neysa Holmes PhD
- *Advantage of Your Body's Natural Healing Power,* by Andrew Weil, M.D.
- *American Cartel,* by Scott Higman and Sari Horwitz
- *Awaken the Giant Within: How to Take Immediate Control of Your Mental, Emotional, Physical and Financial Destiny!* by Tony Mark Sloan
- *Complete Guide to Fasting: Heal Your Body Through Intermittent, Alternate-Day and Extended Fasting,* by Dr. Jason Fung and Jimmy Moore
- *Convict Conditioning: How to Bust Free of All Weakness—Using the Lost Secrets of Supreme Survival Strength,* by Paul Wade
- *Crazy Good Living: Healthy Gums, Healthy Gut, Healthy Life,* by Jennifer Bonetto
- *Eat Fat, Get Thin: Why the Fat We Eat Is the Key to Sustained Weight Loss and Vibrant Health,* by Mark Hyman, M.D.
- *Eat Smarter,* by Shawn Stevenson
- *Eat to Beat Your Diet,* by William W. Li, M.D.
- *Fit for Duty, Fit for Life,* by David B. Wright
- *Forever Young,* by Dr. Mark Hyman, M.D.
- *Going Vegan for Beginners: The Essential Nutrition Guide to Transitioning to a Vegan Diet,* by Pamela Fergusson, R.D., Ph.D.
- *How Emotions Work: In Humans and Computers,* by Sean Webb
- *How to Starve Cancer,* by Jane McLelland
- *In Defense of Food: An Eater's Manifesto,* by Michael Pollan
- *Lies My Doctor Told Me: Medical Myths That Can Harm Your Health,* by Ken D. Berry, M.D., FAAFP
- *Liver and Gallbladder Miracle Cleanse: An All-Natural, At-Home Flush to Purify and Rejuvenate Your Body,* by Andreas Moritz
- *Lymph & Longevity,* by Gerald Lemole, M.D.
- *Making the Cut: The 30-Day Diet and Fitness Plan for the Strongest, Sexiest You,* by Jillian Michaels
- *Maps of Meaning: The Architecture of Belief,* by Jordan B. Peterson
- *Master Your Metabolism: The 3 Diet Secrets to Naturally Balancing*

Your Hormones for a Hot and Healthy Body, by Jillian Michaels

- *Men's Work,* by Connor Beaton
- *Mind Hacking Happiness Volume 1*, by Sean Webb
- *Spontaneous Healing: How to Discover and Embrace Your Body's Natural Ability to Maintain and Heal Itself,* by Andrew Weil, M.D.
- *The 4-Hour Body: An Uncommon Guide to Rapid Fat-loss, Incredible Sex and Becoming Superhuman,* by Tim Ferriss
- *The 4-Hour Workweek: Escape 9-5, Live Anywhere and Join the New Rich,* by Tim Ferriss
- *The American Legion Fitness Handbook,* by the American Legion
- *The Anxiety and Phobia Workbook,* by Edmund J. Bourne, Ph.D.
- *The Blood Sugar Solution: The Ultra Healthy Program for Losing Weight, Preventing Disease and Feeling Great Now!* by Mark Hyman, M.D.
- *The Carnivore Diet of Dr. Jordan Peterson and Mikhaila Peterson:* How meat healed their depression, anxiety and diseases: Revised Transcripts and Blogposts Featuring Dr. Shawn Baker, by Rocko Jay Solid
- *The Carnivore Diet,* by Dr. Shawn Baker
- *The Complete Guide to Fitness for Veterans,* by Bill O'Brien
- *The Complete Guide to Nutrition for Veterans,* by Robert G. Price
- *The Complete Guide to Pilates for Veterans*, by Daniel Loigerot and Karine Charbonneau
- *The Complete Guide to Running for Veterans,* by John F. Kennedy
- *The Complete Guide to Service-Disabled Veteran Owned Business,* by Jay DeShaw
- *The Complete Guide to Veterans' Affairs,* by Darlene Cypser
- *The Complete Guide to Veterans' Benefits,* by Bruce C. Brown
- *The Complete Guide to Veterans' Employment,* by Bruce C. Brown
- *The Complete Guide to Veterans' Health,* by Maria Fletcher and Mary Ellen Oliverio
- *The Complete Guide to Women's Health,* by Susan Lark and Karen O'Brien
- *The Complete Guide to Yoga for Veterans,* by Tara Fraser
- *The Essential Guide to Healing Foods,* by Jonny Bowden
- *The Healing Power of Essential Oils,* by Eric Zielinski
- *The Keto Reset Diet: Reboot your Metabolism in 21 Days and Burn Fat Forever,* by Mark Sisson

- *The Military Guide to Financial Independence and Retirement*, by Doug Nordman
- *The Obesity Code – Unlocking the Secrets of Weight Loss,* by Dr. Jason Fung
- *The Omnivore's Dilemma:* A Natural History of Four Meals, by Michael Pollan
- *The Paleo Diet Revised: Lose Weight and Get Healthy by Eating the Foods You Were Designed to Eat,* by Loren Cordain, Ph.D.
- *The Primal Blueprint,* by Mark Sisson
- *The PTSD Solution: The Truth About Your Symptoms and How to Heal,* by Alan Gordon and Alon Ziv
- *The PTSD Workbook for Veterans,* by Mary Beth Williams and Soili Poijula
- *The PTSD Workbook: Simple, Effective Techniques for Overcoming Traumatic Stress Symptoms,* by Mary Bet Williams
- *The Real Mediterranean Diet: A practical guide to understanding and achieving the healthiest diet in the world,* by Dr. Simon Poole
- *The Science of Nutrition,* by Janice Thompson and Melinda Manore
- *The Ultimate Guide to Methylene Blue,* by Mark Sloan
- *The Ultimate Guide to Personal Training for Veterans,* by Jonathan Goodman
- *The Ultimate Guide to Self-Defense for Veterans,* by Martin J. Dougherty
- *The Ultimate Guide to Stretching and Flexibility,* by Brad Walker
- *The Ultimate Guide to the VA Disability Claims Process*, by Chris Attig
- *The Ultimate Guide to VA Disability Claims and Appeals,* by Brad Riley
- *The Ultimate Guide to Weight Training for Veterans,* by Robert G. Price
- *The War on Ivermectin,* by Pierre Kory
- *The Warrior's Guide to the Combat Mindset,* by Dr. Michael Asken
- *The Way of The Iceman: How The Wim Hof Method Creates Radiant, Long Term Health—Using The Science and Secrets of Breath Control, Cold-Training and Commitment,* by Wim Hof, Koen de Jong, et al.
- *The Wim Hof Method: Activate Your Full Human Potential,* by Wim Hof, Elissa Epel, Ph.D., et al.
- *Unlimited Power: The New Science of Personal Achievement,* by Tony Robbins
- *Veteran's Benefits Guidebook,* by Berry Dunster and Tom Philpott
- *Veteran's Guide to Benefits and Services,* by the U.S. Veterans Administra-

tion

- ***Veteran's PTSD Handbook: How to File and Collect on Claims for Post-Traumatic Stress Disorder,*** by John D. Roche
- ***Why We Sleep,*** by Matthew Walker
- ***World Without Cancer,*** by G. Edward Griffin

Annex H – Books I Have Personally Read (Erik Lawrence)

- *Becoming Superhuman*, by Joe Dispenza
- *Blink,* by Malcolm Gladwell
- *Brain Concussion,* by Diane Roberts Stoler and Barbara Albers Hill
- *Changing Body Composition Through Diet and Exercise,*
  by Michael Ormsbee
- *Codependent No More,* by Melody Beattie
- *Codependency: No More,* by Chris S. Jennings
- *Complex PTSD,* by Pete Walker
- *Coffee Dialysis,* by Mark Buse, BSC, CT, CWR
- *Concussion Repair Manual,* by Dr. Dan Engle
- *Conquering Concussion,* by Mary Lee Esty, C M Shifflett
- *Conversations with God,* by Neale Donald Walsch
- *Deep Nutrition*, by Catherine Shanahan, M.D. and Luke Shanahan
- *Dr. Kellyann's Bone Broth Diet,* by Dr Kellyann Petrucci
- *Earthing,* by Clinton Ober, Stephen T Sinatra, Martin Zucker
  and James L Oschman
- *Eat Smarter,* by Shawn Stevenson
- *EMF*D,* by Dr. Joseph Mercola
- *Everybody Poops 410 Pounds a Year*, by Deuce Flanagan
- *Existential Kink*, by Carolyn Elliott PhD
- *Farmacology,* by Daphne Miller
- *Genius Foods*, by Max Lugavere
- *Genius Foods,* by Max Lugavere and Paul Grewal, M.D.
- *Gut Balance Revolution,* by Mullin E. Gerard, M.D.
- *Head Strong,* by Dave Asprey
- *Healing with Whole Foods,* by Paul Pitchford
- *Herbal Remedies,* by Andrew Chevallier
- *How To Be an Adult In Relationships,* by David Richo
- *How to Change Your Mind,* by Michael Pollan
- *Intestinal Health is connected to what?,* by Mark Buse, BSC, CT, CWR
- *Keto Clarity,* by Jimmy Moore, Eric C. Westman
- *Keto Diet,* by Josh Axe
- *Ketofast,* by Joseph Mercola and Alan Goldhamer
- *Letting Go,* by David R. Hawkins, M.D.
- *Life Force,* by Tony Robbins

- *Limitless,* by Jim Kwik
- *Lymph and Longevity,* by Dr. Gerald Lemole, M.D.
- *Mating in Captivity,* by Esther Perel
- *Mayo Clinic Book of Alternative Medicine and Home Remedies,* by the Mayo Clinic
- *Mission America, Straight Talk About Military Transition,* by LTC Scott Mann, SF
- *Natural Born Heroes,* by Christopher McDougall
- *PEMF - The Fifth Element of Health,* by Bryant A. Meyers
- *Primal Endurance,* by Mark Sisson
- *Probiotics, Nature's Internal Healer,* by Natasha Trenev
- *Sex at Dawn,* by Christopher Ryan and Cacilda Jetha
- *Sodium Bicarbonate,* by Dr. Mark Sircus
- *Stop Doing That Sh*t,* by Gary John Bishop
- *Super Gut,* by William Davis, MD
- *12 Rules for Life,* by Jordan B. Peterson
- *The Automatic Millionaire,* by David Bach
- *The Body Ecology,* by Donna Gates and Linda Schatz
- *The Body Keeps the Score,* by Bessel A. van der Kolk
- *The Bulletproof Diet,* by Dave Asprey
- *The Clever Gut Diet,* by Michael Mosley
- *The Complete Book of Water Therapy,* by Dian Dincin Buchman
- *The Complete Guide to Fasting,* by Jason Fung, Jimmy Moore
- *The Complete Guide to Fasting Log, Journal and Workbook: Based on Dr. Jason Fung's Principles for Fasting for Health and Weight Loss,* by Dr Jason Fung
- *The Definitive Guide to Colon Hydrotherapy,* by Stephen Holt, MD, DSC
- *The Divided Mind,* by John E. Sarno
- *The Field*, by Lynne McTaggart
- *The 4-Hour Work Week,* by Tim Ferriss
- *The 4-Hour Body,* by Tim Ferriss
- *The Healing Power of Enzymes,* by DicQie Fuller-Looney, PhD
- *The Holographic Universe,* by Michael Talbott
- *The Human Machine, Volume III, Hiatal Hernia Syndrome,* by Phil Selinsky, ND
- *The Keto Reset Diet,* by Mark Sisson
- *The Liver and Gallbladder Miracle Cleanse,* by Andreas Moritz
- *The Meditations,* by Marcus Aurelius and Sam Torode

- *The Mountain is You,* by Brianna West
- *The Oxygen Advantage,* by Patrick McKeown
- *The Power of Now,* by Eckhart Tolle
- *The Rational Male: Preventive Medicine,* by Rollo Tomassi
- *The Sedona Method,* by Hale Dwoskin
- *The Subtle Art of Not Giving a F*ck,* by Mark Manson
- *The Unplugged Alpha,* by Richard Cooper
- *Unfuck Yourself,* by Gary John Bishop
- *What Doesn't Kill Us,* by Scott Carney
- *Why We Sleep,* by Matthew Walker
- *Yoga Body and Mind Handbook,* by Jasmine Tarkeshi

Annex I – 20 Fitness Rules for Men & Women over 40

1. Your focus in the gym is injury prevention first and results second. The older you get, the smarter you must train.

2. Stop trying to burn fat with your workouts. Instead, use them to gain muscle. You will burn more fat by adding more muscle to your frame.

3. Keep your movement smooth and controlled.

4. Stick with the same workouts for 8 to 16 weeks while using progressive overload to make gains in the Gym.

5. Start your workouts with a dynamic warm-up using mobility stretches & muscle activation to keep yourself injury-free.

6. As you age, protein becomes more important. Get at least 1 gram per pound of ideal body weight every day.

7. Get your blood work done every 6 months. You need to know what is happening under the hood.

8. Track your workouts. This may seem annoying at first, but you'll find you'll make faster progress doing this than lifting aimlessly at the Gym.

9. The path to sustainable health is to find a way of eating that works for the body and lifestyle you want to live.

10. One of the best ways to live longer is to increase your lung capacity. Find a form of cardio you enjoy and can see yourself doing for a lifetime.

11. To optimize your brain and body get at least one hour of sun exposure a day. If you can't do that then supplement with Vitamin D3.

12. Keep yourself at a healthy body fat percentage. One thing to note is that this number changes as you age and varies based on gender.

13. Cardio is how you live a long life. Resistance training is how you live a quality life. Sleep is how you recover and regulate your hormones. Marry all three of these together to make a fitness kingdom.

14. Attune your lifestyle to the sun and your circadian rhythms. Over time the body becomes its own alarm clock.

15. Sleep is the best legal performance-enhancing drug on the planet. Do everything you can to get the hours of sleep you need and work to enhance the quality of your sleep. Use a sleep tracker like an Oura ring or Whoop to measure your improvement.

16. Create a habit of walking every day. This is the most underrated exercise for living longer and a better working brain.

17. Creatine should be a staple in most people's supplement cabinets.

18. Your workouts should be centered around pillar movements such as the squat, deadlift, bench press, back row, lat pulldown, overhead press, lunge, and carry. Don't think these are mandatory exercises. Think of them as movements you want to become stronger in.

19. Drinking water is one of the most underrated ways to improve your health and body. Drink it.

20. Never use age as an excuse. Unless you were a pro athlete you can still become the fittest version of yourself past the age of 40 if you know how to do the right things.

- ENDNOTES -

1   Hill, Bradford G,, Rood, Benjamin, Ribble, Amanda, Haberzettl, Petra, "Fine particulate matter (PM$_{2.5}$) inhalation-induced alterations in the plasma lipidome as promoters of vascular inflammtion and insulin resistance", American Physiological Society, American *Journal of Physiology—Heart and Circulatory Physiology*, Vol 320, Issue 5, 2021-05-01, doi: 10.1152/ajpheart.00881.2020; https://doi.org/10.1152/ajpheart.00881.2020

2   "Fort Leonard Wood, Missouri Universities Form Consortium to Battle Traumatic Brain Injury", Association of Defense Communities, Aug 15, 2019, DC360, On Base, https://defensecommunities.org/2019/08/fort-leonard-wood-missouri-universities-form-consortium-to-battle-traumatic-brain-injury/ Ahl, Jonathan, "Fort Leonard Wood And Rolla Are At The Center Of Cutting-Edge Research On Traumatic Brain Injury", St Louis Public Radio [Internet], Dec 6, 2019, https://news.stlpublicradio.org/health-science-environment/2019-12-06/fort-leonard-wood-and-rolla-are-at-the-center-of-cutting-edge-research-on-traumatic-brain-injury

3   "Monoamine oxidase inhibitors (MAOIs)", Mayo Clinic Staff, https://www.mayoclinic.org/diseases-conditions/depression/in-depth/maois/art-20043992?

4   "Selective serotonin reuptake inhibitors (SSRIs)", Mayo Clinic Staff, https://www.mayoclinic.org/diseases-conditions/depression/in-depth/ssris/art-20044825

5   Ozdowski L, Gupta V. Physiology, Lymphatic System. [Updated 2022 May 8]. In: StatPearls [Internet]. Treasure Island (FL): StatPearls Publishing; 2022 Jan-. Available from: https://www.ncbi.nlm.nih.gov/books/NBK557833/

6   Ahl, J

.

7   "Joe Rogan Experience #1139 – Jordan Peterson", https://www.youtube.com/live/9Xc7DN-noAc?feature=share&t=3757, July 2, 2018.

8   https://www.myplate.gov/myplate-plan

9   https://www.healthline.com/health/hot-tub-benefits#health-benefits

10   Skar GL, Simonsen KA. Lyme Disease. [Updated 2022 May 6]. In: StatPearls [Internet]. Treasure Island (FL): StatPearls Publishing; 2022 Jan-. Available from: https://www.ncbi.nlm.nih.gov/books/NBK431066/

11   https://www.cdc.gov/lyme/treatment/index.html

12   https://www.mayoclinichealthsystem.org/hometown-health/speaking-of-health/grocery-store-tour-shopping-the-perimeter

13   Holdiness M. R. (1991). Clinical pharmacokinetics of N-acetylcysteine. *Clinical pharmacokinetics*, 20(2), 123–134. https://doi.org/10.2165/00003088-199120020-00004

14   Smaga, I., Frankowska, M., & Filip, M. (2021). N-acetylcysteine as a new prominent ap-

proach for treating psychiatric disorders. *British journal of pharmacology*, *178*(13), 2569–2594. https://doi.org/10.1111/bph.15456

15   Samuni, Y., Goldstein, S., Dean, O. M., & Berk, M. (2013). The chemistry and biological activities of N-acetylcysteine. *Biochimica et biophysica acta*, *1830*(8), 4117–4129. https://doi.org/10.1016/j.bbagen.2013.04.016

16   Chughlay, M. F., Kramer, N., Spearman, C. W., Werfalli, M., & Cohen, K. (2016). N-acetylcysteine for non-paracetamol drug-induced liver injury: a systematic review. *British journal of clinical pharmacology*, *81*(6), 1021–1029. https://doi.org/10.1111/bcp.12880

17   Izquierdo-Alonso, J. L., Pĭrez-Rial, S., Rivera, C. G., & Peces-Barba, G. (2022). N-acetylcysteine for prevention and treatment of COVID-19: Current state of evidence and future directions. *Journal of infection and public health*, *15*(12), 1477–1483. https://doi.org/10.1016/j.jiph.2022.11.009

18   National Institutes of Health, Office of Dietary Supplements, Niacin Health Professional Fact Sheet[Internet], accessed Mar 15, 2023 at https://ods.od.nih.gov/factsheets/niacin-healthprofessional/

19   Shade C. The Science Behind NMN—A Stable, Reliable NAD+Activator and Anti-Aging Molecule. Integr. Med. 2020;19:12–14. - PMC - PubMed

20   "Feel-good hormones: How they affect your mind, mood and body" Stephanie Watson, Harvard Women's Health Watch, Harvard Health Publishing [Internet], Jul 20, 2021 at https://www.health.harvard.edu/mind-and-mood/feel-good-hormones-how-they-affect-your-mind-mood-and-body
        "Endorphins: The brain's natural pain reliever" Stephanie Watson, Harvard Women's Health Watch, Harvard Health Publishing [Internet], Jul 20, 2021 at https://www.health.harvard.edu/mind-and-mood/endorphins-the-brains-natural-pain-reliever
        "Serotonin: The natural mood booster", Stephanie Watson, Harvard Women's Health Watch, Harvard Health Publishing [Internet], Jul 20, 2021 at https://www.health.harvard.edu/mind-and-mood/serotonin-the-natural-mood-booster

21   Avci, P., Gupta, A., Sadasivam, M., Vecchio, D., Pam, Z., Pam, N., & Hamblin, M. R. (2013). Low-level laser (light) therapy (LLLT) in skin: stimulating, healing, restoring. *Seminars in cutaneous medicine and surgery*, *32*(1), 41–52.

22   Clijsen R, Brunner A, Barbero M, Clarys P, Taeymans J. Effects of low-level laser therapy on pain in patients with musculoskeletal disorders: a systematic review and meta-analysis. Eur J Phys Rehabil Med 2017;53:603-10. DOI: 10.23736/S1973-9087.17.04432-X

23   Chaves, M. E., Araҍjo, A. R., Piancastelli, A. C., & Pinotti, M. (2014). Effects of low-power light therapy on wound healing: LASER x LED. *Anais brasileiros de dermatologia*, *89*(4), 616–623. https://doi.org/10.1590/abd1806-4841.20142519

24   Valverde, A., Hamilton, C., Moro, C., Billeres, M., Magistretti, P., & Mitrofanis, J. (2023). Lights at night: does photobiomodulation improve sleep?. *Neural regeneration research*, *18*(3), 474–477. https://doi.org/10.4103/1673-5374.350191
Zhao, J., Tian, Y., Nie, J., Xu, J., & Liu, D. (2012). Red light and the sleep quality and endurance performance of Chinese female basketball players. *Journal of athletic training*, *47*(6), 673–678. https://doi.org/10.4085/1062-6050-47.6.08

25   Zhao, 2012.

26   Salehpour, F., Mahmoudi, J., Kamari, F., Sadigh-Eteghad, S., Rasta, S. H., & Hamblin, M. R. (2018). Brain Photobiomodulation Therapy: a Narrative Review. *Molecular neurobiology*, *55*(8), 6601–6636. https://doi.org/10.1007/s12035-017-0852-4

27   Li-Xue Zhang, Chang-Xing Li, Mohib Ullah Kakar, Muhammad Sajjad Khan, Pei-Feng Wu, Rai Muhammad Amir, Dong-Fang Dai, Muhammad Naveed, Qin-Yuan Li, Muhammad Saeed, Ji-Qiang Shen, Shahid Ali Rajput, Jian-Hua Li,Resveratrol (RV): A pharmacological review and call for further research, Biomedicine & Pharmacotherapy, Volume 143, 2021, 112164, ISSN 0753-3322, https://doi.org/10.1016/j.biopha.2021.112164.(https://www.sciencedirect.com/science/article/pii/S0753332221009483)

28   Salehi, B., Mishra, A. P., Nigam, M., Sener, B., Kilic, M., Sharifi-Rad, M., Fokou, P. V. T., Martins, N., & Sharifi-Rad, J. (2018). Resveratrol: A Double-Edged Sword in Health Benefits. *Biomedicines*, *6*(3), 91. https://doi.org/10.3390/biomedicines6030091
29   https://www.healthline.com/health/rife-machine-cancer

On Point
Veterans Foundation

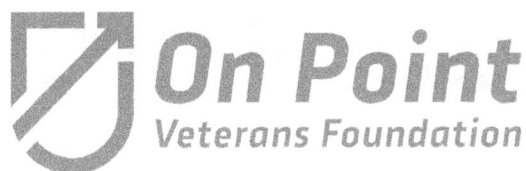

Supporting veterans and their families in times of need by providing financial assistance to access medical care, mental health counseling, and other supplemental services.

On Point Veterans Foundation is a non-profit organization founded by US Army Special Forces veteran Erik Lawrence. Our mission is simple, to provide our veterans with top-notch support and services that aid in transitioning into successful post-service lives. We are passionate about guiding veterans toward a brighter future, with services like healthy lifestyle support and counseling for mental health. Your service to the country has given us the freedom we cherish, and we feel it's our duty to give you the support you deserve.

onpointvets.org

VSS BOOKS

Visit vssbooks.com to see our full listing of available titles.

VSS Books is a website that showcases books authored and published by Erik Lawrence. Lawrence is a U.S. Army Special Forces (Green Beret) veteran that has authored over 50 books in a variety of categories.

CATEGORIES:
  » Preparedness & Personal Protection
  » Veteran Wellness
  » Firearms Training & Handbooks
  » Firearms Owner's Manuals
  » AR-15 Rifle Assembly
  » Paper Targets

Books showcased on vssbooks.com are linked to their listings on Amazon.com to purchase.

vssbooks.com

www.ingramcontent.com/pod-product-compliance
Lightning Source LLC
Chambersburg PA
CBHW080642270326
41928CB00017B/3159